W9-CAZ-027

# Problems with Geriatric Anesthesia Patients

*Guest Editor*

JEFFREY H. SILVERSTEIN, MD

ANESTHESIOLOGY CLINICS

www.anesthesiology.theclinics.com

*Consulting Editor*
LEE A. FLEISHER, MD, FACC

September 2009 • Volume 27 • Number 3

SAUNDERS an imprint of ELSEVIER, Inc.

**W.B. SAUNDERS COMPANY**
*A Division of Elsevier Inc.*

1600 John F. Kennedy Boulevard, Suite 1800 • Philadelphia, PA 19103-2899

http://www.theclinics.com

**ANESTHESIOLOGY CLINICS Volume 27, Number 3**
**September 2009 ISSN 1932-2275, ISBN-13: 978-1-4377-1288-9, ISBN-10: 1-4377-1288-6**

Editor: Rachel Glover

Developmental Editor: Donald Mumford



*Anesthesiology Clinics* (ISSN 1932-2275) is published quarterly by Elsevier Inc., 360 Park Avenue South, New York, NY 10010-1710. Months of issue are March, June, September, and December. Periodicals postage paid at New York, NY and at additional mailing offices. Subscription prices are $122.00 per year (US student/resident), $244.00 per year (US individuals), $298.00 per year (Canadian individuals), $372.00 per year (US institutions), $461.00 per year (Canadian institutions), $172.00 per year (Canadian and foreign student/resident), $338.00 per year (foreign individuals), and $461.00 per year (foreign institutions). To receive student and resident rate, orders must be accompanied by name of affiliated institution, date of term, and the *signature* of program/residency coordinator on institutions letterhead. Orders will be billed at individual rate until proof of status is received. Foreign air speed delivery is included in all *Clinics'* subscription prices. All prices are subject to change without notice. POSTMASTER: Send address changes to *Anesthesiology Clinics,* Elsevier Health Sciences Division, Subscription Customer Service, 3251 Riverport Lane, Maryland Heights, MO 63043. Customer Service (orders, claims, online, change of address): Elsevier Health Sciences Division, Subscription Customer Service, 3251 Riverport Lane, Maryland Heights, MO 63043. Tel: 1-800-654-2452 (U.S. and Canada); 314-447-8871 (outside U.S. and Canada). Fax: 314-447-8029. E-mail: journalscustomerservice-usa@elsevier.com (for print support); journalsonlinesupport-usa@elsevier.com (for online support).

*Reprints*. For copies of 100 or more of articles in this publication, please contact the Commercial Reprints Department, Elsevier Inc., 360 Park Avenue South, New York, NY 10010-1710. Tel.: 212-633-3812; Fax: 212-462-1935; E-mail: reprints@elsevier.com.

*Anesthesiology Clinics,* is also published in Spanish by McGraw-Hill Inter-americana Editores S. A., P.O. Box 5-237, 06500 Mexico D. F., Mexico.

Anesthesiology *Clinics*, is covered in *MEDLINE/PubMed (Index Medicus), Current Contents/Clinical Medicine, Excerpta Medica, ISI/BIOMED*, and *Chemical Abstracts*.

Printed in the United States of America.

# Contributors

## CONSULTING EDITOR

**LEE A. FLEISHER, MD, FACC**
Robert D. Dripps Professor and Chair of Anesthesiology and Critical Care, Department of Anesthesiology and Critical Care, University of Pennsylvania School of Medicine, Philadelphia, Pennsylvania

## GUEST EDITOR

**JEFFREY H. SILVERSTEIN, MD, CIP**
Professor, Departments of Anesthesiology, Surgery, and Geriatrics & Adult Development; and Vice Chair for Research, Department of Anesthesiology; and Associate Dean for Research; and Director, Program for the Protection of Human Subjects, Mount Sinai School of Medicine, New York, New York

## AUTHORS

**SHAMSUDDIN AKHTAR, MD**
Associate Professor, Department of Anesthesiology, Yale University School of Medicine, New Haven, Connecticut

**ZIRKA H. ANASTASIAN, MD**
Assistant Professor of Anesthesiology, Division of Neurosurgical Anesthesiology, Department of Anesthesiology, Columbia University, New York, New York

**SHEILA RYAN BARNETT, MD**
Associate Professor of Anesthesiology, Harvard Medical School, Department of Anesthesiology, Critical Care and Pain Medicine, Beth Israel Deaconess Medical Center, Boston, Massachusetts

**DANIELA M. DARRAH, MD**
Resident in Anesthesiology, Department of Anesthesiology, Mount Sinai School of Medicine, New York, New York

**STACIE DEINER, MD**
Assistant Professor of Anesthesiology, Department of Anesthesiology, Mount Sinai School of Medicine, New York, New York

**MICHAEL DUDLEY, MD**
Fellow, Cardiothoracic Anesthesiology, Department of Anesthesiology, Wake Forest University School of Medicine, Medical Center Boulevard, Winston-Salem, North Carolina

**PATTI M. EDELSTEIN, MD, FAAP, FAAMA**
Department of Anesthesia, Shaare Zedek Medical Center, Jerusalem, Israel

**GREGORY W. FISCHER, MD**
Associate Professor, Department of Anesthesiology and Cardiothoracic Surgery, Mount Sinai School of Medicine, Mount Sinai Medical Center, One Gustave L. Levy Place, New York, New York

**TOMAS L. GRIEBLING, MD, MPH**
John P. Wolf 33° Masonic Distinguished Professor of Urology, Department of Urology, University of Kansas School of Medicine; The Landon Center on Aging, University of Kansas School of Medicine, Kansas City, Kansas

**LEANNE GROBAN, MD**
Associate Professor of Anesthesiology, Department of Anesthesiology, Wake Forest University School of Medicine, Medical Center Boulevard, Winston-Salem, North Carolina

**JOHN HAGEN, MD**
Resident in Anesthesiology, Department of Anesthesiology, Mount Sinai School of Medicine, New York, New York

**ERIC J. HEYER, MD, PhD**
Professor of Clinical Anesthesiology and Clinical Neurology, Division of Neurosurgical Anesthesiology, Department of Anesthesiology, Columbia University, New York, New York

**YULIA IVASHKOV, MD**
Acting Assistant Professor, Department of Anesthesiology and Pain Medicine, Harborview Medical Center, University of Washington, Seattle, Washington

**ARTHUR M. LAM, MD, FRCPC**
Professor of Anesthesiology, Department of Anesthesiology and Pain Medicine, University of Washington, Harborview Medical Center; Medical Director, Cerebrovascular Laboratory, Harborview Medical Center, Seattle, Washington

**STEFAN A. LOMBAARD, MBChB, FANZCA**
Assistant Professor, Department of Anesthesiology and Pain Medicine, University of Washington Medical Center, Seattle, Washington

**JASON MAGGI, MD**
Division of Wound Healing and Regenerative Medicine, Department of Surgery, NYU Langone Medical Center, New York, New York

**JULIA I. METZNER, MD**
Assistant Professor, Department of Anesthesiology and Pain Medicine, University of Washington, Seattle Washington

**DANIEL K. O'NEILL, MD**
Assistant Professor, Department of Anesthesiology, New York University School of Medicine, New York, New York

**EUGENE ORNSTEIN, PhD, MD**
Associate Professor of Clinical Anesthesiology, Division of Neurosurgical Anesthesiology, Department of Anesthesiology, Columbia University, New York, New York

**RAMESH RAMAIAH, MD, FCARCSI, FRCA**
Acting Assistant Professor of Anesthesiology, Department of Anesthesiology and Pain Medicine, University of Washington, Harborview Medical Center, Seattle, Washington

**REINETTE ROBBERTZE, MBChB, FANZCA**
Clinical Assistant Professor, Department of Anesthesiology and Pain Medicine, University of Washington Medical Center, Seattle, Washington

**DAVID SANDERS, MD**
Fellow, Cardiothoracic Anesthesiology, Department of Anesthesiology, Wake Forest University School of Medicine, Medical Center Boulevard, Winston-Salem, North Carolina

**FREDERICK E. SIEBER, MD**
Director of Anesthesiology and Clinical Research, Department of Anesthesiology, Johns Hopkins Bayview Medical Center, Johns Hopkins Medical Institutions; Associate Professor, Anesthesiology and Critical Care Medicine, Johns Hopkins University School of Medicine, Baltimore, Maryland

**JEFFREY H. SILVERSTEIN, MD**
Professor, Departments of Anesthesiology, Surgery, and Geriatrics & Adult Development; and Vice Chair for Research, Department of Anesthesiology; and Associate Dean for Research; and Director, Program for the Protection of Human Subjects, Mount Sinai School of Medicine, New York, New York

**GAIL A. VAN NORMAN, MD**
Professor, Department of Anesthesiology and Pain Medicine, Harborview Medical Center; and Adjunct Professor, Department of Biomedical Ethics, University of Washington, Seattle, Washington

**ALEXANDER A. VITIN, MD, PhD**
Assistant Professor, Department of Anesthesiology and Pain Medicine, University of Washington, Seattle Washington

**CHARLES Z. ZIGELMAN, MD**
Director, Post Anesthesia Care Unit, Department of Anesthesia, Shaare Zedek Medical Center, Jerusalem, Israel

# Contents

Elderly patients are increasingly referred for complex surgery, but are at particular risk for coronary artery disease. One strategy to prevent perioperative cardiac events in elderly patients is to employ perioperative β-blockade, but doing so has the potential to increase the incidence of congestive heart failure, perioperative hypotension, bradycardia, and stroke. This article examines common comorbidities in the elderly who may benefit from the chronic use of β-blockers, prophylactic perioperative use of β-blockers including timing, dosage, and choice of β-blocker, the pharmacologic effects of aging, and recommendations on the use of β-blockers.



Wound patients commonly have multiple comorbidities, which should be optimized before anesthesia. These factors contribute not only to skin breakdown but also other causes of mortality and morbidity. Skin becomes more vulnerable to damage from pressure, friction, shear, and moisture when the skin is dry, less elastic, and less perfused. Careful assessment and implementation of an anesthetic plan using regional or general techniques can improve outcomes. The anesthesiologist plays a vital role in maintaining homeostasis during the surgically stressful perioperative period of the wound patient. Aggressive wound management in the early stages is likely to prevent wound progression to deeper levels. Policies are being implemented to decrease the risk of pressure ulcers by prevention.

## FORTHCOMING ISSUES

***December 2009***

**Preoperative Medical Consultation: A Multidisciplinary Perspective**

Lee A. Fleisher, MD and
Stanley H. Rosenbaum, MD,
*Guest Editors*

***March 2010***

**Anesthesia for Patients Too Sick for Anesthesia**

Benjamin Kohl, MD and
Stanley H. Rosenbaum, MD,
*Guest Editors*

***June 2010***

**Ambulatory Anesthesia**

Peter Glass, MD, *Guest Editor*

## RECENT ISSUES

***June 2009***

**Cutting-Edge Topics in Pediatric Anesthesia**

Ronald Litman, DO and
Arjunan Ganesh, MBBS,
*Guest Editors*

***March 2009***

**Anesthesia Outside the Operating Room**

Wendy L. Gross, MD, MHCM and
Barbara Gold, MD, *Guest Editors*

***December 2008***

**Value-Based Anesthesia**

Alex Macario, MD, MBA,
*Guest Editor*

**RELATED INTEREST**

*Clinics in Geriatric Medicine,* November 2008 (Volume 24, Issue 4)
**Perioperative Management**
Amir K. Jaffer, MD, *Guest Editor*

# Foreword

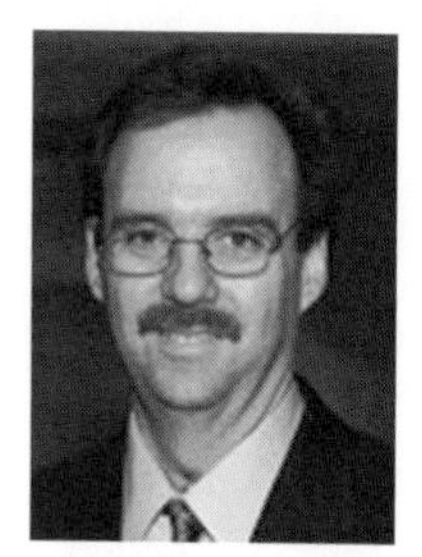

Lee A. Fleisher, MD, FACC
*Consulting Editor*

Anesthesia at the extremes of age has been a topic of interest to anesthesiologists, but much of the focus has been on the very young as opposed to the very old. Anesthesiologists are acquainted with managing patients with multiple comorbidities, which are known to increase with increasing age, but the very old have some unique problems, and the manifestations of the comorbidities have changed. Therefore, there is increasing interest in geriatric patients and their perioperative care, and in this issue of *Anesthesiology Clinics*, the editor has chosen a different format from the traditional monograph, using a problem-based approach. As guest editor for this issue, the *Clinics* is fortunate to have Jeffrey H. Silverstein. Dr. Silverstein is Professor of Anesthesiology, Surgery, and Geriatrics and Adult Development and Associate Dean for Research at the Mount Sinai School of Medicine. He has authored 47 original articles, 13 chapters, and 2 books. He has been a principle or co-investigator on several National Institutes of Health grants and other national grants related to geriatric care and is a member of the Aging Systems and Geriatrics Study Section of the National Institutes of Health. He is, therefore, in an excellent position to provide the readership with a broad array of exciting discussions from world-renowned experts.

Lee A. Fleisher, MD, FACC
Department of Anesthesiology and Critical Care
University of Pennsylvania School of Medicine
6 Dulles, 3400 Spruce Street
Philadelphia, PA 19104, USA

E-mail address:
fleishel@uphs.upenn.edu (L.A. Fleisher)

Anesthesiology Clin 27 (2009) xiii
doi:10.1016/j.anclin.2009.08.001
anesthesiology.theclinics.com
1932-2275/09/$ – see front matter 

# Preface

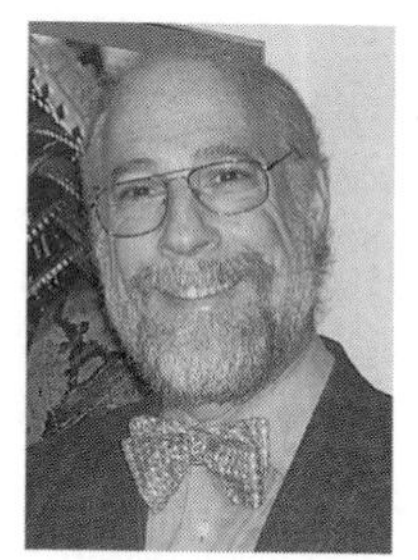

Jeffrey H. Silverstein, MD, CIP
*Guest Editor*

This issue of *Anesthesiology Clinics*, focused on problems encountered in geriatric patients, comes at an interesting and exciting time in modern anesthesia practice. The practices of anesthesiologists in North America are becoming progressively populated by aging patients. Longevity seems to be increasing steadily, and the expectations of a vital elderly population include quality medical care. The quality and diversity of information regarding the perioperative care of the elderly has increased significantly, as can be noted at national meetings, in scientific journals, and by the creation of the subspecialty Society for the Advancement of Geriatric Anesthesia (SAGA). It is a paradoxical irony that the current primary reimbursement system for the elderly surgical patient undervalues anesthesia services at a time when we are encouraging fellow anesthesiologists to spend more time and effort learning about the details of aging patients and their care.

This issue presents a problem-based approach to elderly patients. These problems tend to be complicated, with age-related homeostenosis being an important component. For reviews of the physiology and pharmacology of aging, the reader is referred to recent textbooks on geriatric anesthesiology. In this issue, traditional areas of anesthesia understanding, such as aortic stenosis, atrial fibrillation, and the status of perioperative beta blockade, are attuned to the needs of the elderly patient. Movement disorders tend to manifest in the elderly, making an anesthetic approach to the exciting new technologies used in Parkinson's disease a particularly useful review. Some of our articles address problems that, although not limited to the elderly, such as mesenteric ischemia, delirium, and postoperative cognitive dysfunction, are primarily syndromes of the elderly. Others, such as fat embolism syndrome and diastolic heart failure, may be more physiologically disruptive in the elderly. Some common problems such as polypharmacy, anesthesia for wound care, and postoperative urinary retention are perhaps perceived as problems for other specialties but frequently confront the anesthesiologist in the preoperative holding area, the operating room, and the postanesthesia care unit. The article on issues of informed consent in the elderly is

Anesthesiology Clin 27 (2009) xv–xvi
doi:10.1016/j.anclin.2009.07.019
1932-2275/09/$ – see front matter 

particularly poignant. Finally, every anesthesiologist who cares for elderly patients has waited a while for some patients to emerge from anesthesia. The article on when it is time to be concerned and how to approach the complication of delayed arousal fills a practical niche.

On behalf of all the authors, I thank you for considering this material. We all believe that there remains significant opportunity to improve the perioperative care of the elderly. Thus we hope that many of you will find this information useful in your practice and that a few of you will be encouraged to explore and develop new knowledge, both of which are essential to our goal of improved care for the elderly.

Jeffrey H. Silverstein, MD, CIP
Departments of Anesthesiology, Surgery, and Geriatrics and Adult Development
Mount Sinai School of Medicine
Box 1010
1 Gustave L. Levy Place
New York, NY 10029-6574

E-mail address:
jeff.silverstein@mssm.edu (J.H. Silverstein)

# Polypharmacy and Perioperative Medications in the Elderly

Sheila Ryan Barnett, MD

**KEYWORDS**

- Polypharmacy • Anticholinergic effects
- Anticholinergic properties • Beers criteria
- Adverse drug events • Prescription medications
- Over the counter medications

*Mr. W presents to the hospital with a painful ischemic leg. He is scheduled for a lower extremity angiogram and possible bypass procedure. His family is concerned that over the last 3 weeks, in addition to increasing leg pain, he has also become more confused. On arrival, neurology and geriatric consults are obtained. After bedside neuropsychological testing, it is felt that in addition to baseline cognitive deficits, his mental status is impaired by pain and additional medications. Medical history is remarkable for multiple significant comorbidities including ischemic heart disease, prior myocardial infarct and a coronary artery bypass, poorly controlled diabetes mellitus complicated by neuropathy, retinopathy, and blindness, and peripheral vascular disease. He had a left-sided cerebrovascular accident 3 years previously, and has a carotid stent. He is known to have atrial fibrillation at baseline. Medications at time of the hospitalization include aspirin, atorvastatin, clopidogrel bisulfate, duoxetine, furosemide, quinapril, metoprolol, potassium, warfarin, and sliding-scale insulin. For pain he receives multiple analgesics at different times including gabapentin, hydrocodone acetaminophen, tramadol, and oxycodone.*

*The morning following admission he undergoes a lower extremity angiogram and attempted stent placement; this is scheduled with monitored anesthesia because of significant comorbidities. For the procedure he receives fentanyl 50 μg and midazolam 1.5 mg. He appears to tolerate the procedure well, but later that evening he becomes progressively more agitated and combative. During the next 2 hours he develops some bleeding around the sheath site and his hematocrit drops to 24% from 34% preprocedure. The bleeding abates with pressure, and he receives 2 units of packed red blood cells. However, there*

Harvard Medical School, Department of Anesthesiology, Critical Care, and Pain Medicine, Beth Israel Deaconess Medical Center, 330 Brookline Avenue, FD 407, Boston, MA 02215, USA
*E-mail address:* sbarnett@bidmc.harvard.edu

Anesthesiology Clin 27 (2009) 377–389
doi:10.1016/j.anclin.2009.07.004 **anesthesiology.theclinics.com**
1932-2275/09/$ – see front matter 

*is further concern that he will bleed from the femoral sheath site, and over the next few hours he receives 25 mg of haloperidol in divided doses. By morning he is extremely sedated and minimally responsive, although vital signs remain stable. A medical workup is performed to rule out any unstable conditions. His laboratory workup is significant for a sodium of 131, hematocrit is 32%, and other electrolytes including creatinine are normal; his examination is consistent with excessive haloperidol. He remains hospitalized for the following 10 days; however, surgery is not performed due to his poor mental status. He is discharged to a rehabilitative facility, and scheduled to return for a femoral popliteal bypass in 4 weeks.*

## POLYPHARMACY AND ANESTHESIA

Geriatric patients presenting for surgery carry an increasing burden of disease so it is not surprising that older patients are also on a substantial number of medications, both prescribed and over the counter.[1,2] Polypharmacy is the term applied to describe patients receiving multiple medications. Polypharmacy is a substantial health care problem, and has been shown to contribute to an increase in adverse drug events and subsequent hospitalizations.[3] Estimates in the United States suggest that prescription polypharmacy (using 5 or more prescription medications at the same time) has increased in the adult population in recent years from 7% to 12%, and if all medications are considered (ie, prescription and over the counter) the prevalence of polypharmacy has increased from 23% to 29% of adults.[1,4] Although it may occur within any age group, polypharmacy is particularly relevant to older patients: results from recent surveys revealed that more than 90% of persons older than 65 years use at least one drug per week, 40% take 5 or more drugs, and 12% to 19% % use 10 or more medications in a week.[1,4]

It is estimated that one-third of the population older than 65 years will undergo at least one surgical procedure before death, thus it is important that anesthesiologists have an understanding of the problems associated with the multiple medications prescribed for chronic conditions and their potential interactions. It is not possible to list all possible interactions and side effects, so this article highlights some of the larger issues surrounding polypharmacy in geriatric patients (**Box 1**).

*Mr. W presents with several classic polypharmacy-related issues: he is on at least 15 medications when he enters the hospital and has multiple significant comorbidities. A major concern is his mental status; it is not surprising he develops delirium following his procedure. It is not known if the delirium could have been*

**Box 1**
**Factors predisposing elderly patients to adverse drug events**

1. Multiple comorbidities
2. Polypharmacy
3. Drug-drug interactions
4. Age-related reductions in metabolism and excretion
5. Increased sensitivity of central nervous system to side effects of medications
6. Complicated medication regimens
7. Multiple providers

*prevented; however, addressing the polypharmacy surrounding his pain preoperatively with a more organized regimen may have been beneficial.*

## MEDICATIONS IN OLDER PATIENTS

Qato and colleagues[1] surveyed more than 3000 older Americans (age 57 to 85 years) and reported the weighted prevalence estimates of all medication usage, including prescription and over-the-counter (OTC) drugs and supplements used on a regular basis. The results of this survey indicated that only 9% of this population was not taking any medication, 81% took at least one prescription drug, 42% regularly used OTC medications, and 49% used dietary supplements. Twenty-nine percent of all respondents and 36% of women older than 75 years were taking 5 medications. Among those taking prescriptions, 46% used concurrent OTC medications and 52% used dietary supplements. Of note, 90% of the oldest patients (>75 years) took at least one prescription medication regularly.

It is not unexpected that this group of older patients also suffered from significant comorbid diseases. The most common comorbidities encountered in this survey included cardiovascular disease (60%), arthritis (51%), diabetes (20%), thyroid problems (15%), ulcers (13%), chronic obstructive pulmonary disease or emphysema (11%), and asthma (10%). In the oldest patients (>75 years), the prevalence of cardiovascular disease increased to 70%, and in general thyroid disease was more common in women. The prevalence of pain medications and psychotropic medications was surprisingly low in this study; however, in a study by Gurwitz and colleagues[5] that included more than 27,000 Medicare enrollees, the percentage of patients taking nonopioid and opioid medications was 19% to 22%, and 12% to 14% of this population were taking antidepressants, sedatives, or nutrient supplements. Cardiovascular or diuretic medications, however, were still the most common medications, prescribed in 53% and 30% of the Medicare enrollees, respectively.

In the report by Qato and colleagues,[1] the most commonly prescribed and OTC medications are the cardiovascular agents, including aspirin, hydrochlorthiazide, atorvastatin, lisinopril, metoprolol, simvastatin, atenolol, amlodipine, furosemide, ezetimide, vasarten, warfarin, and clopidogrel. When examining the risk from patient medication interactions these investigators found that 4%, or roughly 1 in 25, older Americans were at risk of a major drug interaction; more than half of these involved a nonprescription medication, and many involved either warfarin or an antiplatelet medication. Common potential interactions in this study included the combined use of lisinopril and potassium, increasing the risk of hyperkalemia, or a combination of b-agonists and antagonists (eg, albuterol/atenolol), potentially decreasing the effectiveness of both treatments.

Potential drug-drug interactions are a concern, as often physicians may not be aware of a patient's nonprescription medication usage in the preoperative period. Although there is limited literature on medications in the perioperative period, as the population continues to expand and require surgery it is possible that these types of interactions may become more relevant clinically. At a minimum, the anesthesiologist should review all medications and be aware of potential interactions (see **Box 1**).

## ADVERSE EVENTS RELATED TO MEDICATIONS IN OLDER PATIENTS

Adverse events from medications are a major source of health care costs, impacting millions of patients each year, and contributing to lengthy hospitalizations and increased morbidity. National surveillance data on of adverse drugs events over a 2-year period found that older patients were twice as likely to be treated in an emergency room for an adverse drug event compared with younger patients, and almost 7 times more likely to require hospitalization after an emergency department visit for a drug-related event.[6] Almost one-third of all emergency room visits for adverse drug events in these older patients were due to toxicity related to insulin, digoxin, or warfarin. These survey results exposed significant inadequate therapeutic monitoring for desirable and adverse effects in these three commonly administered medications. The perioperative period provides an opportunity to review therapeutic end points as well as medication compliance.[6]

Juurlink and colleagues[3] examined the prevalence of "preventable" drug-drug interactions in patients admitted to hospital over a period of approximately 6 years. These investigators looked specifically at patients receiving glyburide, digoxin, or an angiotensin-converting enzyme (ACE) inhibitor, who were admitted with hypoglycemia, digoxin toxicity, or hyperkalemia, respectively. On review of the medical history, the introduction of a second drug in the week preceding admission increased the likelihood of an adverse event. For glyburide, administration of cotrimoxazole increased the risk by 6 times, patients on digoxin receiving clarithromycin were 12 times more likely to develop toxicity, and patients on ACE inhibitors were 20 times more likely to have had a potassium-sparing diuretic added the prior week. Although not directly relevant to anesthesia, this type of study illustrates how risky medication changes can be in vulnerable older patients, yet duration of medication usage is rarely included in the preoperative medication history. It is important perioperatively to be aware of all medications, including those that may have been recently added.

In a similar study, Gurwitz and colleagues[5] report the incidence of preventable adverse drug events occurring in a cohort of Medicare enrollees during a 12-month period. These investigators identified 1523 adverse drug events in this population; the events were considered preventable in 27% of incidences. The results indicated that preventable error occurred most commonly with cardiovascular medications (25%), diuretics (22%), nonopioid analgesics (15%), hypoglycemic agents (11%), and anticoagulants (10%). The most common "preventable" events were: electrolyte or renal imbalance (27%), gastrointestinal tract side effects (21%), hemorrhagic events (16%), metabolic disorders (eg, hyponatremia or hypoglycemia) (14%), and neuropsychiatric disorders (9%).

Anesthesiologists have the opportunity to review the patient's medications at the time of the preoperative visit. With future developments in electronic medical record systems, it may be possible that the anesthesia preoperative medication list will provide a significant automated safety check against preventable drug-drug interactions. In addition, sophisticated electronic interfaces may ultimately diminish the need for repetitive and time-consuming medication reconciliation requirements between anesthesia, nursing, and surgery services. Van den Bemt and colleagues[7] describe a pharmacy-led review of all medications in the preoperative clinic. In this small prospective study, a dedicated pharmacy technician reconciled all medication or allergy discrepancies, and checked for compliance on antithrombotic perioperative requirements. It was found that the pharmacy technician reconciliation check reduced errors significantly. These data, albeit preliminary, hold promise for further future studies in this area.

*On admission Mr. W was at risk of several drug-drug interactions. His risk of bleeding was increased through the additive effects of aspirin and clopidogrel and warfarin. He was on an ACE inhibitor and potassium that has led to an increase in hyperkalemia in poorly monitored outpatients.*

## INAPPROPRIATE PRESCRIBING IN THE ELDERLY: BEERS CRITERIA

"Inappropriate" is used to describe drugs for which the potential risk of an adverse event outweighs the benefit. In 1981 Beers developed a set of criteria for inappropriate medication usage in geriatric institutionalized patients. The original Beers criteria have undergone several revisions, and now provide some guidance for prescribing appropriately in the elderly population.[8] In the perioperative period relevant "inappropriate" medications identified using the Beers criteria include drugs with significant anticholinergic activity such as diphenhydramine, hydroxyine, and promethazine. Other inappropriate medications according to the Beers criteria include the longer-acting benzodiazepines such as diazepam and flurazepam, as well as higher doses of lorazepam.[9,10] Using the Beers criteria, recent studies have found a 20% prevalence of inappropriate use of medications in older hospitalized patients, although the contribution to adverse drug events and emergency visits was much smaller and accounted for less than 3% of emergency department visits.[11,12] Significant associated risk factors for inappropriate prescribing include age older than 85 years, living alone, poor economic situation, polypharmacy (defined as >6 drugs), anxiolytic medications, and depression. The potential for inappropriate drug use was additive by number of factors identified (**Box 2**).

## ANTICHOLINERGIC ACTIVITY

As described by Beers, medications with anticholinergic properties have been associated with significant adverse events in older patients; delirium and confusion is a particular concern for anesthesiologists in the perioperative period. Aging is associated with a decrease in cholinergic central transmission; this renders even healthy older patients sensitive to the central effects of anticholinergic medications. Many of the drugs listed in the Beers criteria have significant anticholinergic properties, for example, the tricyclic antidepressant amitriptyline and the antiarrhythmic agent disopyramide.[2,13,14]

More recently, Rudolf and colleagues[13] have developed an Anticholinergic Risk Scale (ARS) that they used to rank common medications according to anticholinergic

**Box 2**
**Selected agents from Beers criteria divided into categories**

Inappropriate/always avoid
- Flurazepam (Dalmane)
- Pentozocine (Talwin)
- Meperidine (Demerol)

Risky: avoid if possible
- Long-acting benzodiazepines: diazepam (Valium)
- Limit doses: intermediate-acting benzodiazepines: lorazepam (Ativan)

Ineffective or a better alternative exists
- Diphenhydramine (Benadryl)
- Chlorpheniramine (Chlor-trimeton)
- Ketorolac (Toradol)
- Clopidogrel (Plavix)

*Data from* Refs.[8–11]

properties. These investigators demonstrated that in a group of older outpatients, a higher ARS score was associated with an increase in adverse anticholinergic effects reported by patients or their practitioners. Anticholinergic effects in the perioperative period can be significant and lead to increased delirium and instability, and it is important for the anesthesiologist to recognize high-risk medications. In certain instances a substitution with a lower-risk medication may be appropriate, for instance, avoiding diphenhydramine for sedation or chlorpromazine for nausea prophylaxis (**Box 3**).

*Fortunately Mr. W was not on medications with strong anticholinergic properties. Haloperidol, a butyrophenone antipsychotic, has some anticholinergic activity but at low doses it is generally well tolerated; however in the doses Mr. W ultimately received intravenously the anticholinergic and extra pyramidal effects are more pronounced, contributing to his extreme sedation.*

## DRUG CASCADES

Prescribing cascades is the term used to describe the prescription of a second medication to treat potentially unrecognized side effects of the original medication. Older patients on multiple medications with significant comorbidities are at particular risk. In anesthesia there is a risk of cascading when considering the treatments for delirium in patients with cognitive side effects from anticholinergic medications that may have been avoided initially.[2]

**Box 3**
**Anticholinergic Risk Scale**

*Points are associated with increased adverse anticholinergic effects*

1 point
- Haloperidol (Haldol)
- Metoclopramine (Reglan)
- Paroxetine HCl (Paxil)

2 points
- Baclofen
- Prochlorperazine maleate (Compazine)
- Cyclobenzaprine HCl (Flexeril)

3 points
- Atropine-like medications
- Chlorpheniramine maleate (Chlor-trimeton)
- Diphenhydramine HCl (Benadryl)
- Promethazine HCl (Phenergan)
- Fluphenazine HCl (Prolixin)
- Chlorpromazine (Thorazine)

*Data from* Rudolph JL, Salow MJ, Angelini MC, McGlinchey RE. The Anticholinergic Risk Scale and anticholinergic adverse effects in older persons. Arch Intern Med 2008;168(5):508–13.

## MEDICATION HISTORIES

Accurate medication histories are an important part of the preoperative evaluation. One small prospective study examined the concordance between anesthesia and surgical medication lists in patients admitted to a surgical intensive care unit following surgery.[15] Of the 79 charts reviewed, they found that 53% had at least one discrepancy, 23% had different allergies noted, 56% had different preoperative medications, and 43% had different dosing or frequency instructions.[16] To avoid inaccurate reporting it may be necessary to request that geriatric patients bring all their medications or a complete list for review preoperatively.

Another disadvantage of polypharmacy is the impact on medication adherence. Certain characteristics lead to poor adherence, including old age, side effects, cost, dosing greater than daily, and multiple medications and complex schedules. This situation can make preoperative instructions particularly challenging, and written preoperative instructions should be used to improve compliance with instructions.

*On admission it was noted that Mr. W was taking 4 different opioids and pain medications (tramolol, gabapentin, oxycodone, hydromorphone, acetaminophen). An important part of history would have been to establish which medications he was actually taking regularly and the doses. His family described increasing pain, but it was not clear if he was on a regular pain regimen. Also following his procedure it was not apparent that his regular pain medications were continued or substituted in an intravenous form, and his pain may have significantly contributed to his confusion.*

## OVER-THE-COUNTER AND HERBAL REMEDIES

Herbal medications present a particular challenge to anesthesiologists, and patients underreport herbal use in the perioperative period.[17] In the survey by Qato and colleagues[1] almost 50% of older patients were taking alternative medications. The Slone survey[4] indicates that 60% of women older than of 65 years take at least one vitamin product per week.

There is limited information on the actual impact of herbs and vitamins on anesthetic administration. Many of these substances have the potential to alter the metabolism or impact of other drugs, but the clinical relevance is not well established, especially in the older population. In general, the American Society of Anesthesiologists has recommended that all herbs and supplements be discontinued at least 2 weeks before surgery when possible; again, when working with older and potentially frail patients these instructions should be clearly written down.

Chondroitin and glucosamine are amongst the most commonly reported alternative medicines. Reports suggest that between 5% and 9% of the older population are taking these medications. These medications seem to be safe in the perioperative period, although the data are limited.[1,17]

A few herbs and supplements, such as ginkgo and garlic, are particularly popular in older patients. Ginkgo, from *Ginkgo biloba*, is reported to potentially improve cognition. Perioperatively there have been isolated cases of spontaneous hemorrhage due to ginkgo, and bleeding is a potential concern. Garlic contains several active ingredients including alliin, allicin, and ajoene, and is purported to have beneficial effects on cardiovascular disease. Garlic inhibits platelet aggregation and may potentate other platelet inhibitors; another potential effect is lowering of blood pressure, but of little clinical relevance. A major concern with herbs is the potential for drug-drug interactions, especially with platelet and anticoagulant medications.[17]

## PHARMACOLOGIC CONSIDERATIONS IN THE ELDERLY

### *Narrow Therapeutic Range and Low Therapeutic Index*

Certain drugs have a narrow therapeutic index, and this increases the potential for drug-drug interactions. This group includes commonly administered medications such as oral hypoglycemics, calcium channel blockers, antiarrhythmics, tricyclic antidepressants, anticoagulants such as warfarin, digoxin, phenytoin, and theophylline.

### *Physiologic Alterations*

Aging is associated with a steady decline in organ function that predisposes the older patient to adverse drug events, and this vulnerability is increased significantly in the presence of common comorbid conditions such as diabetes mellitus and renal disease. As a group, the older population is heterogeneous, and it may be difficult to predict how aging and disease has impacted the physiologic reserve of an individual patient, and thus how a patient will handle a single medication or multiple combination drugs. However, certain predictable changes in renal and metabolic systems do occur, and these are briefly reviewed.[16,18,19]

### *Pharmacokinetics and Pharmacodynamics*

Plasma concentration and drug distribution are critical elements in predicting the response and duration of medications. Aging leads to alterations in body compartments, with a decrease in total body water and relative increase in body fat. Specifically, water-soluble agents such as most induction agents are distributed in a smaller initial compartment, resulting in increased exposure of receptors and potentially augmented impact. These age-related alterations impact the distribution and effect of drugs. Initial plasma concentration of hydrophilic medications is higher, and this may account for part of the initial exaggerated responses observed with propofol boluses. In contrast, lipophilic drugs are distributed within a greater volume, potentially leading to more prolonged elimination, as with long-acting benzodiazepines such as diazepam. This elimination is clinically most relevant when repeated doses are administered and metabolites accumulate.

Protein binding is a major factor in establishing drug distribution in older patients, and quantitative, such as reduced albumin, as well as qualitative factors may contribute, leading to unexpected increased free fraction of drugs. Given the importance of protein binding for a medication such as warfarin and the narrow therapeutic index of the drug, it is not surprising that it is responsible for some of the most commonly reported adverse drug events in the elderly patient.

Renal function, as measured by glomerular filtration rate (GFR), decreases with aging, and a 25% to 50% decline in GFR is observed between the age of 20 and 90 years. Furthermore, serum creatinine in the older patient may not provide an accurate estimate of actual creatinine clearance, and it is possible to underestimate the degree of baseline impairment by the serum blood urea nitrogen and creatinine alone. There is substantial variability, with some patients actually maintaining good renal function, so an actual measure of GFR may be superior to measuring creatinine. Patients with additional risk factors such as diabetes, hypertension, vascular disease, and recent dye studies are at high risk from renal insufficiency. In older patients dosages of renally excreted medications should be reduced. Aging results in a slow but steady decline in hepatic blood flow and by age 65 years, hepatic blood flow is reduced by approximately 40% compared with a 25-year-old. The reduction in flow is primarily responsible for a reduction in the high extraction medications such as lidocaine, and common opioid medications such as fentanyl and remifentanil. Aging is also associated with increased sensitivity to medications such as the opioids and benzodiazepine midazolam, the latter reflecting the pharmacodynamic changes within the g-butyric acid type receptor.[16,18,19]

## PERIOPERATIVE CONSIDERATIONS FOR CHRONIC MEDICATION USE IN THE ELDERLY PATIENT

One of the challenges for the anesthesiologist taking care of elderly patients is understanding the indications and potential interactions of the older patient's medications.[2] It is not possible to review every potential interaction or medication, but a few of the more relevant drugs are described here (**Box 4**).

### *Psychotropic Medications*

Psychotropic and antidementia treatments may be particularly relevant as the population ages, and drug-drug interactions can lead to significant issues including the development of delirium, agitation, and cardiovascular collapse. Depression is common in older patients and has been associated with increased risk of delirium after surgery, and tricyclic antidepressant medications have been associated with falls and cognitive decline in geriatric patients.[20–22]

### *Monoamine Oxidase Inhibitors*

Monoamine oxidase inhibitors (MAOIs) are antidepressant medications, generally used for the treatment of difficult to treat or severe depression. MAOIs inhibit the breakdown of norepinephrine and serotonin through inactivation of the monoamine oxidase (MAO) enzyme, thus increasing the available level of these neurotransmitters. Tranylcypromine (Parnate) and phenelzine (Nardil) are nonselective MAOIs, blocking both MAO-A and MAO-B enzymes. The effects on the enzymes lasts at least 30 days, and it takes approximately 14 days to generate adequate new enzymes. In contrast, moclobemide is a reversible MAOI. Moclobemide is more selective, inhibiting 80% of MAO-A and 30% of MAO-B, leading to the accumulation of norepinephrine and serotonin and, to a more limited degree, dopamine.

**Box 4**
**Medications strongly recommended to avoid in the elderly patient**

Meperidine (Demerol)

- Increased risk of delirium

Diphenhydramine (Benadryl)

- Strong anticholinergic properties, may lead to delirium

Long-acting benzodiazepines

- Diazepam: increased falls and confusion

Disopyramide

- Strong anticholinergic properties

Indomethacin

- Central nervous system side effects

Chlorpropramide (Diabinese)

- Has caused prolonged hypoglycemia

Patients on MAOIs may exhibit exaggerated hypertensive responses following the administration of indirect-acting sympathomimetic agents such as ephedrine, and to a lesser degree direct-acting agents. In general, hypotension should be avoided if possible, and treated cautiously with direct acting agents such as phenylephrine.

Meperidine should not be administered with any MAOIs; these medications block the neuronal reuptake of serotonin, and concurrent administration can lead to the development of serotonin overdose. Serotonergic crisis is potentially fatal, and is characterized by headache, agitation, delirium, convulsions, and hyperthermia. Concurrent administration of MAOIs and a selective serotonergic reuptake inhibitor (SSRI) or dextromethorphan may also lead to reduction in the metabolism of serotonin, leading to the development of a potentially lethal serotonergic syndrome, as described earlier.[2,20]

### *Serotonergic Reuptake Inhibitors*

These medications inhibit the reuptake of neuronal serotonin, thus increasing available levels of serotonin. SSRIs do not have anticholinergic side effects, in contrast to the tricyclic antidepressants, and are used to treat depression as well as other syndromes such as panic, and phobic and obsessive compulsive disorders. Commonly encountered SSRI medications include citalopram (Celaxa), escitalopram (Lexapro), fluoxetine (Prozac), paroxetine (Paxil), and sertraline (Zoloft). MAOIs may reduce metabolism of the serotonin, and coadministration could lead to the development of serotonergic syndrome. Duloxetine (Cymbalta) is a selective serotonin and norepinephrine reuptake inhibitor prescribed for major depression and painful diabetic peripheral neuropathy, and also should not be combined with MAOIs.[20,23]

### *Antiparkinson Medication*

Levodopa is the mainstay of treatment of Parkinson's disease, but unfortunately has a short half-life and multiple side effects, for example, orthostatic hypotension and hypovolemia. Patients with Parkinson's disease carry a high risk of postoperative delirium and can be challenging to manage perioperatively. Interruption of levodopa around the time of surgery can lead to a significant increase in Parkinsonian features such as rigidity, and even lead to difficulty with ventilation. Dopamine antagonists such as metoclopramide and phenothiazines like prochlorperazine (Compazine) can worsen Parkinson's disease and should be avoided in these patients.[2,20]

### *Haloperidol (Haldol)*

Haloperidol is an antipsychotic medication, frequently used for treatment of emergency psychotic events. It is a butyrophenone, and its effects are similar to phenothiazine medications, although it is has less profound anticholinergic effects. It has become popular for the treatment of agitation and delirium in low doses in elderly patients. In higher doses it may exhibit significant extrapyramidal side effects.

### *Meperidine*

Meperidine is a popular opioid, frequently used for postoperative analgesia and conscious sedation. In elderly patients the excretion of both meperidine and its active metabolite, normeperidine, is delayed, potentially leading to toxicity with repeated doses. Meperidine has been associated with an increased risk of delirium, and normeperidine accumulation may lead to seizures. Potential negative cardiovascular events related to meperidine include depressed cardiac output secondary to negative inotropic properties, and tachycardia secondary to anticholinergic effects. Meperidine combined with MAOIs can result in the occurrence of a potentially lethal serotonergic crisis. In general, meperidine should be avoided in older patients, especially in repeated doses. The only caveat is that the very low dose (12.5 mg) administered to treat postoperative shivering is unlikely to result in harm.[24]

### *Cholinesterase Inhibitors and Alzheimer Disease*

Alzheimer is a devastating disease, potentially impacting the lives of millions of older patients and their families. In recent years there has been substantial interest in the pharmacologic treatment of these patients early in the course of the illness. Current research suggests that early treatment with acetylcholinesterase inhibitors, such as revastigmine and donepezil, may stabilize or reduce the rate of progression of early Alzheimer dementia. Several of these medications have the potential to interfere with cholinesterase-related metabolism of muscle relaxants, and there are a few reports of prolonged paralysis after succinylcholine. Memantine is the first in a novel class of Alzheimer disease medications that act on the glutamatergic system by blocking *N*-methyl-D-aspartate glutamate receptors. This class of drug is generally reserved for patients with moderate disease progression. At present there are limited data on the significance of the anesthesia interactions; however, dementia itself carries the risk of increased delirium following surgery.[25–27]

### *Cardiovascular Medications*

Given the high incidence of cardiovascular disease and hypertension in the elderly population, it is not surprising that cardiovascular medications and ACE inhibitors in particular are among the most commonly administered medications to persons older than 65 years. In general, it is recommended that patients continue therapy that may offer myocardial protection through the perioperative period. This treatment includes the b-blockers and calcium channel blockers. Medications with potential for rebound after withdrawal, such as the a2-adrenoreceptor agonists, should also be continued. The management of renin angiotensin aldosterone system antagonists is more controversial, and is discussed briefly here.

The ACE inhibitors, generally of the -pril family, block the formation of the potent vasoconstrictor angiotensin II from angiotensin I, and the angiotensin receptor blockers (ARBs), recognized as -sartans, block the angiotensin type I receptor, blocking the action of angiotensin II. ACE inhibitors also block the breakdown of bradykinins, resulting in further vasodilation. The angiotensin II receptor subtype 1 antagonists (ARAs) and ACE inhibitors have both been found to improve cardiovascular outcomes when used to treat hypertension, congestive heart failure, and diabetic nephropathy. However, several studies have demonstrated that these medications may be associated with prolonged and sometimes refractory hypotension following the induction of anesthesia.[28–31]

Comfere and colleagues[28] studied 267 patients receiving ACE inhibitor/ARA treatment that was administered within 10 hours or longer than 10 hours, and found that patients receiving ACE inhibitor/ARA within 10 hours were more likely to become hypotensive after induction of general anesthesia. Kheterpal and colleagues[30] performed a large, prospective, observational study that included more than 9000 patients on ACE inhibitor/ARB therapy. The results demonstrated that patients receiving ACE inhibitor/ARA therapy and concomitant diuretic therapy had more episodes of hypotension intraoperatively. These data suggest that hypovolemia may play a role in the hypotension observed during surgery.

In general, patients with hypertension arrive for surgery on multiple medications, and withholding ACE inhibitors for 10 hours before surgery may result in less intraoperative hypotension. However, further randomized studies will be needed to identify any impact on cardiac events postoperatively.[28–30]

*Mr. W will return to the operating room in a few weeks for a bypass reconstruction under general anesthesia. On return, the anesthesiologist will need to pay particular attention to his medications, to reduce his risk of an adverse event related to his polypharmacy. It will be important to hold his ACE inhibitor for 10 hours but to continue his b-blocker. His risk of delirium is very high, and avoiding any anticholinergic medications such as diphenhydramine or the antiemetics such as promethazine will be necessary. Following the bypass there may be an opportunity to reduce some of his medications if his pain from ischemia abates.*

## SUMMARY

Polypharmacy is a significant and complex problem in the geriatric population. More than 40% of older patients referred for surgery will be taking at least one prescription drug and another OTC remedy at the same time. Accurate preoperative histories of medication usage are critical and should include nonprescription remedies. A working understanding of medications that are contraindicated in the elderly, such as those with strong anticholinergic properties, may reduce predictable adverse events in this vulnerable population.

## REFERENCES

1. Qato DM, Alexander GC, Conti RM, et al. Use of prescription and over-the-counter medications and dietary supplements among older adults in the United States. JAMA 2008;300(24):2867–78.
2. Hayes B, Klein-Schwartz W, Barrueto F. Polypharmacy and the geriatric patient. Clin Geriatr Med 2007;23:371–90.
3. Juurlink DN, Mamdani M, Kopp A, et al. Drug-drug interactions among elderly patients hospitalized for drug toxicity. JAMA 2003;289(13):1652–8.
4. Available at: http://www.bu.edu/slone/SloneSurvey/AnnualRpt/SloneSurveyReport2006.pdf.
5. Gurwitz JH, Field TS, Harrold LR, et al. Incidence and preventability of adverse drug events among older persons in the ambulatory setting. JAMA 2003;289(9):1107–16.
6. Budnitz DS, Pollock DA, Weideenback KN, et al. National surveillance of emergency department visits for outpatients adverse drug events. JAMA 2006;296:1858–66.
7. van den Bemt PM, van den Broek S, van Nunen AK, et al. Medication reconciliation performed by pharmacy technicians at the time of preoperative screening. Ann Pharmacother 2009;43(5):868–74.
8. Beers M. Explicit criteria for determining potentially inappropriate medication usage by the elderly. An update. Arch Intern Med 1997;157:1531–6.
9. Jano E, Aparasu RR. Healthcare outcomes associated with Beers' criteria: a systematic review. Ann Pharmacother 2007;41:438–48.
10. Aparasu RR, Mort JR. Inappropriate prescribing for the elderly: Beers criteria-based review. Ann Pharmacother 2000;34:338–46.
11. Gallagher PF, Barry PJ, Ryan C, et al. Inappropriate prescribing in an acutely ill population of elderly patients as determined by Beers' criteria. Age Ageing 2008;37(1):96–101.
12. O'Mahoney D, Gallagher PF. Inappropriate prescribing in the older population: need for new criteria. Age Ageing 2008;37(2):138–41.

13. Rudolph JL, Salow MJ, Angelini MC, et al. The Anticholinergic Risk Scale and anticholinergic adverse effects in older persons. Arch Intern Med 2008;168(5): 508–13.
14. Gallagher P, O'Mahony D. STOPP (Screening Tool of Older Persons' potentially inappropriate Prescriptions): application to acutely ill elderly patients and comparison with Beers' criteria. Age Ageing 2008;37(6):673–9.
15. Burda SA, Hobson D, Pronovost PJ. What is the patient really taking? Discrepancies between surgery and anesthesiology preoperative medication histories. Qual Saf Health Care 2005;14(6):414–6.
16. Heaver JE. Polypharmacy. In: Sieber FE, editor. Geriatric anesthesia. The McGraw-Hill Companies, Inc. 2007. p. 163–72.
17. Ang-Lee MK, Moss J, Yuan CS. Herbal medicines and perioperative care. JAMA 2001;286(2):208–16.
18. Szabo TE, Warters D. Anesthetic implications of chronic medications. In: Silverstein JH, Rooke GA, Reves JG, editors. Geriatric anesthesiology. 2nd edition. New York: Springer; 2007. p. 197–208.
19. Rivera R, Antognini JF. Perioperative drug therapy in elderly patients. Anesthesiology 2009;110:1176–81.
20. Huyse FJ, Touw DJ, van Schijndel RS, et al. Psychotropic drugs and the perioperative period: a proposal for a guideline in elective surgery. Psychosomatics 2006; 47(1):8–22.
21. Ensrud KE, Blackwell T, Mangione CM, et al. Study of osteoporotic fractures research group. Central nervous system active medications and risk for fractures in older women. Arch Intern Med 2003;163(8):949–57.
22. Cao YJ, Mager DE, Simonsick EM, et al. Physical and cognitive performance and burden of anticholinergics, sedatives, and ACE inhibitors in older women. Clin Pharmacol Ther 2008;83(3):422–9.
23. Westanmo AD, Gayken J, Haight R. Duloxetine: a balanced and selective norepinephrine- and serotonin-reuptake inhibitor. Am J Health Syst Pharm 2005;62(23): 2481–90.
24. Shafer SL, Flood P. The pharmacology of opioids. In: Silverstein JH, Rooke GA, Reves JG, editors. Geriatric anesthesiology. 2nd edition. New York: Springer; 2007. p. 209–22.
25. Farlow MR, Cummings JL. Effective pharmacologic management of Alzheimer's disease. Am J Med 2007;120(5):388–97.
26. Fodale V, Quattrone D, Trecroci C, et al. Alzheimer's disease and anaesthesia: implications for the central cholinergic system. Br J Anaesth 2006;97(4):445–52.
27. Jones PM, Soderman RM. Intra-operative bradycardia in a patient with Alzheimer's disease treated with two cholinesterase inhibitors. Anaesthesia 2007; 62(2):201.
28. Comfere T, Sprung J, Kumar MM, et al. Angiotensin system inhibitors in a general surgical population. Anesth Analg 2005;100(3):636–44.
29. Augoustides JG. Angiotensin blockade and general anesthesia: so little known, so far to go [editorial]. J Cardiothorac Vasc Anesth 2008;22(2):177–9.
30. Kheterpal S, Khodaparast O, Shanks A, et al. Chronic angiotensin-converting enzyme inhibitor or angiotensin receptor blocker therapy combined with diuretic therapy is associated with increased episodes of hypotension in noncardiac surgery. J Cardiothorac Vasc Anesth 2008;22(2):180–6.
31. Rosenman DJ, McDonald FS, Ebbert JO, et al. Clinical consequences of withholding versus administering renin-angiotensin-aldosterone system antagonists in the preoperative period. J Hosp Med 2008;3(4):319–25 [review].

# Parkinson's Disease and Deep Brain Stimulator Placement

Stacie Deiner, MD, John Hagen, MD

**KEYWORDS**

- Parkinson's disease • Deep brain stimulation • Anesthesia
- Scalp nerve blocks • Airway management

A 72-year-old man with long-standing Parkinson's disease presents for deep brain stimulaton (DBS) electrode placement. He was first diagnosed more than 15 years ago. After many years of medical management with diminishing results, worsening quality of life, and disabling tremor, he was referred by his neurologist for surgical intervention. His medical history is significant for controlled hypertension, prior myocardial infarction, percutaneous transluminal coronary angioplasty with stenting, permanent pacemaker (PPM) placement, and depression. He is scheduled for unilateral ventralis intermedius deep brain stimulation (Vim-DBS). The patient is extremely concerned that he is supposed to be awake during brain surgery.

## PARKINSON'S DISEASE

Parkinson's disease (PD) is a common, chronic, progressive neurodegenerative disease. PD is typified by four cardinal motor manifestations, at least two of which are necessary for diagnosis: postural instability, rigidity, bradykinesia (or slowing of movement), and tremor at rest, which is present in about 70% of patients.[1] In addition, there are many nonmotor features that are common to PD, such as depression, anxiety, cognitive impairment, sleep disturbances, sensory abnormalities (eg, akathesia), anosmia, and autonomic dysfunction. The clinical diagnosis of PD is made based on medical history and neurologic examination, as there is currently no laboratory test that can definitively establish a diagnosis. In people older than 65 years, the incidence is about 0.1%[2] and the prevalence is about 1%.[3] There seems to be no difference in distribution by gender. As of yet, there is no definitive etiology in PD, although one study points to possible neurotoxin involvement,[4] whereas another suggests a possible genetic predisposition.[5]

Department of Anesthesiology, Mount Sinai School of Medicine, 1 Gustave L. Levy Place, New York, NY 10029-6574, USA
*E-mail address:* Stacie.deiner@mountsinai.org (S. Deiner).

Anesthesiology Clin 27 (2009) 391–415
doi:10.1016/j.anclin.2009.07.005
1932-2275/09/$ – see front matter. Published by Elsevier Inc.
anesthesiology.theclinics.com

### Pathophysiology

Movement is a complex process mediated in the central nervous system (CNS) by the basal ganglia (caudate, putamen, nucleus accumbens, globus pallidus, substantia nigra, subthalamic nucleus), the cerebral cortex, the cerebellum, and thalamus. Under normal conditions, the motor cortex sends information to the cerebellum and the basal ganglia, and both structures send information back to the cortex via the thalamus. The balance between these two systems allows for smooth, coordinated movement. A disturbance in either will manifest as a movement disorder. In PD, the symptoms result from the loss of dopaminergic cells in the pars compacta region of the substantia nigra reticulata (SNr). This loss upsets the normal balance between dopaminergic inhibition and cholinergic (acetylcholine; ACh) excitation of striatal output ($\gamma$-aminobutyric acid; GABA) neurons. The net effect is to increase GABAergic output from the striatum, eventually leading to excessive inhibition of the thalamic and brainstem nuclei that receive the outflow from the basal ganglia. This excessive thalamic inhibition results in suppression of the cortical motor system, leading to akinesia, rigidity, and tremor, whereas inhibition of brainstem motor areas may contribute to abnormalities of posture and gait.

## TREATMENT OF PARKINSON'S DISEASE

### Medical Management

The goals of therapy in PD are to maintain motor function and preserve quality of life (QoL), while minimizing drug-induced complications. Current medical therapies achieve this by restoring the dopaminergic/cholinergic balance in the striatum by effectively blocking the effect of ACh. This block can be accomplished with anticholinergics or by enhancing dopaminergic transmission, either by increasing the concentration of dopamine in the CNS or by binding to central dopaminergic receptors directly. Motor symptoms respond favorably to symptomatic medical therapy early in the course of the illness, whereas nonmotor symptoms typically respond poorly. Medical intervention is usually initiated when symptoms begin to interfere with function. As of yet, no treatment exists that slows down or significantly improves disability of advanced stages of PD.[6] Current medical therapy is summarized in **Table 1**.[7,8]

### Surgical Management

#### Lesioning

The mean duration of PD at the time of surgical intervention is about 12 to 15 years.[9–12] Surgical intervention historically was limited to lesioning of deeper brain structures. Thalamotomy was used in treating tremor, whereas pallidotomy was used for levodopa-induced dyskinesia/antiparkinsonian effects.[13] The rationale for these surgical interventions was that the pathophysiological manifestations of PD were known to be due to abnormal CNS activity, and permanent lesioning would remove these stimuli. Although beneficial, these interventions were shown to induce several permanent side effects, such as paresis, confusion, quadrantanopsia, gait disturbances, dysarthria, and hypersalivation.[13,14] Furthermore, these surgical procedures are associated with a high risk of complications when bilateral and loss of long-term benefit, with no possibility of decreasing anti-PD drugs.[13] These procedures are uncommon today, although they may be employed in areas where stimulators are not available or in circumstances in which they are contraindicated.

#### Deep brain stimulation

In the late 1980s, it was discovered intraoperatively that high-frequency electrical stimulation was able to induce the same functional effect as lesioning, thus introducing DBS as a treatment modality.[15] This discovery revolutionized the treatment of PD in advanced stages, and has rejuvenated the role of surgery. There are many reports documenting significant and long-term benefits of DBS.[9,11,16,17] Some of the advantages of DBS include its reversibility and that it is safer than lesioning even when bilateral. Also, the flexibility of the parameters of stimulation can optimize benefits while minimizing side effects. Furthermore, there is much less potential for interference with new treatments. However, there are drawbacks. DBS is more expensive and time-consuming than lesioning. DBS requires specialized personnel to perform the procedure and manage the stimulator postoperatively. DBS is associated with an increased risk of infection, as the hardware is indwelling, and postoperative magnetic resonance imaging (MRI) requires special precautions. Furthermore, there is a need for periodic battery replacement.[18]

The targets of DBS include the ventralis intermedius nucleus (Vim), the subthalamic nucleus (STN), and the globus pallidus (GPi). Benabid and colleagues found that 88% of patients treated with Vim-DBS had complete or near-complete tremor relief at 6 months to 8 years postoperatively. However, the effects of Vim-DBS on the other symptoms of PD, such as akinesia, rigidity, bradykinesia, or drug-induced dyskinesias, were either short-lasting or nonexistent.[15] As such, Vim-DBS is usually limited to patients with tremor-predominant symptoms. However, as those other symptoms are often the most disabling signs in advanced PD, another target was needed. Although there has been debate over the superiority of STN versus GPi-DBS, evidence suggests that DBS of the STN is superior to that of GPi.[10,19–21] In a randomized study, there was a 48% improvement in motor Unified Parkinson's Disability Rating Scale (UPDRS) scores in STN patients, as compared with GPi.[20] However, there were more cognitive and behavioral complications in STN group, although the duration of disease and age at time of surgery was higher in the STN group. In a study that looked at 5-year follow-up, there was a dramatic loss of benefit in 6 PD patients with bilateral GPi-DBS. In 4 of 6 of these patients, subsequent STN was able to restore benefit.[22] Thus, STN-DBS seems to be a superior initial procedure, and may even be used as salvage therapy in those patients in whom GPi-DBS has failed.

### *Patient selection for deep brain stimulation*

Patient selection is a complex process, and it is recommended that a multidisciplinary team, including a movement-disorder neurologist specialized in DBS, a neuropsychologist, a psychiatrist, and a stereotactic neurosurgeon should be involved.[18,23] It is still unclear whether there is an ideal duration of PD before transitioning to surgery, although the mean duration of disease at the time of surgery is approximately 12 to 15 years.[9–12] There are many components in the preoperative assessment of those patients considered for DBS surgery, including the Core Assessment Program for Surgical Interventional Therapies in Parkinson's Disease (CAPSIT-PD) protocol, the severity of disease, the levodopa response, and age. As of yet, there are no studies to show that earlier intervention is neuroprotective.[24]

**Core Assessment Program for Surgical Interventional Therapies in Parkinson's Disease** CAPSIT-PD is a protocol developed to establish minimal requirements for a common evaluation protocol of patient candidates for lesions and DBS. This protocol recommends a working diagnosis of PD at least 5 years to avoid misdiagnosis.[25] Components include levodopa responsiveness, QoL, dyskinesia scales, and cognitive/behavioral assessments. Although aiming to achieve some uniformity in assessing patients for DBS, these criteria for selection of PD patients for DBS are being actively

**Table 1**
**Common medications for management of Parkinson's disease**

| Type | Comments | Side Effects | Contraindications |
|---|---|---|---|
| Dopamine agonists | | | |
| Ergot alkaloids<br>Bromocriptine<br>Cabergoline<br>Lisurid<br>Nonergot Alkaloids<br>Pramiprexole<br>Ropinirole<br>Rotigotone | Readily cross BBB<br>Long-acting<br>Less effective than levodopa in:<br>– Relieving signs/symptoms of PD<br>Less likely to cause:<br>– Dyskinesia<br>– "On-Off" phenomenon | Nausea/Vomiting<br>Hypotension<br>Dyskinesias<br>Akathesia<br>Confusion<br>Dysrhythmias<br>Psychiatric:<br>– Delusions<br>– Hallucinations | History of psychotic disorders<br>Relative contraindications:<br>– Recent MI<br>– Severe PVD<br>– Active PUD |
| Dopamine precursors | | | |
| Levodopa | Converted to DA<br>Ameliorates all major clinical features of parkinsonism<br>Often helpful for hyperkinesias | Similar to DA agonists | Narrow-angle glaucoma<br>Psychotic illness<br>Patients on MAOIs |
| Carbidopa | Inhibits Dopa Decarboxylase<br>– enzyme responsible for conversion of levodopa to DA<br>Cannot cross BBB<br>– limits breakdown of levodopa outside CNS<br>– Increases effectiveness of levodopa, while minimizing side effects | Possible rebound HTN | — |
| Sinemet | Combination of carbidopa/ levodopa<br>Fixed proportion<br>– 1:10 or 1:4 | — | — |

| | | | |
|---|---|---|---|
| Anticholinergics | | | |
| Trihexyphenidyl Benzotropine | More helpful for tremor and rigidity<br>Generally less effective than DA drugs | Excessive drowsiness<br>Constipation<br>Dry mouth<br>Urinary retention<br>Defective papillary accommodation<br>Confusion<br>Hallucinations | Relative contraindications:<br>– elderly<br>– cognitive disturbances |
| Antivirals | | | |
| Amantadine | Given for mild parkinsonism<br>Used alone or in combo with anti-ACh<br>Precise MOA is unclear<br>Improves all clinical features of PD | SE relatively uncommon:<br>– restlessness<br>– confusion<br>– rashes<br>– edema<br>– dysrhythmias | — |
| COMT inhibitors | | | |
| Tolcapone<br>Entacapone | ↓ dose and response fluctuations to Sinemet<br>Helps sustain plasma levels of levodopa | Nausea<br>Diarrhea<br>Confusion<br>Dyskinesias<br>Abnormal LFTs<br>Discoloration of the urine | — |
| MAO-B inhibitor | | | |
| Selegeline | Inhibits breakdown of DA<br>Enhances antiparksonian effect of levodopa<br>May reduce mild on-off fluctuations in responsiveness | Diarrhea | Concomitant use with meperidine |

*Abbreviations:* ACh, acetylcholine; BBB, blood-brain barrier; COMT, catechol-*O*-methyltransferase; DA, dopamine; HTN, hypertension; LFT, liver function test; MI, myocardial infarction; MAO, monoamine oxygenase; MOAI, monoamine oxygenase inhibitor; PUD, peptic ulcer disease; PVD, peripheral vascular disease; SE, side effects.

modified.[18,26,27] Furthermore, many surgical centers adopt their own protocols although these protocols generally follow CAPSIT-PD guidelines, especially the diagnosis of PD, responsiveness to dopaminergic therapies, when to consider surgical options, and that there are no cognitive/behavioral deficits that preclude surgery.

**Severity of disease** The UPDRS is a validated clinical scale that evaluates the longitudinal course of disease. Components include mentation, activities of daily living, motor function, and complications of anti-PD therapy. However, UPDRS has not been shown to be predictive of benefit from DBS, although meta-analysis shows greater motor UPDRS score improvement with higher baseline scores.[28,29] In general, parkinsonian signs or specific side effects of medications starting to have an impact on QoL, despite optimized medical therapy, remains a good indication for DBS.

**Levodopa response** Preoperative levodopa responsiveness has been considered predictive of postoperative clinical improvement in multiple studies,[9,25,26,29–31] although a positive correlation at 3- and 12-month follow up was only looked at specifically in two studies.[28,30] All motor signs that are improved by levodopa before surgery are expected to improve after DBS. In contrast, patients with levodopa-resistant signs will have poor clinical benefit after DBS.

**Age** There are many possible reasons why surgical centers might consider elderly patients less eligible, including other age-related comorbidities, a higher risk of surgical complications, and longer postoperative recovery.[18] However, there is currently insufficient evidence to clearly establish a cutoff age for DBS surgery. The average age for patients undergoing DBS is between 50 and 60 years old, ranging from 31 to 81 years.[12] Whereas some studies suggest an age limit of 70,[9,11,32] others say an age less than 75 is suitable for surgery.[17,31] Only a few articles correlated clinical outcome and complications in STN-DBS with age at the time of surgery.[28,29,31,33,34] Two studies showed no correlation at all,[29,34] whereas the others showed better postoperative outcomes for younger patients.[28,31,33] Whether this is confounded by other age-related comorbidities will need to be addressed in future studies.

### *DBS exclusion criteria*

Exclusion criteria include evidence of cognitive impairment and certain medical comorbidities. Cognitive impairment is reported as the most frequent cause of exclusion.[9,11,28] This finding is supported by evidence showing cognitive changes in elderly patients after STN-DBS in those without cognitive impairment before surgery,[35] and a worsening in those patients with preexisting impairment.[36,37] Evidence suggests that there are no consistent cognitive deficits after Vim-DBS,[38–40] which is a major reason the age limit is higher for Vim-DBS more than STN- or GPi-DBS. Several comorbidities often represent major exclusion criteria for DBS surgery. These comorbidities include coagulopathies, severe and uncontrolled hypertension, cerebral vascular disease, severe coronary artery disease and diabetes mellitus, active cancer, and active infection, although no correlation between these comorbidities and surgical risk and outcome has been established.[9,10,32,34,41] A permanent pacemaker is not a contraindication for DBS, although precautions must be taken to limit possible DBS generator-PPM electrical interference,[42] and MRI will not be possible. Diagnoses that are no longer considered exclusion criteria are medication-induced psychosis and depression,[43] as there is currently no clear evidence that preoperative depression is a risk factor for postoperative depression.[44]

## ANESTHETIC MANAGEMENT OF THE PARKINSON'S PATIENT UNDERGOING DBS LEAD PLACEMENT

DBS surgery requires that the patient be secured in a stereographic head frame in a semi-upright position, and be awake enough to respond appropriately to the surgeon, as the actual positioning of the electrodes requires the cooperation of an alert patient.

The anesthetic goals for DBS surgery include ensuring a safe airway, maintaining hemodynamic stability, and providing adequate analgesia and sedation, all the while attempting to have an alert, cooperative patient for intraoperative neurologic assessment. Furthermore, anesthetics, when necessary, must not interfere with electrophysiological brain mapping and clinical testing. Unfortunately, common GABAergic sedative drugs, such as propofol and midazolam, ameliorate tremor or rigidity, and interfere with brain mapping and testing of the implanted DBS electrode lead. Moreover, these medications easily impair the level of consciousness, and may cause disinhibition or inability to cooperate with intraoperative testing, as well as respiratory depression, which can have disastrous complications due to difficult access to the airway secondary to the bulky metal head frame.

### *Preoperative Concerns*

A careful assessment of extent of the disease and coexisting medical conditions should be made. The patient should be assessed for their ability to cooperate. A full explanation to the patient about each step of the procedure is absolutely necessary. If MRI will be used for the procedure, a careful history of implanted ferrous metals, pacemakers, and aneurysm clips should be obtained. If MRI is contraindicated, computed tomography scanning is a viable alternative. The planned intraoperative position should be ascertained and the need for invasive monitoring determined, based on severity of coexisting diseases and patient positioning (eg, monitoring for air embolism). Medications used for treatment of motor symptoms should be held in these patients overnight and on the morning of surgery. Preoperative benzodiazepines, opioids, and other sedatives can interfere with patient cooperation and the interpretation of tremor, and therefore should be avoided. Contraindications to DBS surgery include dementia, extensive brain atrophy, comorbid medical conditions that preclude safe surgery, and patient noncompliance.

## STAGE 1: STEREOTACTIC HEAD-FRAME PLACEMENT AND IMAGING/DBS LEAD IMPLANTATION

Generous local anesthetic infiltration in the scalp is essential, even for patients undergoing general anesthesia (GA). Local anesthetic typically will be given by the neurosurgeon at the pin insertion sites. The scalp blocks may be placed at this time, or any time before start of the craniotomy. Moderate sedation during the imaging may be used when necessary to minimize patient anxiety and decrease movement during the scan. At the author's institution, most patients receive a propofol infusion at about 50 μg/kg/min. Dexmedetomidine infusions may be used as well. After the imaging has been completed, if an awake craniotomy is planned then the anesthetic is discontinued before transport back to the operating room.

DBS lead implantation does not typically require wide exposure. The implantation can be performed with local infiltration of the scalp or with scalp blocks. During burr-hole placement, the placement of a bite block is done to limit possible dental damage from the vibrations of the drill. Once the skull opening has been created safely, the microelectrode is inserted into the brain toward the thalamus and subthalamic region. Ideally, a neurophysiologist participates in the identification of specific brain cells in these regions, the purpose being to map out the area and optimize placement of the electrode. The time for microelectrode recording may take several hours. Once the appropriate area is identified, test stimulation is performed to check that the electrode is in a safe location that will not disturb brain function. When a safe area is identified, the electrode is left in place and clipped to the skull with bone-fastening devices. If both sides of the brain are to be operated on at the same setting, a second incision will be made on the other side and the procedure repeated, which will again take several hours. For most patients, the first stage of the operation (placing electrodes into the brain) will all be performed in 1 day, the scalp incisions will be closed, and the patient will be observed overnight. The patient will return to the hospital 3 to 10 days later for the second stage of the procedure.

The patient must be fully conscious for the recordings and neurologic examination. If sedation or GA is employed, the transition from the asleep to the awake phase can be extremely challenging, due to the potential complications during awakening and manipulation of the airway with the brain exposed, such as coughing, Valsalva maneuvers, vomiting, and movement; this may lead to disastrous complications such as bleeding, brain swelling, venous air embolism, and potentially, death. For these reasons, many anesthesiologists try to avoid airway instrumentation. As mentioned earlier, airway intubation when the patient's head is secured in the head frame to the operating table and covered by the surgical drapes may be difficult, especially if emergency intubation of the trachea is required. When mapping is completed, sedation or analgesia, or both, may be provided.

### *Anesthetic Options for Deep Brain Stimulation Lead Placement*

Numerous techniques have been described: local anesthesia, regional anesthetic techniques (scalp nerve blockade), intravenous sedation, and GA using an asleep-awake-asleep (AAA) technique, with or without airway instrumentation. With no consensus as to the optimal regimen, most institutions have developed their own techniques to suit the needs of their surgeons and individual preference. At the author's institution, an awake craniotomy with local anesthetic supplementation is the preferred anesthetic technique. With adequate preprocedural patient education to minimize anxiety, the procedure is usually well tolerated. This procedure ensures adequate microelectrode recording (MER) signal strength and bedside neurophysiologic evaluation to optimize lead placement. In a recent prospective trial of 200 patients, an awake craniotomy with DBS lead placement was well tolerated, with reduced intensive care time and hospital stay.[45]

### *Regional Anesthesia for Deep Brain Stimulation Lead Placement: Scalp Nerve Blocks*

Skin infiltration with local anesthetic at pin insertion sites and the skin incision, or performance of a scalp nerve block, is essential for pain relief and reducing potential opiate-related complications. Blocks of the auriculotemporal, zygomaticotemporal, supraorbital, supratrochlear, occipital, and greater occipital nerves can allow for pain-free skin incision. Supraorbital and occipital blocks observationally have been found to give adequate pain relief at the author's institution. Infiltration with large volumes of local anesthetic or scalp blocks carries the potential risk of local anesthetic toxicity in patients who are already prone to seizures, although doses of up to 4.5 mg/kg of ropivacaine seem safe.[46] Doses of 2.5 mg/kg levobupivacaine were also acceptable, although levobupivacaine is no longer commercially available.[47] Several studies have measured plasma concentrations of local anesthetics and demonstrated that absorption is rapid, and that whereas potentially toxic plasma concentrations were achieved in some patients, no signs or symptoms of local toxicity were evident.[46–48]

### *Sedation for Deep Brain Stimulation Lead Placement Using Propofol*

Propofol is one of the most frequently used drugs for both sedation and GA in DBS procedures. Propofol provides titratable sedation and a rapid, smooth recovery, decreases the incidence of seizures, and when used with an AAA technique, minimizes interference with electrocortical recordings on awakening before lead placement.[49] Propofol is often used as a target-controlled infusion and may be combined with remifentanil or fentanyl. In a study of 50 patients comparing propofol infusion supplemented with remifentanil or fentanyl for conscious sedation, there was no difference in outcomes among the groups, and most patients were completely satisfied.[50] Furthermore, retrospective analysis of an AAA technique using propofol and remifentanil showed that adequate conditions were obtained in 98% of patients, with a median wake-up time of 9 min.[51] In addition, a case report of 15 patients examined the effects of propofol on MER signals, and found that a propofol infusion titrated until adequate sedation was achieved, with a mean infusion dose of 50 μg/kg/min, did significantly decrease the spontaneous activity of the STN neurons and might therefore interfere with optimal lead placement. However, the effect of propofol was short-lived and neuronal activity returned to baseline in 9.4 ± 4.2 minutes after propofol administration was terminated.[49] A recent retrospective study of 250 DBS patients from the Cleveland Clinic by Khatib and colleagues evaluated the perioperative risk for patients undergoing DBS procedure. In most cases, propofol was used primarily only during the first 30 to 45 minutes of the case to facilitate head-frame placement, with a mean infusion dose of propofol of 67.2 ± 53.2 μg/kg/min.[52] All patients received local anesthetic before scalp incision. The researchers found an adverse-events total complication rate of 11.6%. The most common complications were neurologic, which accounted for 3.6% and included intracranial hemorrhage and seizure, and psychological/psychiatric complications, with an incidence of about 3.2%, with confusion and anxiety being the most frequent. Age was found to be an independent risk factor for complications during surgery. The rate of major complications was found to be 5.6%. There are some limitations to this study: this is one institution's experience using predominately one anesthetic technique, more than 90% of DBS procedures were done under propofol sedation, and only 2.3% of cases were done without supplemental sedatives or anesthetic drugs. At present there are no studies comparing different anesthetic techniques and perioperative risk.

### *Sedation for Deep Brain Stimulation Lead Placement Using Dexmedetomidine*

There is growing research suggesting that dexmedetomidine may the ideal sedative for DBS procedures. Dexmedetomidine is a central-acting α2 agonist that offers sedation and anxiolysis, and helps maintain hemodynamic stability (through its central a-agonist activity).[53] Dexmedetomidine also has an anesthetic-sparing effect and preserves respiration with minimal respiratory depression, even with infusions at the higher end of the dose range.[54,55] Patients can also be awakened easily by verbal stimulation after administration of dexmedetomidine. The cerebral effects are consistent with a desirable neurophysiologic profile, including neuroprotective characteristics.[56–58] Dexmedetomidine is particularly valuable when eloquent areas (those involved in communication) of the brain are stimulated, and an awake, cooperative patient must be capable of undergoing neurocognitive testing. Dexmedetomidine can be used as a sole agent, an adjunct, or a rescue drug for the awake craniotomy.[59–62] In recent retrospective study dexmedetomidine provided patient comfort, did not interfere with electrophysiological mapping, and provided hemodynamic stability, significantly reducing the use of antihypertensive medication, although supplemental antihypertensives were given.[59] The researchers also noted that a dosage range of 0.3 to 0.6 μg/kg/h did not impair intensity of movement disorder in PD, or interfere with mapping using MER. There are currently no randomized trials of this agent in comparison with other anesthetic agents.

### *General Anesthesia*

GA in DBS surgery may be a viable alternative in patients who cannot tolerate local anesthesia or monitored anesthetic care due to massive fear, reduced cooperation, or coughing attacks. In general, there has been a hesitation to resort to GA, as optimal targeting of the STN with intraoperative MERs is usually performed under local anesthesia.[63] Experience in intraoperative microrecording of STN under GA is sparse, and neuronal firing patterns are not well characterized.[64] Furthermore, the use of GA has not been specifically assessed on long-term neuropsychological sequelae and QoL.

Studies are emerging that suggest DBS with MER can be done under GA with some accommodation, with minimal interference. A recent retrospective case report of 10 patients using desflurane as maintenance anesthesia reported that if the minimal alveolar concentration (MAC) level was kept below 1, it did not drastically interfere with microelectrode mapping.[65] An attenuated, but typical firing pattern of STN and SNr neurons was observed. This result is consistent with another study showing that maintaining a MAC greater than 1 depresses the discharge rate of the GPi/external GPi neurons, particularly in patients with PD.[66,67] Furthermore, in those patients in whom light desflurane anesthesia was used, passive movement-related neuronal activity could be observed in a good MER trajectory.[65] Moreover, 6-month follow-up showed a decreased daily levodopa equivalent dose, improvement in UPDRS total and motor scores, significantly lower postoperative off-medication/with DBS state mean UPDRS total and motor scores when compared with preoperative baseline values ($P<.05$). These results are similar to previous studies.[63,64,68] Another much smaller study examined using a propofol-remifentanil technique with a Bispectral Index (BIS) goal during microrecording of 60 to 65 in one patient.[58] It was noted that the spontaneous firing patterns of STN and SNr neurons under GA were similar to the spontaneous neuronal discharges of these nuclei recorded in PD patients who had awake craniotomies.[69] The investigators suggest that this minimal interference is probably because of the light level of general anesthesia under which the recordings were obtained. The researchers found that the patient's motor function improved after the surgery at 12-month follow-up, with a reduction of the duration of "off" periods of about 60%, the off-period dystonia and biphasic dyskinesias practically disappearing, and the dose of antiparkinsonian medication reduced by 40%. Another case-control study of 25 patients compared a nitrous-sevoflurane-opioid technique versus local anesthesia, and found administration of GA did not correlate with lesser postoperative improvements in motor and daily activity scores, except for off-medication bradykinesia.[70]

There is growing evidence to suggest that DBS surgery for advanced PD with MER guidance is possible, with good clinical results under GA, using a variety of techniques. Care must be taken to limit the amount of anesthetic given. Under these settings the typical STN bursting pattern can be identified, although the typical widening of the background noise baseline entering the STN region is typically absent. Although patients receiving local anesthesia showed greater improvement, both groups showed significant improvement when compared with preoperative baseline, which is encouraging in patients for whom this may be the only viable surgical option. **Table 2** lists more information.

**Table 2**
**Anesthetic options in deep brain stimulation lead placement**

| Anesthetic Agents | | Target Dosing Values[a] | Side Effects | Comments |
|---|---|---|---|---|
| Local anesthetics[b] | Bupivacaine | <4.5 mg/kg | — | Sufficient analgesia with combination of:<br>– injection at pin insertion sites<br>– scalp blocks |
| Adjuncts to local anesthesia[c] | Benzodiazepines | — | Amelioration of tremor<br>Interference with MER brain mapping and testing of implanted leads<br>Impairs level of consciousness<br>– inability to cooperate with intraoperative testing<br>– may cause respiratory depression | Remains contraindicated |
| | Opiates<br>– Fentanyl<br>– Remifentanil | — | Rigidity | Used in combination with other agents for sedation or GA with success<br>– care must be taken to secure airway |
| | Propofol | ~50 μg/kg/min | Amelioration of tremor<br>Attenuation of MER signaling<br>– typical firing patterns return to baseline after discontinuation of infusion | Can be used as:<br>– sole agent<br>– in combination with opiates, such fentanyl and remifentanil, with equal success |
| | Dexmedetomidine | 0.3–0.6 μg/kg/h | — | – sedative, although patients can be easily awakened<br>– anxiolytic<br>– helps maintain hemodynamic stability<br>– has an anesthetic sparing effect<br>– preserves respiration with minimal respiratory depression |
| | General anesthesia<br>– Volatiles<br>– IV agents<br>– Combination | BIS score ~60<br>MAC <1 | — | A secure airway is essential |

*Abbreviations:* BIS, Bispectral Index; GA, general anesthesia; MAC, minimal alveolar concentration; MER, microelectrode recording.

[a] For most agents, an ideal dosing range has not been established. These values are from case reports suggesting safe dosing limits with minimal MER interference.

[b] Only ropivacaine has specifically been addressed in scalp block use for DBS lead placement. Please refer to standard reference source for other specific local anesthesia agent maximum doses in general use.

[c] In general, DBS lead placement is not overly stimulating. Sedation, if required, should be aimed at using the minimal amount necessary to achieve patient compliance.

### Airway Management

Intraoperative airway management may be uneventful during sedation. However, the anesthesiologist must be ready for the possibility of hypoventilation or airway obstruction. There must always be a plan for securing the airway if necessary. Patient positioning may limit access and further contribute to airway compromise. Airway instrumentation when the patient's head is in the stereotactic frame and covered by the surgical drapes may be difficult, especially if emergency endotracheal intubation is required.

Various airway adjuncts have been described for the awake craniotomy, including nasal cannula, facemask, awake fiberoptic endotracheal intubation with local anesthetic infiltration, the laryngeal mask airway (LMA), and cuffed oropharyngeal airway. Facemask ventilation may be limited by the head frame. A cooperative patient may be coached to breathe directly into the y-piece connector of the anesthesia circuit. If the front arch of the stereotactic head frame is concave-down, use of a video laryngoscope (eg, GlideScope) may be possible, should intubation become necessary. In recent years, the LMA has become a popular adjunct for craniotomies. LMA is well tolerated at lighter planes of anesthesia, is easy to insert and remove, and enables ventilation to be controlled, thus providing optimal operative conditions. As an alternative to the LMA, Huncke and colleagues found that a cuffed oropharyngeal airway may be safe. In a case series of 20 patients undergoing a craniotomy using the AAA technique with spontaneous ventilation, insertion was accomplished easily at the first attempt in all cases, irrespective of patient position (supine versus lateral), although airway maneuvers were occasionally required when patients were supine.[71–74]

### Hemodynamic Monitoring

A well-known complication of DBS procedures is intracerebral hemorrhage. It has been estimated that the incidence is about 2% to 4%, or about 1.4% per lead implant.[75,76] However, there is little evidence available to guide intraoperative blood pressure management. One study suggests that maintaining a systolic blood pressure of less than 140 mm Hg is associated with a lower risk of intracerebral hemorrhage.[76] This study also found that significant risk factors for intracerebral hemorrhage were chronic arterial hypertension and acute intraoperative hypertension. There are currently no corroborative studies. Furthermore, there are no studies assessing optimal intravenous antihypertensive therapy to accomplish this goal.

### Processed Electroencephalography Monitoring

Previous research has noted that processed electroencephalography (pEEG) (primarily BIS, Aspect Medical) values correspond linearly to the hypnotic dose of intravenous or volatile agents.[77] In general, BIS values of 65 to 85 have been recommended for sedation, whereas values of 40 to 65 are usually employed during GA.[78] With this in mind, BIS monitoring may allow the level of sedation and analgesia to be rapidly adjusted to accommodate specific requirements, in this case intraoperative microrecording. There are a few studies looking at the role of pEEG monitoring in DBS, none of which are randomized controlled studies. Schulz and colleagues[79] investigated whether BIS monitoring would be beneficial in patients receiving AAA, and found no difference between groups with respect to times of arousal, total amount of propofol consumption, and cardiopulmonary stability. In contrast, an earlier study found that pEEG monitoring led to lower propofol infusion rates and a significantly decreased amount of total propofol given.[80] The evidence regarding the utility of pEEG monitoring in DBS is scarce and sometimes conflicting. Although its role continues to evolve, pEEG monitoring may still become a useful adjunct in patients otherwise unable to undergo awake functional neurosurgery, as some investigators have suggested.[81]

## *Intraoperative Complications of the Lead Placement Procedure*

### *Venous air embolism*

Air may be entrained through bone or dural veins causing venous air emboli (VAE), which can result in significant hemodynamic changes, pulmonary edema, respiratory failure, and even death. The incidence of VAE in the recumbent position is estimated at around 3% to 4.5%.[82] Two important predictors to consider in VAE are patient positioning and the occurrence of coughing. The patient typically is positioned with the surgical site above the right atrium, which creates a negative pressure gradient. Unfortunately, the venous sinuses, due to their fixed dural attachment, are unable to collapse under this negative pressure gradient and instead facilitate air entrainment. Clinically significant cases of VAE in subjects that are spontaneously breathing are often preceded by cough. The exact mechanism is still currently unknown. This occurrence is rare, except during the early minutes of the operation when air entrainment most commonly occurs. In addition to coughing, awake patients may also subjectively report experiencing chest pain or nausea. Other risk factors associated with VAE include spontaneous breathing, deep inspiration, and hypovolemia, all of which increase the risk for VAE by precipitating a larger negative intrathoracic pressure that in turn is transmitted to the venous system.[83]

There are many modalities to diagnose VAE. Transesophageal echo (TEE) is the most sensitive monitoring tool available for detection of VAE, and is considered the gold standard. However, it is invasive, expensive, and has a risk of injury. Moreover, it is not a technique tolerated by awake patients. A noninvasive alternative to TEE is precordial Doppler, which can detect turbulent sound reflecting entrained air. The drawback to this technique is its subjectivity, as well as the importance of probe placement, which if not correct may lead to missing subtle VAE. In addition, the noise level of the precordial Doppler can be challenging. Changes in vital signs may also aid in the diagnosis. Hypoxemia, hypercapnia, and decreased end-tidal $CO_2$ may signal an increase in the functional dead space. Also, if available, an increase in end-tidal $N_2$ (nitrogen) may be noticed. If undiagnosed, hypotension, cardiac dysrhythmias, and cardiovascular collapse can occur as air entrainment continues.

Treatment is largely supportive. The surgeon should be informed as soon as the diagnosis is made, after which time the surgical field should be flooded with fluids, open veins cauterized, and exposed bone waxed. If the airway is not secured, placement of an LMA can be used as a bridge until the head frame can be removed. If $N_2O$ is used it should be discontinued, as $N_2O$ diffuses into air bubbles faster than nitrogen can diffuse out, and increases the size of the bubble. $FiO_2$ should be increased to 100%. If significant amounts of air have entered the circulation, the jugular veins should be manually occluded in an attempt to prevent additional air from being entrained while the surgeon obtains hemostasis. The blood pressure should be supported with fluid and vasopressors. If possible, the operative site should be positioned below the level of the heart.[83–85] This move can be accomplished by tilting the table into the Trendelenberg position. A large central venous catheter may be inserted and the right atrium aspirated until no more air can be obtained. Preventive measures include maintaining adequate volume status (as hydration increases central venous pressure [CVP]), which in turn decreases the pressure gradient between the surgical site and CVP. Furthermore, adequate volume status is associated with increased left atrial pressure, which minimizes the risk of paradoxic embolism to the left side of the circulation.

### *Intracerebral hemorrhage*

The incidence of intracerebral hemorrhage after DBS is about 2% to 4%.[76] Possible risk factors include a history of chronic hypertension or acute intraoperative hypertension. Evidence suggests that maintaining a systolic blood pressure of less than 140 mm Hg may be protective. Furthermore, a positive trend between the occurrence of hemorrhage and multiple MER lead passes was noticed.[76] Although not specifically addressed in the literature, rebound hypertension secondary to discontinuation of PD medications the morning before surgery is not uncommon. Patients on Sinemet anecdotally are perceived to be more apt to experience this phenomenon (Dr. Ron Alterman, personal communication). It is postulated that carbidopa, in addition to minimizing levodopa breakdown in the periphery, may also inhibit baseline peripheral catecholamine synthesis, and that discontinuation before surgery may result in increased synthesis and sympathetic response. Restarting PD medications after lead placement may be associated with significant hypotension, especially if the intraoperative antihypertensives are still in effect.

## ANESTHESIA FOR DEEP BRAIN STIMULATION LEAD PLACEMENT. STAGE 2: STIMULATOR PLACEMENT

Most patients will usually return to the operating room a few weeks after DBS lead placement. During this procedure the cables, batteries, and simulator will be inserted into the neck and chest area. As neurologic monitoring is not required, this procedure can be performed safely under GA. Once the device is inserted, the patient will return to the neurology clinic. The neurologist will turn on the stimulators several weeks later.

### *Deep Brain Stimulation Lead Placement: Postoperative Hardware-Related Complications*

Miscellaneous hardware complications include hardware infection, DBS electrode fracture, extension wire failure, generator malfunction, lead migration, skin erosion, foreign body reaction, pain over the generator, and seromas. For some of these complications, such as electrode fracture, generator malfunction, foreign body reaction, or lead migration, a second surgical procedure to reposition or replace malfunctioning equipment is necessary. For others, less invasive modalities may be attempted first. Hardware infection rates vary widely, from less than 1% to as high as 15%.[86] There are several options for dealing with infections once they occur. Superficial infections of the wound and can be treated with intravenous or even oral antibiotics. Deep infections around hardware must be surgically treated, often with device removal.[86] Pain over the generator may be treated with topical analgesics, such as capsaicin cream. Seromas may be safely drained under sterile conditions, although fluid should be sent for pathology for analysis.

## ANESTHETIC CONSIDERATIONS FOR PD PATIENTS WITH IMPLANTED DEEP BRAIN STIMULATION

As DBS is still a young treatment modality, there is little evidence in the literature to guide many of the postoperative considerations, anesthetic or otherwise, that these patients may require after DBS lead and generator placement. The evidence that does exist consists of mainly small case reports with small cohorts. The concerns range from the safety of MRI to specific operative accommodations should additional surgery become necessary.

**Table 3**
**Recommended assessment of the patient with Parkinson's disease**

| Organ System | Signs/Symptoms | Pertinent Questions | Relevant Workup |
|---|---|---|---|
| Respiratory system – particularly prone to upper airway complications | Upper airway dysfunction:<br>– retained secretions<br>– atalectasis<br>– respiratory infections<br>– aspiration pneumonia<br>– most common cause of death<br>Other complications:<br>– post-extubation laryngospasm<br>– postoperative respiratory failure | Dysphagia<br>Sialorrhea<br>Respiratory impairment<br>– rigidity<br>– Bradykinesia or uncoordinated movement of respiratory muscles | Chest radiograph<br>Pulmonary function tests<br>Arterial blood gas |
| Autonomic nervous system | Difficulty with:<br>– salivation<br>– micturition<br>– GI function<br>– temperature regulation<br>Seborrhea | — | — |
| Cardiovascular system | Orthostatic hypotension<br>Cardiac arrhythmias<br>Dependent edema<br>Hypertension | Orthostatic hypotension<br>Arrhythmias<br>Hypertension<br>Hypovolemia | Electrocardiogram<br>Echocardiogram |
| Gastrointestinal system | Dysphagia<br>Esophageal dysfunction<br>Constipation<br>Weight loss<br>Sialorrhea | Weight loss<br>GERD | Serum albumin/ transferrin |
| Endocrine system | Abnormal glucose metabolism | — | Blood glucose concentration |
| Central nervous system | Muscle rigidity<br>Akinesia<br>Tremor<br>Confusion<br>Depression<br>Hallucination<br>Speech impairment | — | — |

*Abbreviations:* GI, gastrointestinal; GERD, gastroesophageal reflux disease.

### *Magnetic Resonance Imaging*

There are several possible adverse events associated with DBS patients and MRI. The safety concerns for electrical stimulation devices include heating, magnetic field interactions, induced electrical currents, image distortion, and the functional disruption of the operational aspects of these devices. Failure to follow manufacturer's MRI

**Table 4**
**Anesthetic options for Parkinson's disease patients having non-Parkinson's disease surgery**

| Anesthetic Agents | | Comments | Complications/Contraindications |
|---|---|---|---|
| Intravenous anesthetics | | | |
| Induction agents | Thiopental | — | Parkinsonian episodes[94,112,113] |
| | Ketamine | — | Theoretically contraindicated<br>– exaggerated sympathetic response<br>– has been used safely[114] |
| | Propofol | Ideal agent while applying head frame<br>– rapid metabolism<br>– predictable emergence profile | Case reports<br>– dykinesia[115]<br>– abolition of tremor[116] |
| NMBDs | Non-depolarizers | Sensitivity to agents is similar to normal patients<br>May mask tremor<br>No reported cases of complications<br>No evidence suggesting preferred NMBD | — |
| | Depolarizers | Not contraindicated in PD | Reported case of hyperkalemia[117]<br>– case complicated by other issues<br>Subsequent case series showed no signs of succinylcholine-induced hyperkalemia[100] |
| Opioids | Fentanyl | — | Muscle rigidity[118,119]<br>– responds to neuromuscular blockade[119] |
| | Morphine | — | Low doses:[120] Reduction in dyskinesias<br>High doses:[120] Increase in akinesia |
| | Alfentanil | — | Acute dystonia[99] |
| | Meperidine | Coadministration of MAOIs should be avoided | Agitation<br>Muscle rigidity<br>Hyperthermia |

| | | | |
|---|---|---|---|
| Inhalational anesthetics[a] | Halothane | — | Sensitizes heart to catecholamines<br>– L-dopa is contraindicated<br>– already arrhythmogenic |
| | Newer agents<br>Isoflurane<br>Sevoflurane | Less arrhythmogenic<br>Hypotension is still a concern due to:<br>– hypovolemia<br>– norepinephrine depletion<br>– autonomic dysfunction | Coadministration with other medications:<br>– bromocriptine or pergolide<br>– prone to excessive vasodilation<br>– further exacerbates hypotension |
| Reversal agents | | | |
| Anticholinesterases | — | Have been used as treatment for certain PD symptoms[121,122]<br>– probably safe<br>– no evidence to suggest one agent over another | — |
| Anticholinergics | Glycopyrrolate | May be anticholinergic drug of choice<br>– it does not cross the blood brain barrier | — |
| Drugs to avoid[b,c] | | | |
| Phenothiazines | Chlorpromazine<br>Promethazine | — | — |
| Butyrophenones | Droperidol<br>Haloperidol | — | — |
| DA receptor antagonist | Metoclopramide | May cause drug-induced PD | — |

*Abbreviation:* NMBD, neuromuscular blocking drugs.

[a] Volatiles have complex effects on central [DA]. They inhibit synaptic reuptake of DA that increases extracellular concentration.[123] This occurs at clinically relevant MAC level.

[b] May precipitate or exacerbate PD.

[c] May precipitate hypotension by causing peripheral vasodilation.

recommendations can result in thermal lesions or device reprogramming, which may result in coma, paralysis, or death.[87] It is essential to check the stimulator manufacturer's Web site or speak to a product representative directly regarding model-specific accommodations, as some models may be less MRI compatible than others.

### *Surgical Considerations for Patients with Deep Brain Stimulation*

#### *Generator protocol*

There is little in the literature to guide intraoperative management of DBS generators. Okajima and colleagues[88] showed that turning off the impulse generator intraoperatively was associated with an uneventful outcome, even for emergency surgery. Transient postoperative Parkinson symptoms were controlled with levodopa. Another case report evaluated a patient for generator battery replacement. The investigators recommended that the DBS generators be activated immediately after replacement, while the patient is still under GA, to prevent a possible akinetic-rigid state that may be refractory to dopaminergic medication.[89]

#### *Electrocautery*

Electrocautery can theoretically damage the generator or DBS leads, potentially causing burns to the CNS, or suppressing or reprogramming the device. A recent literature review by Milligan and colleagues[90] evaluating adverse events associated with electrocautery was unable to find any reports of intraoperative complications. The manufacturers (eg, Medtronic Ltd, Watford, UK) recommend that if use of electrocautery is necessary then, as with pacemakers, bipolar diathermy should be selected.

#### *Recommendations*

MRI seems to be safe, as long as model-specific accommodations are made. For patients with DBS, consulting the primary device specialist before considering inactivation of the device output is recommended, although evidence suggests that even for emergency situations it is safe to turn off the stimulator intraoperatively. Treatment with preoperative anti-PD medication is helpful but not essential. Restarting the generator before emergence may be beneficial, although should parkinsonian symptoms occur they can be treated with anti-PD medication. If electrocautery is to be used intraoperatively, it should be restricted to bipolar. Moreover, placing the dispersion pads as far from the generator and DBS leads without placing them between the cautery source and dispersion pad is essential.

## ANESTHESIA FOR PARKINSON'S DISEASE FOR NON-PARKINSON'S DISEASE SURGERY

### *History of Present Illness and Physical Examination*

There are many preoperative considerations for patients with PD.[91] Patients with PD are particularly prone to respiratory complications, including retained secretions, atelectasis, aspiration, and respiratory infection, with infection being the most common cause of death in these patients.[92] Other potential complications include postextubation laryngospasm and postoperative respiratory failure.[93,94] Patients may complain of difficulty with salivation, micturition, and gastrointestinal function. Seborrhea, a classic feature of Parkinson's disease, is also an autonomic manifestation of the disease.[95] The red, itchy rash and white scales are common on the face and ears, and in areas of skin folds. Specific cardiovascular symptoms about which to inquire include arrhythmias, hypertension, hypovolemia, and orthostatic hypotension, often the most disabling symptom.[96] **Table 3** lists more detailed information.[91,97,98]

### General Considerations

#### Parkinson's disease drug regimen

The patient's usual PD drug regimen should be initiated before surgery and be continued through the morning of surgery, administered as close to beginning of anesthesia as possible. Some medications, like levodopa, have short half-lives and can only be taken parenterally. Such treatment seems to decrease drooling, lowers the potential for aspiration, and minimizes ventilatory weakness.[99–101] Likewise, reinstituting therapy promptly after surgery is crucial.[99–105] If surgery is prolonged and extubation proves difficult, it is possible to administer PD medications via nasogastric tube.

#### Anesthetic techniques: regional versus general

Regional anesthesia has several obvious advantages over GA. Regional anesthesia avoids the effects of GA and neuromuscular blocking drugs (NMBDs), which may mask tremor.[91] In addition, postoperative nausea and vomiting are avoided, which may prevent resumption of oral intake. If sedation is required, diphenhydramine, which has central anticholinergic activity, can be advantageous in those whom tremor can render surgery difficult, particularly for ophthalmic procedures.[106]

During emergence from GA, the transient appearance of a variety of pathologic neurologic reflexes, including hyperreactive stretch reflexes, ankle clonus, the Babinski reflex, and decerebrate posturing, have been reported.[107] Also, shivering is common after GA and should be distinguished from parkinsonian symptoms. Postoperative rigidity, most commonly associated with intraoperative opiates, has also been reported in both high and low doses,[108,109] although it is also seen in patients not treated with opiates. Furthermore, these patients are more prone to postoperative confusion and hallucinations.[110,111] Specific anesthetic agents are listed in **Table 4.**[91,97,124]

#### Drugs to avoid

Drugs to avoid include ones that exacerbate PD symptoms or precipitate hypotension by causing peripheral vasodilation. Culprits include phenothiazines, butyrophenones, and dopamine receptor antagonists, such as metoclopramide. Also, potential drug interactions must also be considered, such as monoamine oxidase inhibitors (MAOIs) and meperidine. The use of potent nonsteroidal anti-inflammatory drugs may avoid the need for narcotic analgesics in patients on MAOIs.

## SUMMARY

DBS has added to the comfort and QoL for an increasing number of Parkinson's disease patients. The anesthesiologist needs to understand the pathophysiology of the disease, the surgical procedure, and its postoperative implications to most effectively manage these patients. In terms of the general anesthetic management of Parkinson's disease patients, it is clear that no simple anesthetic regimen exists. There is a paucity of evidence about the safety of various anesthetic drugs or techniques, and what evidence that does exist is based on single case reports or small case series. Anesthesiologists can provide the best care through preoperative assessment, maintenance of PD drug therapy and, when possible, avoidance of known precipitating agents.

## ACKNOWLEDGEMENT

The author acknowledges Dr. Ronald Alterman, Professor of Neurosurgery and Dr. Irene Osborn, Associate Professor of Anesthesia and Neurosurgery at The Mount Sinai Hospital.

**REFERENCES**


1. Lang AE, Lozano AM. Parkinson's disease. First of two parts. N Engl J Med 1998; 339:1044–53.
2. Bower JH, Maraganore DM, McDonnel SK, et al. Incidence and distribution of parkinsonism in Olmsted County, Minnesota, 1976–1990. Neurology 1999;52: 1214–20.
3. De Rijk MC, Breteler MMB, Graveland GA. Prevalence of Parkinson's disease in Europe: a collaborative study of population-based cohorts. Neurological Disease in the Elderly Research Group. Neurology 2000;54:S21–3.
4. Feldman RG, Ratner MH. The pathogenesis of neurodegenerative disease: neurotoxic mechanisms of action and genetics. Curr Opin Neurol 1999;12:725–31.
5. Zhang Y, Dawson VL, Dawson TM. Oxidative stress and genetics in the pathogenesis of Parkinson's disease. Neurobiol Dis 2000;7:240–50.
6. Lang| AE, Obeso JA. Time to move beyond nigrostriatal dopamine deficiency in Parkinson's disease. Ann Neurol 2004;55:761–5.
7. Aminoff MJ, Greenberg DA, Simon RP. Chapter 7. Movement disorders. Available at: http://www.accessmedicine.com/content.aspx?aID=2082488. Accessed 2009.
8. Lang AE, Lozano AM. Parkinson's disease. Second of two parts. N Engl J Med 1998;339(16):1130–43.
9. Krack P, Batir A, et al. Five-year follow-up of bilateral stimulation of the subthalamic nucleus in advanced Parkinson's disease. N Engl J Med 2003;349(20):1925–34.
10. Rodriguez-Oroz MC, Obeso JA, Lang AE, et al. Bilateral deep brain stimulation in Parkinson's disease: a multicentre study with 4 years follow-up. Brain 2005; 128:2240–9.
11. Schupbach WM, Chastan N, Welter ML, et al. Stimulation of the subthalamic nucleus in Parkinson's disease: a 5-year follow up. J Neurol Neurosurg Psychiatr 2005;76:1640–4.
12. Goodman RR, Kim B, Mclelland S, et al. Operative techniques and morbidity with subthalamic nucleus stimulation in 100 consecutive patients with Parkinson's disease. J Neurol Neurosurg Psychiatr 2006;77:12–7.
13. Lozano Am, Lang AE. Pallidotomy for Parkinson's disease. Arch Neurol 2005;62: 1377–81.
14. Blomstedt P, Hariz MI. Are complications less common in deep brain stimulation than in ablative procedures for movement disorders? Stereotact Funct Neurosurg 2006;84:72–81.
15. Benabid AL, Pollak P, Gervason C, et al. Long-term suppression of tremor by chronic stimulation of the ventral intermediate thalamic nucleus. Lancet 1991; 337:403–6.
16. Kumar R, Lozano AM, Kim YJ, et al. Double-blind evaluation of subthalamic nucleus deep brain stimulation in advanced Parkinson's disease. Neurology 1998;51(3):850–5.
17. Ostergaard K, Sunde N, Dupont E. Effects of bilateral stimulation of the subthalamic nucleus in patients with severe Parkinson's disease and motor fluctuations. Mov Disord 2002;17:693–700.
18. Moro E, Lang AE. Criteria for deep-brain stimulation in Parkinson's disease: review and analysis. Expert Rev Neurother 2006;6(11):1695–705.
19. Krack P, Pollak, Limousin P, et al. Subthalamic nucleus or internal pallidal stimulation in young onset Parkinson's disease. Brain 1998;121(Pt 3):451–7.
20. Anderson VC, Burchiel KJ, Hogarth P, et al. Pallidal versus subthalamic nucleus deep brain stimulation in Parkinson's disease. Arch Neurol 2005;62:554–60.

21. Volkmann J, Allert N, Voges J, et al. Safety and efficacy of pallidal or subthalamic nucleus stimulation in advanced Parkinson's disease. Neurology 2001;56:548–51.
22. Volkmann J, Allert N, Voges J, et al. Long-term results of bilateral pallidal stimulation in Parkinson's disease. Ann Neurol 2004;55:871–5.
23. Houeto JL, Damier P, Bejjani PB, et al. Subthalamic stimulation in Parkinson disease: a multidisciplinary approach. Arch Neurol 2000;57(4):461–5.
24. Hilker R, Portman AT, Voges J, et al. Disease progression continues in patients with advanced Parkinson's disease and effective subthalamic nucleus stimulation. J Neurol Neurosurg Psychiatr 2005;76:1217–21.
25. Defer GL, Widnek H, Marie RM, et al. Core Assessment Program for Surgical Interventional Therapies in Parkinson's disease (CAPSIT-PD). Mov Disord 1999;14:572–84.
26. Lang AE, Widner H. Deep brain stimulation for Parkinson's disease: patient selection and evaluation. Mov Disord 2002;17(Suppl 3):S94–101.
27. Lang AE, Houeto JL, Krack P, et al. Deep brain stimulation: preoperative issues. Mov Disord 2006;21(Suppl 14):S171–96.
28. Welter ML, Houeto JL, Tezenas de Montcel S, et al. Clinical predictive factors of subthalamic stimulation in Parkinson's disease. Brain 2002;125:575–83.
29. Kleiner-Fisman G, Herzog J, Fisman DN, et al. Subthalamic nucleus deep brain stimulation: summary and meta-analysis of outcomes. Mov Disord 2006;(suppl 14):S290–304.
30. Pahwa R, Wilkinson SB, Overman J, et al. Bilateral subthalamic stimulation in patients with Parkinson disease: long-term follow-up. J Neurosurg 2003;99:71–7.
31. Russman H, Ghika J, Villemure JG, et al. Subthalamic nucleus deep brain stimulation in Parkinson disease patients over age 70 years. Neurology 2004;63:1952–4.
32. Gironell A, Kulisevsky J, Rami L, et al. Effects of pallidotomy and bilateral subthalamic stimulation on cognitive function in Parkinson disease. A controlled comparative study. J Neurol 2003;250:917–23.
33. Charles PD, Van Blercom N, Krack P, et al. Predictors of effective bilateral subthalamic nucleus stimulation for Parkinson's disease. Neurology 2002;59(6):932–4.
34. Kleiner-Fisman G, Fisman DN, Sime E, et al. Long-term follow-up of bilateral deep brain stimulation of the subthalamic nucleus in patients with advanced Parkinson disease. J Neurosurg 2003;99:489–95.
35. Morrison CE, Borod JC, Perrine K, et al. Neuropsychological functioning following bilateral subthalamic nucleus stimulation in Parkinson's disease. Arch Clin Neuropsychol 2004;19:165–81.
36. Trepanier LL, Kumar R, Lozano AM, et al. Neuropsychological outcome of GPi pallidotomy and GPi or STN deep brain stimulation in Parkinson's disease. Brain Cogn 2000;42:324–47.
37. Hariz MI, Johansson F, Shamsgovara P, et al. Bilateral subthalamic nucleus stimulation in a parkinsonian patient with preoperative deficits in speech and cognition: persistent improvement in mobility but increased dependency: a case study. Mov Disord 2000;15:136–9.
38. Troster AI, Fields JA, Wilkinson SB, et al. Unilateral pallidal stimulation for Parkinson's disease: neurobehavioral functioning before and 3 months after electrode implantation. Neurology 1997;49:1078–83.
39. Loher TJ, Gutbrod K, Fravi NL, et al. Thalamic stimulation for tremor. Subtle changes in episodic memory are related to stimulation per se and not to a microthalamotomy effect. J Neurol 2003;250:707–13.
40. Caparros-Lefebvre D, Blond S, Pecheux N, et al. Neuropsychological evaluation before and after thalamic stimulation in 9 patients with Parkinson's disease. Rev Neurol 1992;148:117–22.

41. Ondo W, Jankovich J, Schwartz K, et al. Unilateral thalamic deep brain stimulation for refractory essential tremor and Parkinson disease tremor. Neurology 1998;51:1063–9.
42. Capelle HH, Simpson RK, Kronnenbuerger M, et al. Long-term deep brain stimulation in elderly patients with cardiac pacemaker. J Neurosurg 2005;102:53–9.
43. Voon V, Saint-Cyr J, Lozano AM, et al. Psychiatric symptoms in patients with Parkinson disease presenting for deep brain stimulation surgery. J Neurosurg 2005; 103(2):246–51.
44. Berney A, Vingerhoets F, Perrin A, et al. Effect on mood of subthalamic DBS for Parkinson's disease: a consecutive series of 24 patients. Neurology 2002;59(9): 1427–9.
45. Taylor MD, Bernstein M. Awake craniotomy with brain mapping as the routine surgical approach to treating patients with supratentorial intraaxial tumors: a prospective trial of 200 cases. J Neurosurg 1999;90:35–41.
46. Costello T, Cormack JR, Hoy C, et al. Plasma ropivacaine levels following scalp block for awake craniotomy. J Neurosurg Anesthesiol 2004;16:147–50.
47. Costello TG, Cormack JR, Mather LE, et al. Plasma levobupivacaine concentrations following scalp block in patients undergoing awake craniotomy. Br J Anaesth 2005;94:848–51.
48. Audu PB, Wilkerson C, Bartkowski R, et al. Plasma ropivacaine levels during awake intracranial surgery. J Neurosurg Anesthesiol 2005;17:153–5.
49. Raz A, Eimerl D, Bergman H, et al. Propofol induced changes in the neuronal activity of sub-thalamic nucleus neurons. Anesthesiology 2008;109:A838.
50. Manninen PH, Balki M, Lukitto K, et al. Patient satisfaction with awake craniotomy for tumor surgery: a comparison of remifentanil and fentanyl in conjunction with propofol. Anesth Analg 2006;102(1):237–42.
51. Keifer JC, Dentchev D, Little K, et al. A retrospective analysis of a remifentanil/propofol general anesthetic for craniotomy before awake functional brain mapping. Anesth Analg 2005;101:502–8.
52. Khatib R, Ebrahim Z, Rezai A, et al. Perioperative events during deep brain stimulation: the experience at cleveland clinic. J Neurosurg Anesthesiol 2008;20:36–40.
53. Bekker A, Sturaitis MK. Dexmedetomidine for neurological surgery. Neurosurgery 2005;57:1–10.
54. Hsu YW, Cortinez LI, Robertson KM, et al. Dexmedetomidine pharmacodynamics: part I: crossover comparison of the respiratory effects of dexmedetomidine and remifentanil in healthy volunteers. Anesthesiology 2004;101:1066–76.
55. Bustillo MA, Lazar RM, Finck AD, et al. Dexmedetomidine may impair cognitive testing during endovascular embolization of cerebral arteriovenous malformations: a retrospective case report series. J Neurosurg Anesthesiol 2002;14(3):209–12.
56. Hoffman WE, Kochs E, Werner C, et al. Dexmedetomidine improves neurologic outcome from incomplete ischemia in the rat. Reversal by the alpha 2-adrenergic antagonist atipamezole. Anesthesiology 1991;75:328–32.
57. Kuhmonen J, Pokorny J, Miettinen R, et al. Neuroprotective effects of dexmedetomidine in the gerbil hippocampus after transient global ischemia. Anesthesiology 1997;87:371–7.
58. Kuhmonen J, Haapalinna A, Sivenius J. Effects of dexmedetomidine after transient and permanent occlusion of the middle cerebral artery in the rat. J Neural Transm 2001;108:261–71.
59. Rozet I, Muangman S, Vavilala MS, et al. Clinical experience with dexmedetomidine for implantation of deep brain stimulators in Parkinson's disease. Anesth Analg 2006;103:1224–8.

60. Dinsmore J. Anesthesia for elective neurosurgery. Br J Anaesth 2007;99(1):68–74.
61. Mack PF, Perrine K, Kobylarz E, et al. Dexmedetomidine and neurocognitive testing in awake craniotomy. J Neurosurg Anesthesiol 2004;16:20–5.
62. Moore TA, Market JM, Knowlton RC. Dexmedetomidine as rescue drug during awake craniotomy for cortical mapping and tumor resection. Anesth Analg 2006;102:1556–8.
63. Maltete D, Navarro S, Welter ML, et al. Subthalamic stimulation in Parkinson disease: with or without anesthesia? Arch Neurol 2004;61:390–2.
64. Hertel F, Zuchner M, Weimar I, et al. Implantation of electrodes for deep brain stimulation of the subthalamic nucleus in advanced Parkinson's disease with the aid of intraoperative microrecording under general anesthesia. Neurosurgery 2006;59:1138–45.
65. Lin SH, Chen TY, Lin SZ, et al. Subthalamic deep brain stimulation after anesthetic inhalation in Parkinson disease: a preliminary study. J Neurosurg 2008;109(2):238–44.
66. Sanghera MK, Grossman RG, Kalhorn CG, et al. Basal ganglia neuronal discharge in primary and secondary dystonia in patients undergoing pallidotomy. Neurosurgery 2003;52:1358–73.
67. Beric A, Kelly PJ, Rezai A, et al. Complications of deep brain stimulation surgery. Stereotact Funct Neurosurg 2001;77:73–8.
68. Lefaucheur JP, Gurruchaga JM, Pollin B, et al. Outcome of bilateral subthalamic nucleus stimulation in the treatment of Parkinson's disease: correlation with intraoperative multi-unit recordings but not with the type of anesthesia. Eur Neurol 2008;60:186–99.
69. Benazzouz A, Breit S, Koudsie A, et al. Intraoperative microrecordings of the subthalamic nucleus in Parkinson's disease. Mov Disord 2004;17(Suppl 3):S145–9.
70. Yamadaa K, Gotoa S, Kuratsua J, et al. Stereotactic surgery for subthalamic nucleus stimulation under general anesthesia: a retrospective evaluation of Japanese patients with Parkinson's disease. Parkinsonism Relat Disord 2007;13(2):101–7.
71. Huncke K, Van de Wiele B, Fried I, et al. The asleep-awake-asleep anesthetic technique for intraoperative language mapping. Neurosurgery 1998;42:1312–7.
72. Sarang A, Dinsmore J. Anesthesia for awake craniotomy—evolution of a technique that facilitates awake neurological testing. Br J Anaesth 2003;90:161–5.
73. Audu PB, Loomba N. Use of cuffed oropharyngeal airway (COPA) for awake intracranial surgery. J Neurosurg Anesthesiol 2004;16(2):144–6.
74. Hutchinson WD, Lang AE, Dostrovosky JO, et al. Pallidal neuronal activity: implications for models of dystonia. Ann Neurol 2003;53:480–8.
75. Binder DK, Rau G, Starr PA. Hemorrhagic complications of microelectrode-guided deep brain stimulation. Stereotact Funct Neurosurg 2003;80(1–4):28–31.
76. Gorgulho A, De Salles AA, Frighetto L, et al. Incidence of hemorrhage associated with electrophysiological studies performed using macroelectrodes and microelectrodes in functional neurosurgery. J Neurosurg 2005;102:888–96.
77. Hans P, Bonhomme V, Born JD, et al. Target controlled infusion of propofol and remifentanyl combined with bispectral index monitoring for awake craniotomy. Anaesthesia 2000;55:255–9.
78. Johansen JW, Sebel PS. Development and clinical application of electroencephalographic bispectrum monitoring. Anesthesiology 2000;93:1336–44.
79. Schulz U, Keh D, Barner C, et al. Bispectral index monitoring does not improve anesthesia performance in patients with movement disorders undergoing deep brain stimulating electrode implantation. Anesth Analg 2007;104(6):1481–7.

80. Masuda T, Yamada H, Takada K, et al. Bispectral index monitoring is useful to reduce total amount of propofol and to obtain immediate recovery after propofol anesthesia. Masui 2002;51(4):394–9.
81. Duque P, Mateo O, Ruiz F, et al. Intraoperative microrecording under general anesthesia with bispectral analysis monitoring in a case of deep brain stimulation surgery for Parkinson's disease. Letter to the Editor. Eur J Neurol 2008; 15(8):e76–7.
82. Hooper AK, Okun MS, Foote KD, et al. Venous air embolism in deep brain stimulation. Stereotact Funct Neurosurg 2009;87(1):25–30 [Epub 2008 Nov 27].
83. Balki M, Manninen PH, McGuire GP, et al. Venous air embolism during awake craniotomy in a supine patient. Can J Anaesth 2003;50:835–8.
84. Orebaugh SL. Venous air embolism: clinical and experimental considerations. Crit Care Med 1992;20:1169–77.
85. Swartz MA, Munz M, Stern MB. Respiratory failure following stereotactic neurosurgery in a 53-year-old woman. Chest 1997;111:1112–4.
86. Rezai AR, Kopell BH, Gross RE, et al. Deep brain stimulation for Parkinson's disease: surgical issues. Mov Disord 2006;21(suppl 14):S197–218.
87. Rezai AR, Phillips M, Baker KB, et al. Neurostimulation system used for deep brain stimulation (DBS): MR safety issues and implications of failing to follow safety recommendations. Invest Radiol 2004;39:300–3.
88. Okajima H, Ushio M, Higuchi Y, et al. Anesthetic management of a patient with deep brain stimulators. Masui 2007;56(10):1211–3.
89. Dagtekin O, Berlet T, Gerbershagen HJ, et al. Anesthesia and deep brain stimulation: postoperative akinetic state after replacement of impulse generators. Anesth Analg 2006;103(3):784.
90. Milligan DJ, Milligan KR. Deep brain neuro-stimulators and anaesthesia. Anaesthesia 2007;62(8):852–3.
91. Nicholson G, Pereira AC, Hall GM. Parkinson's disease and anesthesia. Br J Anaesth 2002;89(6):904–16.
92. Hoehn MM, Yahr MD. Parkinsonism: onset, progression and mortality. Neurology 1967;17:427–42.
93. Backus WW, Ward RR, Vitkun SA, et al. Postextubation laryngospasm in an unanaesthetised patient with Parkinson's disease. J Clin Anesth 1991;3:314–6.
94. Easdown LJ, Tessler MJ, Minuk J. Upper airway involvement in Parkinson's disease resulting in postoperative respiratory failure. Can J Anaesth 1995;42:344–7.
95. Korczyn AD. Autonomic nervous system disorders in Parkinson's disease. In: Streifler MB, Korczyn AD, Melamed E, editors. Advances in neurology, vol. 53: Parkinson's disease: anatomy, pathology and therapy. New York: Raven Press; 1990. p. 463–8.
96. Gross M, Bannister R, Godwn-Austin R. Orthostatic hypotension in Parkinson's disease. Lancet 1972;1:174–6.
97. Rudra A, Rudra P, Chatterjee S, et al. Parkinson's disease and anaesthesia. Indian J Anaesth 2007;51(5):382–8.
98. Mason LJ, Cojocaru TT, Cole DJ. Surgical intervention and anaesthetic management of the patient with Parkinson's disease. Int Anesthesiol Clin 1996;34:133–50.
99. Mets B. Acute dystonia after alfentanil in untreated Parkinson's disease. Anesth Analg 1991;72:557–8.
100. Muzzi DA, Black S, Cucchiara RF. The lack of effect of succinylcholine on serum potassium in patients with Parkinson's disease. Anesthesiology 1989;71:322.
101. Ngai SH. Parkinsonism, levodopa, and anesthesia. Anesthesiology 1972;37: 344–51.

102. Roberts R. Differential diagnosis of sleep disorders, non-epileptic attacks and epileptic attacks. Curr Opin Neurol 1998;11:135–9.
103. Parkinson Study Group. Impact of deprenyl and tocopherol treatment on Parkinson's disease in DATA TOP patients requiring levodopa. Ann Neurol 1996;39: 37–45.
104. Goetz CG, Olanow CW, Koller WC, et al. Multicenter study of autologous adrenal medullary transplantation to the corpus striatum in patients with advanced Parkinson's disease. N Engl J Med 1989;320:337–41.
105. Wiklund RA, Ngai SH. Rigidity and pulmonary edema after Innovar in a patient on levodopa therapy: report of a case. Anesthesiology 1971;35:545–7.
106. Stone DJ, Difazio CA. Sedation for patients with Parkinson's disease undergoing ophthalmic surgery. Anesthesiology 1988;68:821.
107. Rosenberg H, Clofine R, Bialik O. Neurologic changes during awakening from anesthesia. Anesthesiology 1981;54:125–30.
108. Fearnley JM, Lees AJ. Ageing and Parkinson's disease: substantia nigra regional selectivity. Brain 1991;114:2283–301.
109. Lunn JK, Stanley TH, Eisele J, et al. High dose fentanyl for cardiac surgery. Anesth Analg 1979;58:390–5.
110. Golden WE, Lavender RC, Metzer WS. Acute postoperative confusion and hallucinations in Parkinson's disease. Ann Intern Med 1989;111:218–22.
111. Zornberg GL, Alexander Bodkin J, Cohen BM. Severe adverse interaction between pethidine and selegiline. Lancet 1991;337:554.
112. Muravchick S, Smith DS. Parkinsonian symptoms during emergence from general anesthesia. Anesthesiology 1995;82:305–7.
113. Mantz J, Varlet C, Lecharny JB, et al. Effects of volatile anaesthetics, thiopental and ketamine on spontaneous and depolarization-evoked dopamine release from striatal synaptosomes in the rat. Anesthesiology 1994;80:352–63.
114. Hetherington A, Rosenblatt RM. Ketamine and paralysis agitans. Anesthesiology 1980;52:527.
115. Krauss JK, Akeyson EW, Giam P, et al. Propofol-induced dyskinesias in Parkinson's disease. Anesth Analg 1996;83:420–2.
116. Anderson BJ, Marks PV, Futter ME. Propofol—contrasting effects in movement disorders. Br J Neurosurg 1994;8:387–8.
117. Gravlee GP. Succinylcholine-induced hyperkalaemia in a patient with Parkinson's disease. Anesth Analg 1980;59:444–6.
118. Klausner JM, Caspi J, Lelcuk S, et al. Delayed muscle rigidity and respiratory depression following fentanyl anesthesia. Arch Surg 1988;123:66–7.
119. Wand P, Kuschinsky K, Sontag KH. Morphine-induced muscle rigidity in rats. Eur J Pharmacol 1973;24:189–93.
120. Berg D, Becker G, Reiners K. Reduction of dyskinesia and induction of akinesia induced by morphine in two parkinsonian patients with severe sciatica. J Neural Transm 1999;106:725–8.
121. Maidment I, Fox C, Boustani M. Cholinesterase inhibitors for Parkinson's disease dementia. Cochrane Database Syst Rev 2006;(1):CD004747.
122. Brown JC, Charlton JE. Study of sensitivity to curare in certain neurological disorders using a regional technique. J Neurol Neurosurg Psychiatr 1975; 38(1):34–45.
123. El-Maghrabi EA, Eckenhoff RG. Inhibition of dopamine transport in rat brain synaptosomes by volatile anesthetics. Anesthesiology 1993;78:750–6.
124. Burton DA, Nicholson G, Hall GM. Anaesthesia in elderly patients with neurodegenerative disorders: special considerations. Drugs Aging 2004;21(4):229–42.

# Atrial Fibrillation in the Elderly

Gregory W. Fischer, MD*

**KEYWORDS**

• Atrial fibrillation • Elderly • Anesthesia

A 78-year-old man is admitted to the cardiothoracic intensive care unit after coronary artery bypass grafting and mitral valve repair. Medical history is significant for coronary artery disease, myocardial infarction, congestive heart failure, renal insufficiency, arterial hypertension, and diabetes mellitus. The left ventricular ejection fraction (LVEF) is 30% by transesophageal echocardiogram (TEE). The intraoperative course is uncomplicated. The patient arrives in the intensive care unit in sinus rhythm with stable vital signs on an epinephrine infusion at 0.1 μg/kg/min. After eight uneventful hours the patient's blood pressure is 73/40 mm Hg and shows the rhythm shown in **Fig. 1**.

1. What rhythm is present?
2. How often does this occur after cardiac surgery?
3. Why did such a precipitous decline in blood pressure occur?

**CASE**

One liter of normal saline was administered to the patient, which did not lead to any improvement in systemic blood pressure (70/40 mm Hg). Central venous pressure (CVP) and pulmonary artery (PA) pressure increased, however, from 8 to 18 mm Hg and 40/14 mm Hg to 60/29 mm Hg, respectively. The patient remains intubated with adequate gas exchange.

1. How should we proceed?
2. If electrical cardioversion is decided, does a TEE need to be preformed to rule out intracardiac thrombus?
3. What would be the pharmacologic management of this patient if blood pressure responded to volume challenge?

**CASE**

After starting an amiodarone infusion the patient's heart rate slowed down considerably and is now consistently less than 90/min. Blood pressure, CVP, and PA pressure

Department of Anesthesiology and Cardiothoracic Surgery, Mount Sinai School of Medicine, Mount Sinai Medical Center, One Gustave L. Levy Place, Box 1010, New York, NY 10029, USA
* Corresponding author.
*E-mail address:* Gregory.Fischer@mountsinai.org

Anesthesiology Clin 27 (2009) 417–427
doi:10.1016/j.anclin.2009.07.006 anesthesiology.theclinics.com
1932-2275/09/$ – see front matter 

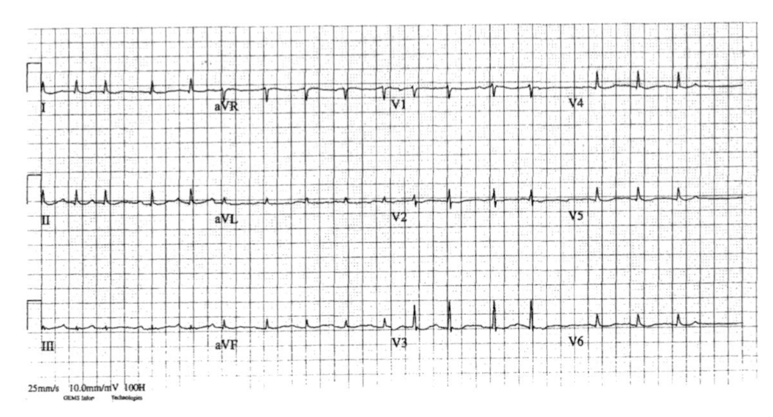


**Fig. 1.** Patient's 12 lead EKG.

have improved. Urine output is 1 ml/kg/h. Lactate levels are less than 2 mmol/L. After 48 hours of therapy the patient remains in atrial fibrillation (AF).

Questions:

1. Will you attempt electrical cardioversion?
2. Will you continue amiodarone or change to another drug class?
3. When will you start anticoagulation and what agent will you use?

## CASE

The patient is successfully rate controlled, extubated, and hemodynamically stable. Prophylactic subcutaneous heparin is administered and warfarin therapy started on postoperative day 2.

1. The patient inquires what else needs to be done regarding the AF.
2. Should electrical cardioversion be attempted?
3. If yes, when?

AF is the most commonly encountered cardiac rhythm disorder seen in adults, associated with an increased risk of morbidity and mortality, leading to a substantial cost burden on society.[1–3] The prevalence in the United States exceeds 2 million people and continues to increase with the aging population.[4] Risk factors for the development of AF include advancing age, increased systolic blood pressure, diabetes, hypertension, heart failure, valvular heart disease, myocardial infarction, and obesity.[5,6]

AF is also frequently encountered after cardiac surgery, with an incidence reported between 25% and 50%.[7] The risk profile is similar to that seen in the general population. Postoperative AF is associated with an increased incidence of congestive heart failure (CHF), renal insufficiency, and stroke[8]; this in turn leads to prolonged hospitalization as well as increased rates of rehospitalization after discharge.[9,10]

This article provides an overview of the pathophysiology, clinical course, and treatment of patients with AF, with special emphasis on the perioperative period.

## INCIDENCE AND PREVALENCE

AF is an illness of aging. Whereas it is rarely encountered in patients younger than 40 years old, the prevalence of the disease increases dramatically with progressing age.

AF has a prevalence of 5% in patients in their 70s and 10% in the population older than 80. Fifteen percent of adults older than 85 years suffer from this most common form of cardiac dysrhythmia.

AF is, according to the Framingham Heart Study, not just an electrophysiological nuisance but increases morbidity and mortality as well. Women with AF are 3 times as likely to suffer a stroke as women without AF. Men with AF have a 2.5 times higher risk of acquiring a cerebrovascular event. Stewart and colleagues showed that subjects younger than 60 years had a 1.5% higher likelihood of having a stroke compared with the same age group without AF. In the aging population between 80 and 89 years a 23.5% higher likelihood of developing a stroke was shown. In addition, patients with AF, irrelevant of gender, are 3.5 times more likely to suffer symptoms of CHF.

## ETIOLOGY AND PATHOPHYSIOLOGY

Fibrosis and loss of muscle mass of the left atrium play a major role in the development of AF. The etiology is multifactorial. Genetic defects like lamin AC gene mutations might explain the idiopathic development of AF.[11] Conditions leading to atrial stretch (eg, mitral stenosis, arterial hypertension) have been identified as being associated with the development of atrial fibrosis by activating neurohumoral pathways including the renin-angiotensin-aldosterone system (RAAS).[12] Systemic disease (eg, inflammatory processes,[13] sarcoidosis,[14] autoimmune disorders[15]) has also been linked to the development of AF. Once activated, rapid heart rates and increased transmural pressures across the wall of the left atrium can lead to a self-sustaining process that cannot be halted even if the initial triggering substrate is removed. This process explains the difficulty in treating patients with chronic persistent AF.

The fibrotic development within the atrium is not continuous but patchy, leading to conduction disturbances and facilitating reentry phenomena. For AF to occur, an initiating focus site must develop. The tissue around the ostium of the pulmonary veins is believed to be the most common site where rapid impulses that are necessary to initiate an episode of AF develop.[16]

The pathophysiological consequences of AF on the cardiovascular system are loss of synchronous atrial mechanical activity, irregular ventricular response, rapid heart rate, and impaired coronary arterial blood flow. The loss of atrial contractility in the setting of diastolic dysfunction (eg, mitral stenosis, obstructive cardiomyopathy, restrictive cardiomyopathy) can lead to as much as a 20% to 50% reduction in cardiac output. This loss of "atrial kick" is especially deleterious in the geriatric population, in whom a decline in ventricular compliance is physiologic. Experimental studies have shown that AF leads to a decrease in coronary blood flow.[17,18] These findings may explain the chest discomfort frequently described by patients undergoing the onset of AF.

## MANAGEMENT

To appropriately manage a patient with new-onset AF, his or her hemodynamic status must first be evaluated. Hemodynamic instability as a consequence of rapid ventricular rates represents a true medical emergency requiring electrical cardioversion. In general, patients with hemodynamic compromise have underlying structural heart disease with severe diastolic dysfunction, resulting in a pronounced loss of preload once atrial contraction is lost.

### Electrical Cardioversion

Direct current cardioversion can be performed with either monophasic or biphasic defibrillators. Regardless of which pattern of energy delivery is used, a synchronized mode must be employed to avoid delivering energy to the heart during the vulnerable phase, potentially causing ventricular fibrillation. In randomized trials success rates were higher when biphasic shocks were administered compared with monophasic patterns. In addition, less energy was required to achieve this higher success rate. Consequently, a biphasic shock represents the present standard for cardioversion of AF resulting in fewer shocks delivered, lower energy requirements, and less dermal injury.[19]

Recent data also support the immediate application of higher energies due to fewer shocks and less cumulative energy being delivered compared with the traditional ascending technique (100, 200, 360 J).[20,21]

### Pharmacologic Interventions

To understand the likelihood of achieving a successful intervention (meaning the patient will not only convert into sinus rhythm, but remain in it as well) the clinician must first identify the temporal pattern of its occurrence. Recurrent AF is defined in a patient who develops two or more episodes of AF. Paroxysmal AF is defined once an episode lasts for more than 7 days. If electrical or pharmacologic cardioversion is required or if the dysrhythmia persists for more than 7 days, the term persistent AF is used. This classification can be useful for the perioperative physician, because it can be used as a guide for determining the further management of the patient. Patients presenting with a first-time episode of AF will usually convert back to sinus rhythm spontaneously without the need for further medical interventions. Patients with known preoperative AF will generally not respond successfully to attempts at cardioversion, whether electrical or pharmacologic. In this case adequate ventricular rate control should be prioritized.

The discussion of how aggressively a physician should be in restoring sinus rhythm is a controversial one, and has led to much academic debate over the course of the last decade. Prospective studies like RAate Control versus Electrical cardioversion for persistent AF (RACE)[22] and Atrial Fibrillation Follow-up Investigation of Rhythm Management (AFFIRM)[23] were able to show, especially for the geriatric population, that rate control was just as effective as rhythm conversion.

### Rate Control

For the initial management, rate control can be achieved in the hemodynamically stabile patient with a variety of rate-controlling medications (**Table 1**). For the perioperative patient requiring ventricular rate control, intravenous administration of pharmaceutical agents is recommended due to uncertain gastrointestinal function. Intravenous β-blockers (eg, esmolol, metoprolol) and nondihydropyridine calcium channel antagonists (eg, verapamil, diltiazem) are effective for control of the rate of ventricular response to AF.

Although still frequently used clinically, digoxin should no longer be considered a first-line agent for ventricular rate control unless the patient shows concurrent signs of congestive heart failure. The geriatric population characterized by multiple comorbidities in combination with digoxin's narrow therapeutic window should prompt for frequent checks of digoxin serum levels to avoid toxic side effects.

Intravenous amiodarone is hemodynamically well tolerated even in critically ill patients, providing both sympatholytic and calcium antagonistic properties.

**Table 1**
**Pharmacologic agents for heart rate control**

| Drug Class | Example | Dosage | Advantage | Side Effects | Caution |
|---|---|---|---|---|---|
| β-Blocker | Esmolol | Bolus: 0.5 mg/kg<br>Maintenance: 50–200 μg/kg/min | Short half-life, easily titratable | Expensive, excessive volume load (esmolol) | Bronchoconstriction, hypoglycemia |
| | Metoprolol | Bolus: 1–5 mg IV | | | |
| Ca channel antagonists | Diltiazem | Bolus: 20 mg IV<br>Maintenance: 5–15 mg/h | | Bradycardia, hypotension | Reduces digoxin elimination and increases levels |
| | Verapamil | Bolus: 5–15 mg<br>Maintenance: 5–15 mg/h | | | |
| Aminoglycoside | Digoxin | Load: 1 mg over 24 h in 4 doses<br>Maintenance: 0.125–0.25 mg/d | Positive inotropic effects for patients in CHF | Long half-life, difficult to titrate | Low therapeutic index. Requires frequent serum levels |
| Amiodarone | Amiodarone | Load: 150 mg over 10 min<br>Infusion: 1 mg/min for 6 h, then 0.5 mg/min for 18 h | Safe in patients with structural heart disease | ARDS, pulmonary fibrosis, thyroid and hepatic dysfunction | Not FDA approved for rate control |

*Abbreviations*: ARDS, acute respiratory distress syndrome; FDA, Food and Drug Administration.

Amiodarone is considered a suitable alternative agent for heart rate control when conventional measures are ineffective. It must be noted that amiodarone solely for the purposes of rate control represents an unapproved (off-label) use in the United States, and the potential benefit must be carefully weighed against the considerable potential toxicity of this drug (see **Table 1**).

### *Rhythm Control*

As previously discussed, the indication to rhythm control (cardiovert) a patient is no longer absolute. Advantages of maintaining sinus rhythm (increased cardiac output, lack of anticoagulation) must be carefully weighed against the long-term sequelae of antiarrhythmic therapy. Patients who are in AF for only a short period of time will generally convert spontaneously or pharmacologically, especially once the precipitating problem has been alleviated (eg, hypoxia, volume overload). However, once AF has persisted for more than a week, electrical cardioversion is recommended due to higher success rates. Cardioverting the patient into sinus rhythm is generally successful; however, up to 50% of patients will return to AF unless chronically placed on antiarrhythmic drug therapy.[24]

Consequently, patients who are symptomatic while in AF will require long-term pharmacologic support after successful electrical cardioversion. Amiodarone is frequently used in this setting due to its efficacy and safety in patients with underlying heart disease. Unfortunately, the drug has been associated with multiple extracardiac adverse effects. Pulmonary fibrosis, hepatic and thyroid dysfunction are the most common. In addition, amiodarone has been described to interact with the metabolism of other drugs, leading to altered plasma levels.[25]

Dronedarone is a noniodinated derivative of amiodarone, which is supposed to have a lower extracardiac risk profile. However, the efficacy of the drug compared with amiodarone is questionable, especially in populations with severe systolic left ventricular dysfunction in whom the mortality rate is increased.[26]

Along the same lines, it has been appreciated since the CAST trial (Cardiac Arrhythmia Suppression Trial) that for patients with structural heart disease caution must be used when prescribing flecainide.[27] Antiarrhythmic agents from the Vaughan Williams classification Ic have been associated with an increase in mortality due to malignant ventricular dysrhythmias in patients with structural heart disease.

### *Nonpharmacologic Approaches*

#### *MAZE procedure*

For patients presenting to the operating room for cardiac surgery in conjunction with chronic persistent AF, a MAZE procedure is frequently concurrently performed. First described by Cox, the procedure entails excluding the focus site responsible for initiating and supporting the dysrhythmia by encircling the pulmonary veins, and creating a mazelike pathway throughout the left and right atria.[28] Whereas the original procedure used a cut-and-sew technique that took many hours to complete, advances in technology have now made it possible for the surgeon to use radiofrequency, laser, or cryoablation techniques to create similar pathways. This advance has decreased the time of the operation considerably, without any change in success rates (80%–90%).[29]

#### *Pacing*

Evidence is emerging to support the use of physiologic pacing (atrial pacing, atrioventricular pacing) to reduce the rate of AF.[30] Although these data were not obtained from postoperative patients, it would still seem prudent to insert atrial pacing wires in all high-risk cardiac surgical patients and pace atrially, especially if premature atrial contractions are telemetrically documented.

***Echocardiography***

If a patient remains in AF for longer than 48 hours or if the starting point of the current episode is unknown, a TEE is obtained to rule out thrombus formation within the left side of the heart. Although interrogation using a transthoracic echocardiogram (TTE) can initially be attempted, the ability to visualize left-sided cardiac structures (left atrial appendage; LAA) is greatly inferior with this method compared with TEE. Clots are frequently found in the LAA due to stasis of blood (see **Figs. 2** and **3**). Alternatively, patients that have been therapeutically anticoagulated for a minimum of 3 weeks can be cardioverted without prior TEE.

***Anticoagulation***

Loss of atrial contraction leads to a changes in flow patterns within the left atrium resulting in an increased risk of thrombus generation, which in turn can lead to embolic complications. Patients who have device-documented recurrent episodes of AF lasting for longer than 24 hours have a three-fold increased risk of suffering a stroke.[31] Lip and colleagues report the results from a large meta-analysis consisting of more than 14,000 patients.[32] Warfarin therapy significantly reduced the risk of ischemic stroke or systemic thromboembolism compared with placebo (relative risk: 0.33). Specifically in the geriatric population, where the incidence of AF is especially high, there is mounting evidence to support the liberal use of oral anticoagulation in the setting of AF. The Birmingham Atrial Fibrillation Treatment of the Aged Study (BAFTA) showed that warfarin therapy, with a goal international normalized ratio (INR) of 2 to 3, was more effective that 75 mg of daily aspirin in stroke prevention in patients older than 75 years in a primary-care setting.[33] No significant differences in major bleeding events were found between the warfarin and aspirin groups. Other studies, however, urge for caution to be used when orally anticoagulating the elderly. If target INR values (2–3) are difficult to maintain, a marked increase in risk of intracerebral hemorrhage is found in this population.[34] Consequently, this subgroup of geriatric patients as well as elderly patients with increased risk of falling should not receive warfarin therapy, but aspirin therapy. Although not as effective as warfarin in reducing stroke, aspirin has been shown to reduce the risk by 22%.[35]

In patients presenting for surgery or other invasive procedures, a temporary discontinuation of their oral anticoagulation therapy may be necessary. In this setting, it is

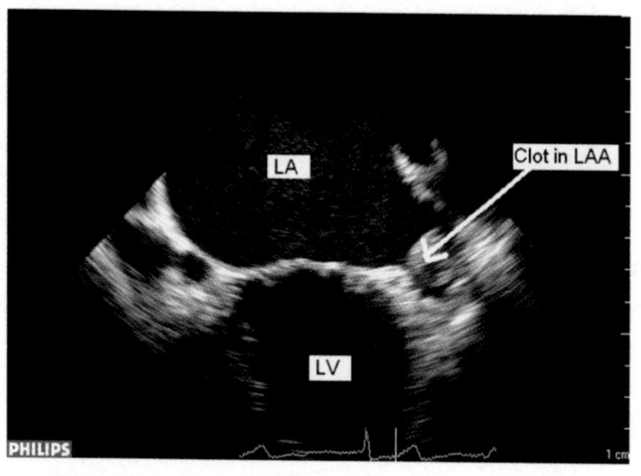


**Fig. 2.** Left atrial appendage clot, transesophageal echocardiogram.

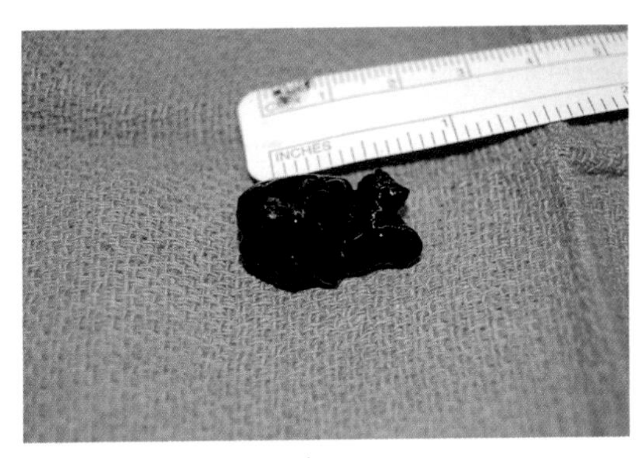


Fig. 3. Clot from Fig 2 after surgical removal.

important for the clinician to determine the indication for the anticoagulation. Although warfarin can be paused, with only minimal risk, 4 to 7 days before a surgical procedure, patients with mechanical heart valves will require a bridging therapy (low molecular weight heparin or unfractionated heparin) to safely clear the effects of warfarin from their system.

In patients developing AF as a first-time event during the perioperative period, anticoagulation (heparin, warfarin) should be started if spontaneous or iatrogenic cardioversion does not occur after 48 hours.

***Catheter ablation***

As a direct result of the success seen in the surgical MAZE procedure, interventionalists developed catheter-based techniques with the goal of excluding arrhythmogenic foci within the atria. As opposed to the surgical technique, catheter-based techniques enter the patient from an endovascular route, passing catheters into the left atrium, generally perforating and crossing the intra-atrial septum. Radiofrequency incisions or cryoincisions are subsequently made from the endocardium into the myocardium. To guarantee proper placement of these burns, the patient must be mapped. A preprocedural cardiac computed tomography scan is required.

Patients in whom pharmacologic or interventional treatment was unsuccessful can become candidates for atrioventricular nodal ablation.[36] Although this procedure can lead to symptomatic relief of rapid atrioventricular conduction, it has the disadvantage of making the patient permanently pacemaker dependent.

***Specific scenarios arising during the perioperative period***

The anesthesiologist caring for patients experiencing an episode of AF during the perioperative period will have to answer several questions, the first of which are: does this patient have chronic AF? If yes, is the AF rate controlled?

In patients with chronic and rate-controlled AF (heart rate 60–100/min) there is no reason to postpone surgery. Special consideration must be taken regarding the coagulation status. Many patients will be on warfarin therapy, which potentially could preclude them from obtaining neuraxial anesthetic techniques. The decision on which INR is safe for the operation to proceed is dependent on procedure and preference of the surgeon.

Patients experiencing a first-time episode of AF during the perioperative procedure will primarily need their hemodynamic status evaluated. Once blood pressure and heart rate are stable a workup to exclude an acute coronary syndrome (ACS) should be started. Although ischemia per se is rarely the cause of AF, changes in diastolic function resulting from myocardial ischemia can lead to increased filling pressure, which in turn is a common cause of AF. In general, these patients are hemodynamically unstable, providing additional clues that something more serious is underlying. Serial electrocardiograms and troponins are sufficient to rule out an ACS in a stable patient, whereas a TTE can be obtained in the operating room or postanesthesia care unit if the patient remains hemodynamically unstable after initial treatment.

The question of whether a case should be cancelled if a first-time episode of AF is detected preoperatively can only be answered on a case-to-case basis. How urgent is the procedure? If completely elective, a cardiology consultation should be obtained to rule out thrombus in the LAA. In addition, some form of rate control therapy should be started preoperatively because the neurohumeral response to surgery (catecholamine release) can potentially lead to a more rapid ventricular response.

After successful surgery the question arises as to the timing of restarting warfarin therapy. This question needs to be addressed by all disciplines taking care of the patient. Although AF carries the risk of embolic stroke, the danger of postponing warfarin therapy during the perioperative period is not to be viewed in the same context as in a patient with a mechanical heart valve. In general, no anticoagulation therapy will be started in patients with AF still exposed to the risk of postoperative bleeding. Once on the floor warfarin therapy can then be restarted. If no other indication for anticoagulation (mechanical heart valves, know thrombus in LAA) is present, therapeutic heparinization is not necessary. Prophylactic heparin (low molecular weight heparin, subcutaneous heparin) can be administered according to institutional protocols.

## SUMMARY

AF remains the most common form of cardiac arrhythmia seen in man. Therapeutic options for patients suffering from AF are constantly evolving. Pharmacologic therapies that modulate the endocrine/inflammatory axis are showing preliminary promise. Can the administration of statins and steroids reduce the incidence of AF in the post-operative period? Initial work is promising; however, still more needs to be learned.

AF is too common and often requires acute interventions. Consequently, the anesthesiologist must be aware of the causes, consequences, and therapies of patients developing AF during the perioperative period as well as patients presenting to the operating room with chronic AF.

## REFERENCES

1. Stewart S, Hart CL, Hole DJ, et al. A population-based study of the long-term risks associated with atrial fibrillation: 20-year follow-up of the Renfrew/Paisley Study. Am J Med 2002;113:359–64.
2. Benjamin EJ, Wolf PA, D'Agostino RB, et al. Impact of atrial fibrillation on the risk of death: the Framingham Heart Study. Circulation 1998;98:946–52.
3. Wolf PA, Abbott RD, Kannel WB. Atrial fibrillation as an independent risk factor for stroke: the Framingham Study. Stroke 1991;22:983–8.
4. Miyasaka Y, Barnes ME, Gersh BJ, et al. Secular trends in incidence of atrial fibrillation in Olmsted County, Minnesota, 1980 to 2000, and implications on the projections for future prevalence. Circulation 2006;114:119–25.
5. Psaty BM, Manolio TA, Kuller LH, et al. Incidence of and risk factors for atrial fibrillation in older adults. Circulation 1997;96:2455–61.
6. Benjamin EJ, Levy D, Vaziri SM, et al. Independent risk factors for atrial fibrillation in a population-based cohort: the Framingham Heart Study. JAMA 1994;271:840–4.

7. Ivanov J, Weisel RD, David TE, et al. Fifteen-year trends in risk severity and operative mortality in elderly patients undergoing coronary artery bypass graft surgery. Circulation 1998;97:673–80.
8. Almassi GH, Schowalter T, Nicolosi AC, et al. Atrial fibrillation after cardiac surgery: a major morbid event? Ann Surg 1997;226:501–11.
9. Borzak S, Tisdale JE, Amin NB, et al. Atrial fibrillation after bypass surgery: does the arrhythmia or the characteristics of the patients prolong hospital stay? Chest 1998;113:1489–91.
10. Mathew JP, Parks R, Savino JS, et al. Atrial fibrillation in coronary artery bypass grafting surgery: predictors, outcomes, and resource utilization. JAMA 1996; 276:300–6.
11. van Berlo JH, de Voogt WG, van der Kooi AJ, et al. Meta-analysis of clinical characteristics of 299 carriers of LMNA gene mutations: do lamin A/C mutations portend a high risk of sudden death? J Mol Med 2005;83:79–83.
12. Goette A, Staack T, Rocken C, et al. Increased expression of extracellular signal-regulated kinase and angiotensin-converting enzyme in human atria during atrial fibrillation. J Am Coll Cardiol 2000;35:1669–77.
13. Pokharel S, van Geel PP, Sharma UC, et al. Increased myocardial collagen content in transgenic rats overexpressing cardiac angiotensin-converting enzyme is related to enhanced breakdown of N-acetyl-Ser-Asp-Lys-Pro and increased phosphorylation of Smad2/3. Circulation 2004;110:3129–35.
14. Sharma OP, Maheshwari A, Thaker K. Myocardial sarcoidosis. Chest 1993;103: 253–8.
15. Maixent JM, Paganelli F, Scaglione J, et al. Antibodies against myosin in sera of patients with idiopathic paroxysmal atrial fibrillation. J Cardiovasc Electrophysiol 1998;9:612–7.
16. Konings KT, Kirchhof CJ, Smeets JR, et al. High-density mapping of electrically induced atrial fibrillation in humans. Circulation 1994;89:1665–80.
17. Wichmann J, Ertl G, Hohne W, et al. Alpha-receptor restriction of coronary blood flow during atrial fibrillation. Am J Cardiol 1983;52:887–92.
18. Kochiadakis GE, Skalidis EI, Kalebubas MD, et al. Effect of acute atrial fibrillation on phasic coronary blood flow pattern and flow reserve in humans. Eur Heart J 2002;23:734–41.
19. Page RL, Kerber RE, Russell JK, et al. Biphasic versus monophasic shock waveform for conversion of atrial fibrillation: the results of an international randomized, double-blind multicenter trial. J Am Coll Cardiol 2002;39:1956–63.
20. Joglar JA, Hamdan MH, Ramaswamy K, et al. Initial energy for elective external cardioversion of persistent atrial fibrillation. Am J Cardiol 2000;86:348–50.
21. Wozakowska-Kaplon B, Janion M, Sielski J, et al. Efficacy of biphasic shock for transthoracic cardioversion of persistent atrial fibrillation: can we predict energy requirements? Pacing Clin Electrophysiol 2004;27:764–8.
22. Van Gelder IC, Hagens VE, Bosker HA, et al. Rate Control versus Electrical Cardioversion for Persistent Atrial Fibrillation Study Group. A comparison of rate control and rhythm control in patients with recurrent persistent atrial fibrillation. N Engl J Med 2002;347(23):1834–40.
23. Wyse DG, Waldo AL, DiMarco JP, et al. Atrial Fibrillation Follow-up Investigation of Rhythm Management (AFFIRM) Investigators. A comparison of rate control and rhythm control in patients with atrial fibrillation. N Engl J Med 2002;347(23):1825–33.
24. Lip GYH, Tse HF. Management of atrial fibrillation. Lancet 2007;370:608–18.
25. Goldschlager N, Epstein AE, Naccarelli G, et al. Practical guidelines for clinicians who treat patients with amiodarone. Practice Guidelines Subcommittee, North

American Society of Pacing and Electrophysiology. Ann intern Med 2000;160: 1741–87.
26. Køber L, Torp-Pedersen C, McMurray JJ, et al. Dronedarone Study Group. Increased mortality after dronedarone therapy for severe heart failure. N Engl J Med 2008;358(25):2678–87.
27. Echt DS, Liebson PR, Mitchell LB, et al. Mortality and morbidity in patients receiving encainide, flecainide or placebo: the Cardiac Arrhythmia Suppression Trial. N Engl J Med 1991;324:781–8.
28. Cox JL. Cardiac surgery for arrhythmias. J Cardiovasc Electrophysiol 2004;15: 250–62.
29. Khargi K, Hutten BA, Lemke B, et al. Surgical treatment of atrial fibrillation; a systematic review. Eur J Cardiothorac Surg 2005;27:258–65.
30. Healey JS, Toff WD, Lamas GA, et al. Cardiovascular outcomes with atrial-based pacing compared with ventricular pacing: meta-analysis of randomized trials, using individual patient data. Circulation 2006;114:11–7.
31. Capucci A, Santini M, Padeletti L, et al. Italian AT500 Registry Investigators. Monitored atrial fibrillation duration predicts arterial embolic events in patients suffering from bradycardia and atrial fibrillation implanted with antitachycardia pacemakers. J Am Coll Cardiol 2005;46:1913–20.
32. Lip GY, Edwards SJ. Stroke prevention with aspirin, warfarin and ximelagatran in patients with nonvalvular atrial fibrillation: a systematic review and meta-analysis. Thromb Res 2006;118:321–33.
33. Mant J, Hobbs FDR, Fletcher K, et al. Warfarin versus aspirin for stroke prevention in an elderly community population with atrial fibrillation (the Birmingham Atrial Fibrillation Treatment of the Aged Study, BAFTA): a randomised controlled trial. Lancet 2007;370:493–503.
34. Hylek EM, Evans-Molina C, Shea C, et al. Major hemorrhage and tolerability of warfarin in the first year of therapy among elderly patients with atrial fibrillation. Circulation 2007;115:2689–96.
35. Antithrombotic Trialists' Collaboration. Collaborative meta analysis of randomised trials of antiplatelet therapy for prevention of death, myocardial infarction, and stroke in high risk patients. BMJ 2002;324:71–86.
36. Wood MA, Brown-Mahoney C, Kay GN, et al. Clinical outcomes after ablation and pacing therapy for atrial fibrillation: a meta-analysis. Circulation 2000;101: 1138–44.

# Delayed Arousal

Zirka H. Anastasian, MD*, Eugene Ornstein, PhD, MD,
Eric J. Heyer, MD, PhD

**KEYWORDS**

- Delayed arousal • Elderly • Geriatric • Management
- Pharmacology

## CASE REPORT

A 78-year-old female with a 6-month history of rapid progressive loss of equilibrium, coordination, balance gait, and hearing of the left ear presented for suboccipital craniotomy for acoustic neuroma. Her past medical history was significant for hypertension, diabetes, and depression, complicated by a 6.8-kg (15-lb) weight loss in the past 3 months.

After application of standard monitors, including a blood pressure cuff, pulse oximeter, and EKG, the patient was induced with midazolam, fentanyl, propofol and succinylcholine. Hemodynamics were originally labile, but stabilized after several boluses of crystalloid. Isoflurane and a fentanyl infusion were used for maintenance of anesthesia. After the end of an 8-hour surgical procedure, the patient remained unresponsive 45 minutes after the discontinuation of all anesthetic agents.

## WHAT IS DELAYED AROUSAL IN STATES OF CONSCIOUSNESS?

Multiple terms are used to describe altered states of consciousness. The term that neurologists and neurosurgeons use to describe a mild state of impaired consciousness is "clouding of consciousness," which refers to a defect in attention. A more severe state of impairment is called "confusional state," in which stimuli are misinterpreted. As attention becomes progressively more impaired and stimuli become increasingly misinterpreted, patients may be called "delirious," and in the extreme "obtunded," "stuporous" or "comatose." The term "coma," describes a state of unresponsiveness to intensely painful stimulation. So, where does "delayed arousal" fit into this spectrum of clouding of consciousness? Clearly, one may consider patients under general anesthesia as experiencing "coma," and under monitored anesthesia care (MAC) as experiencing clouding of consciousness. Here, we define the term "delayed arousal" as referring to a delay in the transition from a state of anesthetic-induced coma to clouding of consciousness, and finally, to fully awake and

EJH was supported in part by Grant No. RO1-AG16404 from the National Institutes of Health.
Division of Neurosurgical Anesthesiology, Department of Anesthesiology, Columbia University, 622 West 168th Street, New York, NY 10032, USA
* Corresponding author.
*E-mail address:* zh2114@columbia.edu (Z.H. Anastasian).

Anesthesiology Clin 27 (2009) 429–450
doi:10.1016/j.anclin.2009.07.007
1932-2275/09/$ – see front matter. Published by Elsevier Inc.
anesthesiology.theclinics.com

aware. For the purposes of our discussion, we define "arousal" as the ability of a patient to follow simple one-step commands that produce simple motor actions or have simple cognitive responses. More elaborate test performance, such as might be required for sensory or detailed cognitive responses, are not required.

## WHAT ARE THE PHYSIOLOGIC COMPONENTS OF CONSCIOUSNESS?

The physiologic components that define levels of consciousness are based on the capability to attain a state of arousal by the central nervous system, the existence and experience of stimuli necessary to stimulate arousal, and the mental functions that can be performed in the aroused state.

## THE ELDERLY

Elderly patients, defined as patients 65 years and older, are clearly different from younger patients. One of these differences is reflected in the common observation that elderly patients often experience delayed arousal. In examining why, the changes that patients experience with aging must be examined. Changes usually occur in the physiology of patients with normal aging. Therefore, medications that are given to younger patients will have different effects on the elderly. Often, medical and psychological conditions develop, which affect multiple organ systems. These conditions can also alter the effect of medications. In addition, some medical problems, for example cerebral infarcts, may not be evident and remain hidden without a previous neurologic workup. With all of these changes, an administered anesthetic may simply uncover previous neurologic deficits.[1] In addition, elderly patients are frequently taking multiple medications, which may affect the pharmacokinetics and pharmacodynamics of medications administered during the course of anesthesia.

## STRUCTURE OF THE ARTICLE

This article is divided into three parts. In the first, the anatomic areas of the brain that are involved in consciousness, and the neurochemical transmitters and modulators associated with these areas are discussed. The functional changes in these areas that occur with normal aging are discussed, in addition to their possible implications in delayed arousal. In the second part, the pharmacology of medications associated with the aging brain are discussed to the extent that it is known. In the third part, an algorithm to determine the cause of delayed arousal is presented, with the previous two components in mind.

## ANATOMIC CORRELATES OF CONSCIOUSNESS: AROUSAL PATHWAYS AND THE EFFECT OF NORMAL AGING

Historically, consciousness was believed to be a product of the summation of the activity of the human cerebral hemispheres. However, unilateral dysfunction of the cerebral hemispheres does not cause impairment of consciousness, except if the size of the lesion affects other cortical areas or the diencephalon. In the early 1900s, Von Economo noted a type of encephalitis, encephalitis lethargica, that attacked regions of the brain, specifically the midbrain and diencephalon, and disturbed sleep and arousal.[2] This is consistent with the current view that there are discrete regions of the central nervous system that are essential for consciousness. In the 1940s, Moruzzi and Magoun experimentally localized the ascending arousal system to the paramedian reticular formation in cats. They found that cats were clinically unresponsive even though they could record cortical evoked potentials in response to electrical stimulation from these areas. Subsequent work demonstrated that electrical stimulation of the midbrain reticular formation and central thalamus desynchronized the large-amplitude slow waves recorded by the electroencephalogram (EEG) induced in anesthetized cats.[3] These areas have extensive ramifications throughout the cerebrum. Similar mechanisms are believed to exist in humans.

The ascending arousal system in the brainstem consists of two branches: the first is an ascending pathway to the thalamus and cerebral cortex, and the second bypasses the thalamus, activating neurons in the lateral hypothalamic area and basal forebrain, and throughout the cerebral cortex.[2] It is associated with specific neurotransmitters (**Fig. 1**).[4]

In this section the known neurobiology of arousal, consciousness, and the effect of aging is discussed.

### *Thalamic Branch of the Ascending Arousal System*

Neuroimaging techniques reveal that there is a decrease in regional activity in the thalamus for all anesthetic classes except for propofol, when compared with awake patients (**Fig. 2**). This observation, in addition to clinical observations that midline

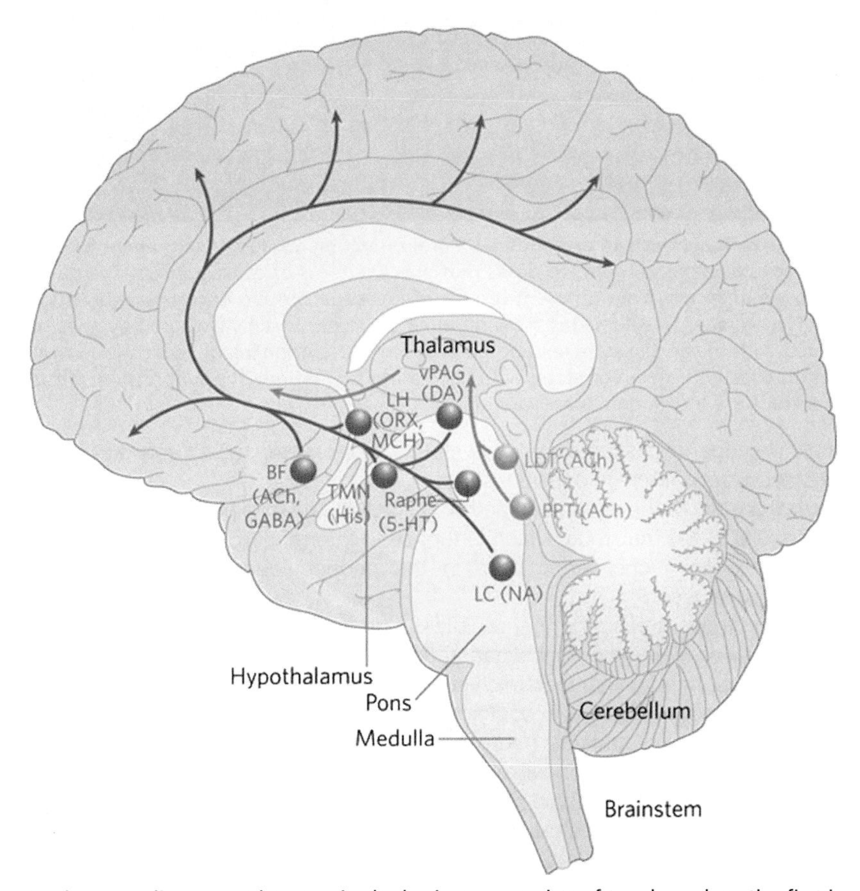


**Fig. 1.** The ascending arousal system in the brainstem consists of two branches: the first is an ascending pathway to the thalamus and cerebral cortex (*yellow*), and the second bypasses the thalamus, activating neurons in the lateral hypothalamic area and basal forebrain, and throughout the cerebral cortex (*red*).

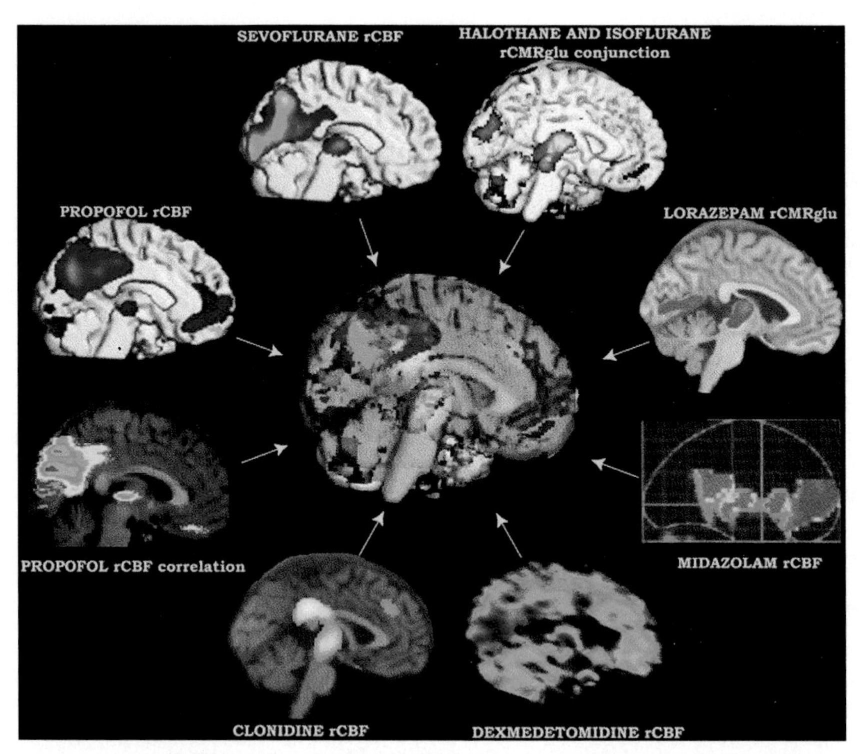


**Fig. 2.** The regional effects of anesthetics on brain function are shown in humans who were given various anesthetic agents at doses that produced loss of consciousness. The data are a composite of results from different groups of investigators and encompass the study of eight different agents. All images show regional decreases in activity caused by anesthesia compared with the awake state, except the propofol correlation image, which shows where increasing anesthetic dose correlates with decreasing blood flow. The suppressive effects on the thalamus are a common anesthetic effect.

thalamic damage results in a vegetative state,[5] supports the hypothesis that the thalamus plays a critical role in consciousness.[6]

The first branch of the ascending pathway involves the midline nuclei and the intralaminar nuclei of the thalamus, which in turn send information to the cerebral cortex. Their input is from cholinergic cells in the pedunculopontine and laterodorsal tegmental nuclei (see **Fig. 1**).[7]

Neurons in these areas fire most rapidly during wakefulness and rapid eye movement (REM) sleep.[8] Action potential generation is effected by the state of wakefulness and anesthetics. Intralaminar thalamic neurons show excitability during wakefulness.[9] Volatile anesthetics decrease acetylcholine levels in the thalamus, reflecting decreased activation of thalamic neurons.[10] The effects of anesthetics in the thalamic region can be experimentally localized: $\gamma$-aminobutyric acid (GABA) agonists injected into the intralaminar nuclei cause rats to rapidly fall asleep and slow the EEG,[11] and rats under anesthetic concentrations of sevoflurane can be awakened by a minute injection of nicotine into the intralaminar nucleus of the thalamus.[12]

### *Nonthalamic Branch of the Ascending Arousal System*

The second branch of the ascending arousal system bypasses the thalamus (see **Fig. 1**). It originates from monoaminergic neurons in the upper brainstem and caudal hypothalamus, including the noradrenergic locus coeruleus, serotoninergic dorsal (DR) and median raphe nuclei, dopaminergic ventral periaqueductal gray matter, and histaminergic tuberomammillary neurons. This pathway activates neurons in the lateral hypothalamic area and basal forebrain, and throughout the cerebral cortex. The input to the cerebral cortex is augmented by lateral hypothalamic peptidergic neurons (containing melanin-concentrating hormone or orexin/hypocretin), and basal forebrain neurons (containing acetylcholine or GABA).[2]

Clinically, lesions in the lateral hypothalmus and rostral midbrain cause profound sleepiness and coma.[13] Similar to the neurons in the thalamic pathway of arousal, neurons in the basal forebrain, including most cholinergic neurons, are active during wake and REM sleep.[14–16] The monoaminergic nuclei that contribute to the nonthalamic arousal pathway fire most rapidly during wakefulness and slowly during non-REM (NREM) sleep. However, they do not fire during REM sleep.[17–19] Melanin-concentrating hormone neurons are active during REM sleep.

The orexin peptides, discovered in 1998, are produced in the posterior lateral hypothalamus and are a critical part of the nonthalamic arousal pathway. The orexin system has recently been of particular interest in the anesthesia literature in the understanding of arousal. These neurons are most active during wakefulness[13,20,21] and play a significant role in narcolepsy (narcoleptic patients have few orexin neurons and low orexin levels in the cerebral spinal fluid).[22–24] Orexin-producing neurons have processes that project to the cerebral cortex, and to all the monoaminergic and cholinergic cell groups of the arousal systems.[25] Two receptors exist for orexins: orexin receptor 1 preferentially binds orexin A over orexin B, whereas orexin receptor 2 binds both ligands with equal affinity.[26]

Orexin agonists decrease the duration or depth of anesthesia as monitored by activation of the EEG in rats anesthetized with isoflurane, and administration of an orexin receptor 1 antagonist increases anesthetic duration.[27,28] Mice bearing a transgene, which results in a degeneration of orexin neurons, lead to delayed emergence from anesthesia but do not change loss of consciousness at induction. In addition to orexin playing a key role in clinical anesthetic emergence, anesthetic administration is associated with decreased orexin neuron activation.[29] Anesthetics affect orexin receptor function directly,[26] and the function of orexin targets. Full understanding of the nonthalamic arousal pathway, and specifically the role of orexin in emergence from anesthesia, and thus arousal, is still under investigation.

### *The Ventrolateral Preoptic Nucleus: A Sleep System*

Von Economo noted that a small percentage of patients with encephalitis lethargica had a paradoxic response; rather than being sleepy, they became insomniac. These patients had lesions involving the basal ganglia and adjacent anterior hypothalamus. Using animal studies, researchers identified a hypothalamic site involving the lateral preoptic area where lesions caused similar insomnia.[30] This region is called the ventrolateral preoptic nucleus (VLPO). Neurons located here send outputs to multiple cell groups in the hypothalamus and brainstem involved in arousal (**Fig. 3**).[31] These neurons have increased activity during sleep, and contain the inhibitory neurotransmitters, galanin and GABA,[2] which innervate diffuse areas of the brainstem.[2,20,32–34]

In turn, these ventrolateral preoptic nucleus neurons receive afferent input from monoaminergic systems.[34] Both noradrenaline and serotonin inhibit these neurons.[35] In addition, GABA and several other potentially inhibitory peptides, such as galanin and endomorphin[36] from tuberomammillary neurons,[37] inhibit ventrolateral preoptic nucleus neurons. However, ventrolateral preoptic neurons do not have histamine receptors or orexin receptors.[38] Because the ventrolateral preoptic neurons can be

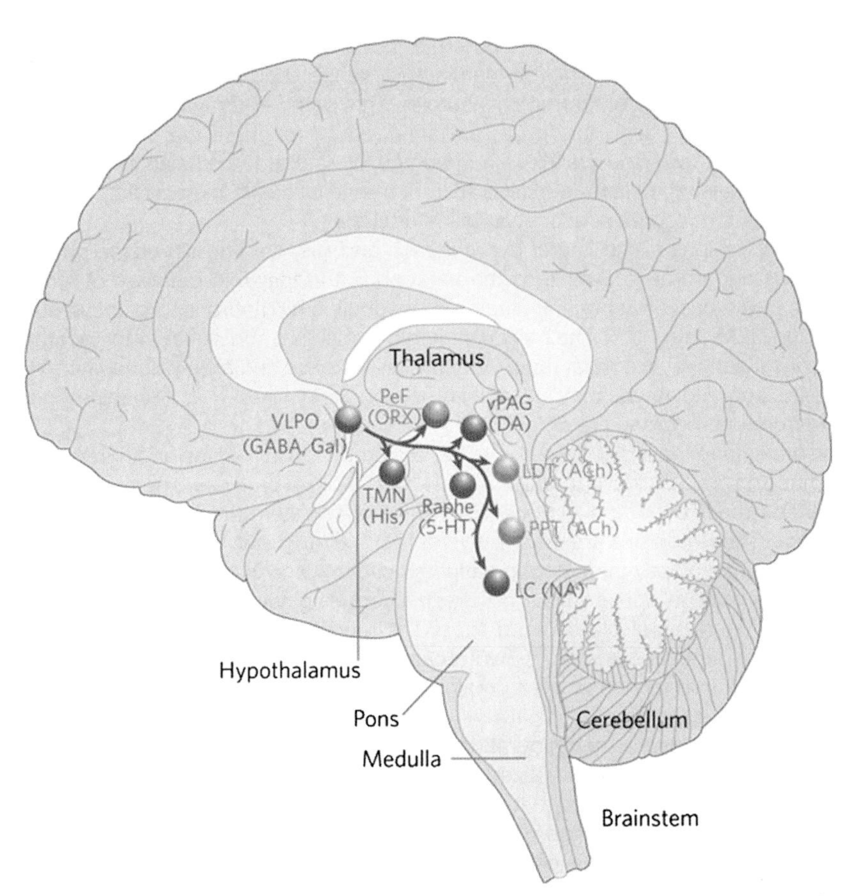


**Fig. 3.** The ventrolateral preoptic nucleus projects to the monoaminergic nuclei (*red*), including the tuberomammillary nucleus (TMN), the raphe cell groups and the locus coeruleus (LC). It also innervates neurons in the lateral hypothalamus (*green*), including the perifornical (PeF) orexin (ORX) neurons, and interneurons in the cholinergic (ACh) cell groups (*yellow*), the pedunculopontine (PPT), and laterodorsal tegmental nuclei (LDT).

inhibited by the very monoaminergic and GABA arousal systems that they inhibit during sleep, Saper has described this as a flip-flop relationship, in which the ventrolateral preoptic nucleus and the arousal system inhibit each other; the ventrolateral preoptic nucleus inhibits the orexin system, thereby inhibiting the arousal system.[2]

## *The Cortex: The Site of End-effect*

Whereas the ascending arousal system with its widespread projections to the thalamus and the cortex is clearly important in arousal and the effects of anesthesia, the cortex also plays an important role in arousal and consciousness. Anesthetics slow cortical oscillatory activity in in-vitro studies independently of subcortical activity.[39] In rats, inhaled agents at concentrations inducing hypnosis directly decrease discharge rates of cortical neurons by 50%.[40] In humans, during induction of general anesthesia, slowing of the EEG occurs earlier and is more prominent, compared with the electrical activity of the midbrain.[41] Even with light anesthesia (0.7% isoflurane), the cortical somatosensory response may be suppressed without reducing the thalamic response to painful stimulation.[42] Spontaneous thalamic firing during anesthesia is largely driven by feedback from cortical neurons, thus modulating the response of the ascending arousal system.[43]

### *Aging*

The speed of arousal is known to decline with aging. The mechanism behind this phenomenon is multifactorial, but most likely it involves physiologic changes in the cortical, brainstem and diencephalic systems. The lateral hypothalamus affects orexin neurons, and the basal forebrain complex affects cholinergic, histaminergic, and serotoninergic transmission.

Age-related cognitive decline is understood to be accompanied by changes in cortical neuronal morphology.[44] The complexity of apical dendrites decreases with age: there is a loss in the total number (28%–37%) and density (~23%) of spines.[45] In humans, neocortical synaptic density declines at a constant rate starting during early adulthood.[46] Although the exact consequence of these changes is still under investigation, dendritic changes are believed to alter the postsynaptic effects of neurotransmitters,[47] and precede other histologic changes found in neurocognitive diseases such as Alzheimer disease.[48]

Similar to the loss in complexity of dendrites in the cortex, the orexin neurons of the arousal system show a decrease in complexity with normal aging. Downs and colleagues[49] studied the number of orexin neurons in the lateral hypothalamus of rhesus macaques across their life span, from prepubertal development to old age. Similar to the primate studies of the cortex, they did not find a decreased number of orexin neurons, but did find a significant loss of orexin axonal density within the locus coeruleus of old macaques, and a concomitant decrease in tyrosine hydroxylase mRNA expression.[49] These data suggest that age-related decreases in excitatory orexin innervation to the noradrenergic locus coeruleus may contribute to poor sleep and delayed arousal in the elderly, specifically with implications for emergence from anesthesia.[29]

During aging, cholinergic neurons of the basal forebrain complex undergo degenerative changes, including cell atrophy, downregulation of choline acetyltransferase activity (ChAT), and mild cellular loss, resulting in cholinergic hypofunction. Neuropharmacologic manipulations that increase or decrease the excitability of basal forebrain cholinergic projections systematically affect attentional performance and cortical acetyl choline (ACh) efflux.[50] There are several human brain conditions, notably Alzheimer disease, in which degeneration of basal forebrain cholinergic neurons have been documented. Therefore, cholinergic changes are important in the arousal system and changes with age likely affect emergence from anesthesia.

Histaminergic neurons play an excitatory role in arousal. The levels of histamine and its metabolites are known to increase in human cerebrospinal fluid (CSF) with age. In addition, there is a age-related decline in histamine-1 receptor binding in the normal human brain,[51] which is believed to be a result of downregulation of receptors caused by high endogenous histamine.[52]

There are limited and conflicting data in the literature regarding changes in the serotonin (5-HT) system in normal aging. Serotonin receptors are more dense at birth than in the mature brain, and may regulate the maturation of cortical neurons.[53] In addition, several postmortem human studies have reported a reduction in the number of cortical 5-$HT_{1A}$, 5-$HT_{1B/D}$, and 5-$HT_{2A}$ binding sites with age in frontal lobe, occipital lobe, and hippocampus.[50,54] Age-related decline in cortical 5-$HT_{2A}$ binding was also found in living healthy subjects demonstrated by positron emission tomography (PET) imaging with [$^{11}$C]*N*-methylspiperone, a ligand with affinity for both 5-$HT_{2A}$ and dopamine $D_2$

receptors.[50,55] Age-related decrease in excitatory ascending arousal pathway stimulation would correlate with a decrease in arousal, and possibly a slower emergence from anesthesia.

In addition to the decreases in size and activity of the excitatory components of the arousal system, the inhibitory ventrolateral preoptic nucleus is significantly reduced in size with aging.[56,57] Degeneration of the ventrolateral preoptic nucleus with age could account for the diminished efficiency and depth of sleep in elderly humans. This difference could be marked, as there is a reported 60% loss of galaninergic neurons in aged versus younger rats in a region that seems to include the ventrolateral preoptic nucleus cluster.[58]

The explanation as to why there are changes with aging in specific cellular populations remains unknown. The perturbation of neuronal calcium homeostasis is a possible explanation.[59] Calcium conductance and the number of calcium channels of the L-type in CA1 pyramidal neurons increase with aging.[60] This high intracellular calcium concentration can activate proteases and induce reactive oxygen species production, which may be neurotoxic.[61]

## PHARMACOLOGY

Delayed arousal may also be caused by altered responses to pharmacologic agents in the geriatric population. This delay may arise from drug-specific pharmacokinetic or pharmacodynamic changes commonly reported in these patients. Whether these differences in pharmacologic parameters are truly age-related independent factors or primarily manifestations of coexistent diseases and/or polypharmacy more frequently seen in the elderly is inconsequential. The net result is the same. Exaggerated pharmacologic responses and prolonged duration of action are often seen following the administration of drugs in dosages that seem appropriate for the age and gender of the patient.

Pharmacokinetic alterations can be characterized by changes in initial and steady state volumes of distribution, clearance rates, redistribution and elimination half-times. The decrease in initial volume of distribution, $V_i$, reflects the age-associated decrease in blood volume, which may result in a higher than expected initial concentration of drug following an intravenous bolus injection. Changes in steady state volumes of distribution, $V_d$, are less consistent, such that the increase in body fat, decrease in lean body mass and decreased total body water result in an increased $V_d$ for lipophilic drugs and a decrease for hydrophilic drugs. Although an increased $V_d$ is associated with a lower concentration of drug, the elimination of drug is likely to be more prolonged. In addition, the decreased plasma protein binding in the elderly results in an increase in the free plasma concentration for drugs such as midazolam, fentanyl, and propofol, which are highly protein bound.[62]

The aging process is generally accompanied by a gradual decline in organ function.[63] Whereas the decrease in renal function resulting from diminished renal blood flow, glomerular filtration, and tubular secretion predictably leads to increased serum concentration and prolonged presence of drugs dependent on renal excretion, the disposition of drugs dependent on hepatic metabolism is less consistent. Phase II metabolic pathways do not seem to be much affected by age, whereas the effect of age on phase I metabolism is unclear.[64] The decrease in liver mass and blood flow in the elderly would predict a delay in the elimination of drugs with a high extraction ratio, such as midazolam, fentanyl, and sufentanil. However, clinical studies have not consistently demonstrated an increased elimination half-life.[65]

With the exception of a few drugs, the behavior of which can be described by a one-compartment model, classic pharmacokinetic parameters are not accurately predictive of the rate of decrease of drugs from the central compartment. Thus, although the elimination half-life of sufentanil is much greater than fentanyl (9.5 vs 3.7 hours), sufentanil is more rapidly cleared from the circulation, at least after prolonged (>2 hours) infusions. The triexponential function derived from three-compartment models characterizing the elimination of most agents administered in the course of anesthesia are descriptive of a scenario where distribution-redistribution between the fast and slow compartments may be the primary factor affecting the disappearance of drug from the central compartment. The complex interaction between compartment sizes, clearance, and intercompartmental rate constants is well characterized by the context-sensitive half-time.[66] The premise of the context-sensitive half-time is that, with large doses or long infusions, drug eliminated from the central compartment may be rapidly replaced by drug redistributing from the slow peripheral compartments, thus hindering the decline in central compartment drug concentration. Thus, context-sensitive half-time estimates the amount of time for the concentration of drug to decrease by 50% in the context of the duration of the drug infusion.

Despite providing an improvement over elimination half-life, context-sensitive half-time does not fully explain recovery from anesthesia.[67] Contributory factors to this problem include the fact that any selected infusion regimen is likely not to reliably yield a constant targeted plasma concentration. In addition, it is unlikely that recovery occurs at exactly 50% of the concentration at the end of the infusion.

Although the pharmacokinetics of anesthetic drugs in the elderly has been studied extensively, pharmacodynamics in the elderly has not received equal attention. The presence of pharmacodynamic alteration is often surmised by the observation of an exaggerated or prolonged effect for a drug for which pharmacokinetic studies failed to discern any difference between age groups. There is a paucity of studies that have examined the relationship between measured plasma concentration or modeled effect compartment concentration and clinical effect.[68] Nonetheless, clinical experience has demonstrated that the elderly are more sensitive to anesthetics, with the consensus opinion that for most agents this effect is primarily, or at least in part, caused by pharamcodynamic changes.

Factors invoked to explain pharmacodynamic changes include altered receptor density and binding, changes in signal transduction and impaired cellular responses.[69] As a result of or in addition to these factors, the elderly exhibit a decrease in homeostatic mechanisms. Any drug-induced perturbation may be longer lasting, requiring a greater length of time for restoration of the steady state.[70]

For drugs such as anesthetics where the primary effect is binary, that is, awake versus asleep, or movement versus no movement, the pharamcodynamic response is best defined by the Hill equation:

$$P = \frac{100 \times C^{\delta}}{(C^{\delta} + C_{50}^{\delta})}$$

where $P$ is the probability of effect (0%–100%), $C$ is the plasma concentration and $C_{50}$ is the concentration at which 50% of subjects exhibit the desired effect. A plot of the Hill equation, dose or plasma concentration against probability of the desired effect, yields a sigmoid curve. The steepness of the curve is defined by the variable delta ($\delta$). When delta is large, as for example, alfentanil and sufentanil, the curve is steep, such that most patients can be expected to respond at doses near the $C_{50}$.

Conversely, smaller values of delta, as for example, propofol and midazolam, are associated with greater variability, with the therapeutic response and the termination of the therapeutic effect occurring at a more variable and less predictable plasma concentration (**Fig. 4**).[71]

Combining pharmacokinetics and pharmacodynamics, intuition would dictate that for a drug with a steep delta, one would know with relative certainty what concentration of drug would be required for the desired effect. Presumably, it might, for illustrative purposes, be assumed that 50% of this concentration could be associated with a 5% probability of this effect, thereby implying that 95% of patients will have recovered at that point. In this simplified example, context-sensitive half-time and $C_{50}$ could give a good approximation as to how long recovery should take. The true situation is more complicated. $C_{50}$ might be greatly decreased in the elderly patient, whereas delta might be smaller, consistent with the wide variability of response that can be seen in this group. For example, $C_{50}$ for propofol is 47% lower in elderly patients compared with young adults, in conjunction with a lower value for delta.[72] Similarly, it has been demonstrated that elderly patients require approximately 40% less propofol to maintain a constant predetermined EEG endpoint.[73] Thus, the selected dose may be inappropriately large, such that recovery might not occur until plasma concentration falls by 90%. In this situation the context-sensitive half-time is not clinically significant. A more accurate predictor in this situation would be the 90% decrement time in the context of the length of drug infusion.[74]

Recovery from inhaled anesthetics may be used as an illustrative example, in that context-sensitive half-time has been used to describe the pharmacokinetics of these

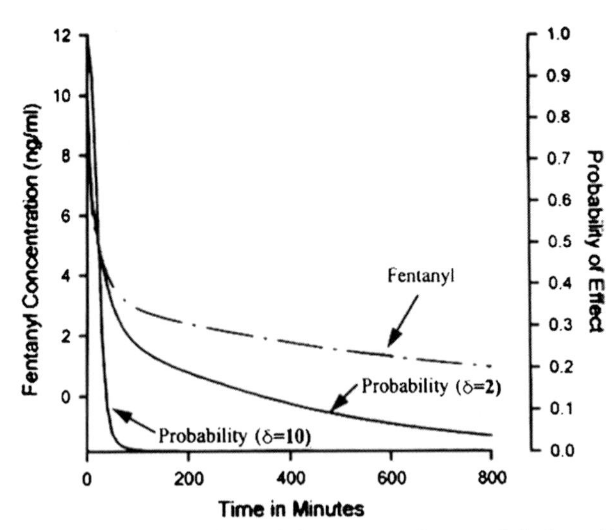


**Fig. 4.** The relationship between delta and the recovery from an infusion of fentanyl maintaining a constant concentration of 10 ng/mL for 60 minutes. Recovery in 50% of patients ($C_{50}$) is assumed to occur at concentration of 5 ng/mL. If delta = 10, almost all patients recover at a concentration of 5 ng/mL at roughly the context-sensitive half-time (approximately 23 minutes). However, when delta = 2, the mean effect time, derived by integrating the probability of effect curve rises to 130 minutes, with approximately 10% of patients not recovering for 5 hours. (*From* Bailey JM. Technique for quantifying the duration of intravenous anesthetic effect. Anesthesiology 1995;83:1095–103; with permission.)

agents.[75] In addition, at least in the steady state, the measured alveolar concentration provides a readily measured estimate of the effect of compartment concentration.

The minimal alveolar concentration of potent inhalational agents at which 50% of patients do not respond to surgical stimulation (MAC) decreases roughly 6.7% per decade from the MAC value of 40-year-old adults. The concentration required to attain a given EEG end point is similarly decreased.[76] MAC-awake, the alveolar concentration at which patients obey commands, also decreases with age, although the ratio of MAC-awake to MAC seems to remain the same throughout different age groups. MAC-awake, on average is approximately one-third of MAC (**Fig. 5**).[77] Clearly in a situation where the inspired or end-tidal concentration of inhaled anesthetic is set for 1 MAC, as displayed by most anesthesia machines (not age-adjusted), a decrement of 50% predicted by the context-sensitive half-time has little relevance to the expected time for awakening. In this situation, the 90% decrement time, the time for the anesthetic concentration to decrease by 90%, would be a more appropriate predictor. It should be noted however, that the effect of context, that is, length of drug administration, has a greater effect on the 90% decrement time than it does for the context-sensitive half-time. Although the context-sensitive half-time is small and relatively unchanged throughout a wide range of exposure times for all inhalational agents, as seen in **Fig. 6**, the changes in 90% decrement time are quite remarkable.[75] Even with the shorter acting agent, sevoflurane, for which there is little change in decrement times during the first 90 minutes of exposure, additional exposure results in a marked increase in 90% decrement times. As a result, awakening times in excess of 1 hour may occur after a 6-hour exposure.

Hence, the combined effects of pharmacokinetic and pharmacodynamic changes in elderly patients may variably and unpredictably prolong arousal time.

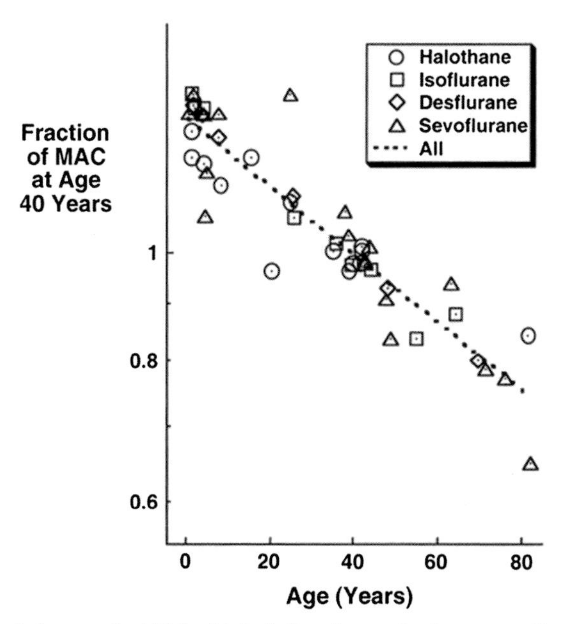


**Fig. 5.** Age-related changes in MAC of inhalational anesthetics, normalized to MAC at 40 years of age. (*From* Eger 2nd EI. Age, minimum alveolar anesthetic concentration, and minimum alveolar anesthetic concentration-awake. Anesth Analg 2001;93:947–53; with permission.)

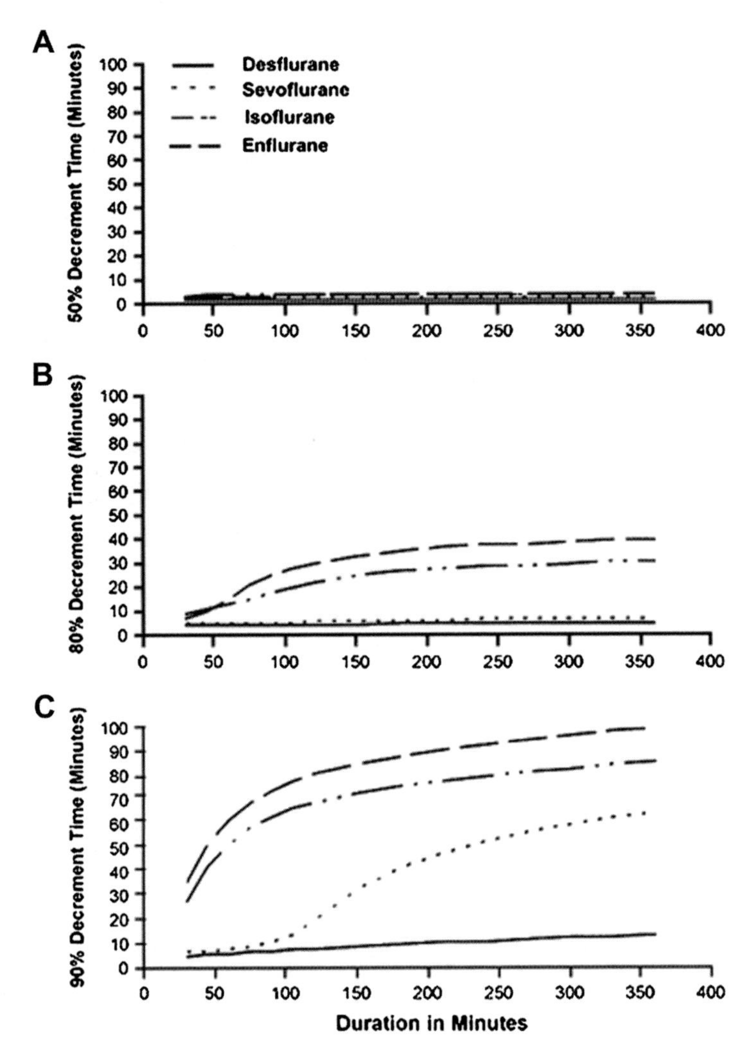


**Fig. 6.** Context-sensitive 50%, 80%, and 90% decrement times for inhalational anesthetics. Note that context-sensitive half-time is analogous to context-sensitive 50% decrement time. (*From* Bailey JM: Context-sensitive half-times and other decrement times of inhaled anesthetics. Anesth Analg 1997;85:681–6; with permission.)

## ALGORITHM FOR APPROACHING A PATIENT WITH DELAYED AROUSAL

The workup for delayed arousal must address the multiple possible causative factors: functional abnormalities that occur naturally with aging, structural abnormalities such as focal lesions in specific areas of the brain or diffuse cortical problems such as multifocal injuries, and metabolic disturbances of common electrolytes or pharmacologic agents. These metabolic problems may be caused by toxic effects or by changes in pharmacokinetic or pharmacodynamic issues. Workup of each of these problems requires a different solution.

Determining the cause of delayed arousal requires clinical, chemical, and structural tests. We are using the term "structural" to refer to physical processes such as hemorrhage, either subarachnoid or epidural, ischemia, or infarction. In this section, the tools to diagnose the cause of delayed arousal are reviewed.

In general, focal or multifocal lesions can be identified by instruments that define structural abnormalities. Therefore computerized tomography (CT), or magnetic resonance imaging (MRI), or derivatives of MRI such as diffusion-weighted imaging (DWI), are useful to define the area of injury, because ischemia can be detected within 5 to 10 minutes.

### *Computerized Tomography*

CT is a medical imaging method employing x-ray radiation and tomography. Digital geometry processing is used to generate a three-dimensional image of the inside of an object from a large series of two-dimensional radiograph images taken around a single axis of rotation.

A CT scan of the head without contrast can be useful to determine whether the patient has had an intracranial hemorrhage. Unfortunately, cerebral ischemia is poorly visualized by CT scan with contrast because it takes 5 to 7 days to become manifest.

### *Magnetic Resonance Imaging*

MRI scans can determine old and new focal infarcts and even ischemia within minutes using DWI.[78,79] A negative CT scan or MRI image may rule out a large mass lesion produced by intracerebral hemorrhage or areas of ischemia when viewed by DWI. Should there be evidence of cerebral ischemia; then it may be necessary to perform a cerebral angiogram to re-establish cerebral perfusion.

MRI does not use x-ray radiation. MRI is based on aligning the proton of the hydrogen ion in water in the presence of a strong magnetic field. A second magnetic field is used to perturb this orientation and energy is released as a photon when the field is turned off. Gradient fields are turned on and off and complicated sequences can be performed to reveal structural and chemical properties of areas of the brain. The basic parameters of image acquisition are produced by varying particular values of the echo time (TE) and the repetition time (TR), which can take on the property of T2-weighting. On a T2-weighted scan, water- and fluid-containing tissues are bright and fat-containing tissues are dark. The reverse is true for T1-weighted images. With an additional radio frequency pulse and additional manipulation of the magnetic gradients, a T2-weighted sequence can be converted to a FLAIR sequence, in which free water is now dark, but edematous tissues remain bright.

There are also specialized MRI scans. Diffusion MRI produces images in which the contrast between tissues is dependent on differences in microscopic water diffusion. In free space, water diffuses at random by Brownian motion. But in biologic tissue, it is restricted in its free motion. In the brain, water diffusion rates are lowest in white matter, higher in gray matter and highest in CSF. White matter also shows prominent diffusion anisotropy, with more rapid diffusion parallel to the orientation of axons along white matter tracts. In pathologic tissue, the lowest diffusion rates are seen in acute infarction (restricted intracellular diffusion), with higher rates in chronic infarcts and reactive interstitial edema such as that associated with tumors, infection, or trauma (more freely diffusing extracellular water), and highest rates in CSF-filled cystic collections such as surgical cavities or arachnoid cysts (unrestricted diffusion in unstructured water). These different water diffusion properties are depicted in two ways. The directly acquired DWI show low diffusion rates as high signal and high diffusion rates as low signal. After processing these images, quantitative apparent diffusion coefficient (ADC) maps are created, which show low diffusion rates as low signal and high diffusion rates as high signal.[80]

## SEIZURES

Status epilepticus may impair consciousness. Elderly patients have increased probability of having previous cerebral infarcts that may not even be evident to the patient, or new ischemic events arising intra-operatively. These events may predispose them to have either seizures that may be focal with secondary generalization or seizures that are generalized in nature. Some of these seizures may not have a motor component (nonconvulsive) and therefore are manifest solely as impaired consciousness. These seizures can be precipitated by metabolic abnormalities that lower seizure threshold and predispose patients to status epilepticus.

### *Electroencephalography*

Functional tests such as electroencephalography can determine rhythms such as burst suppression consistent with persistent sedative-hypnotic medication, or cerebral rhythms associated with hepatic encephalography that may narrow the differential diagnosis.

The electroencephalogram can also be used to evaluate altered states of consciousness.[81–83] However, this evaluation should be performed by a trained electroencephalographer using a full EEG montage because many artifacts including muscle action potentials, which are of the order of a thousand-fold larger in amplitude than cortical activity recorded from the scalp, can confuse interpretation of the electrophysiologic signal. Diffuse slowing of background rhythms and the presence of triphasic waves suggest metabolic dysfunction, particularly hepatic (**Fig. 7**) or renal; spindle coma patterns are believed to indicate dysfunction at the brainstem level.[83] Generalized fast activity may be seen with drug intoxication. Most significantly, nonconvulsive status epilepticus can be diagnosed under conditions when it is least expected. There are several

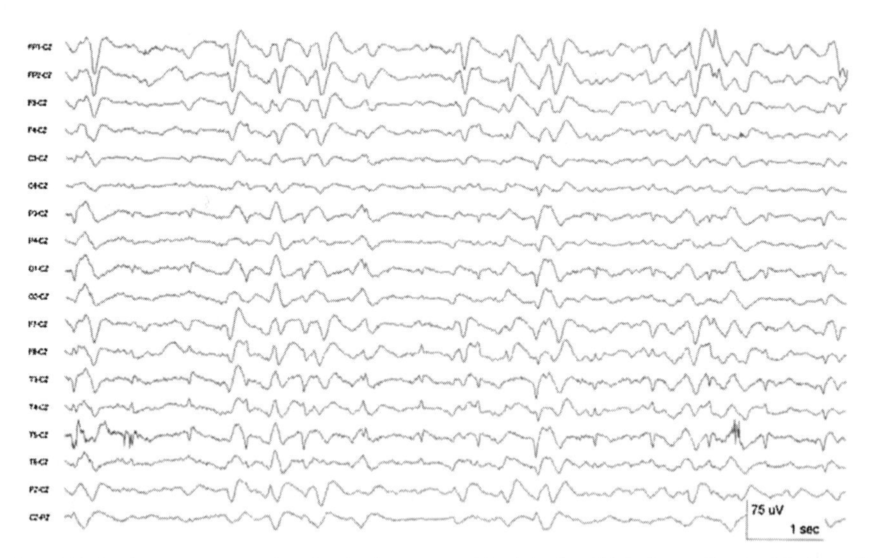


**Fig. 7.** Triphasic waves occurring in clusters are evident in the EEG of a patient with hepatic encephalopathy. Electrodes are placed in the 10–20 international electrode convention. All electrodes are referred to $C_Z$. The electrode positions are in pairs, left then right, from midline anterior to posterior in the upper 10 traces, and from lateral anterior to posterior in the lower 8 traces. (*Reprinted from* Brenner RP. EEG in encephalopathy and coma. Am J Electroneurodiagn Technol 2003;43(3):164–84; with permission.)

electroencephalographic patterns for nonconvulsive status epilepticus (**Figs. 8** and **9**).[81] Many of these patterns are controversial: periodic lateralized epileptiform discharges (PLEDs), bilateral independent PLEDS (BIPLEDs) (see **Fig. 8**), periodic epileptiform discharges (PEDs) which can be focal or generalized, and generalized triphasic waves. Unfortunately, most of these patterns are not specific for a single etiology. For example, both hypoxia and the commonly used sedative-hypnotic medications, such as propofol, etomidate, or thiopental, can produce burst suppression.[81]

### *Metabolic*

Several metabolic abnormalities impair consciousness. Most should be evident before surgery, but can be exacerbated during the course of surgery. By definition, these disorders are diffuse, however, some present with focal findings. One example is diabetes mellitus. Elderly patients are more likely to develop type 2 diabetes mellitus. A high percentage of patients with diabetes are poorly controlled.[80,84] Patients who present out of control with high serum glucose concentrations may be in diabetic ketoacidosis. Some of these patients may develop focal neurologic findings by mechanisms that are not completely understood.[85,86] On the other hand, because there is increasing use of insulin infusions to control serum glucose levels during surgery, it is likely that more and more patients will become hypoglycemic during surgery. Hypoglycemia has become a bigger problem as treatment protocols for diabetes mellitus have attempted to control serum glucose levels closer to normal.[87] Both of these extremes, hyper- and hypoglycemia can impair consciousness.

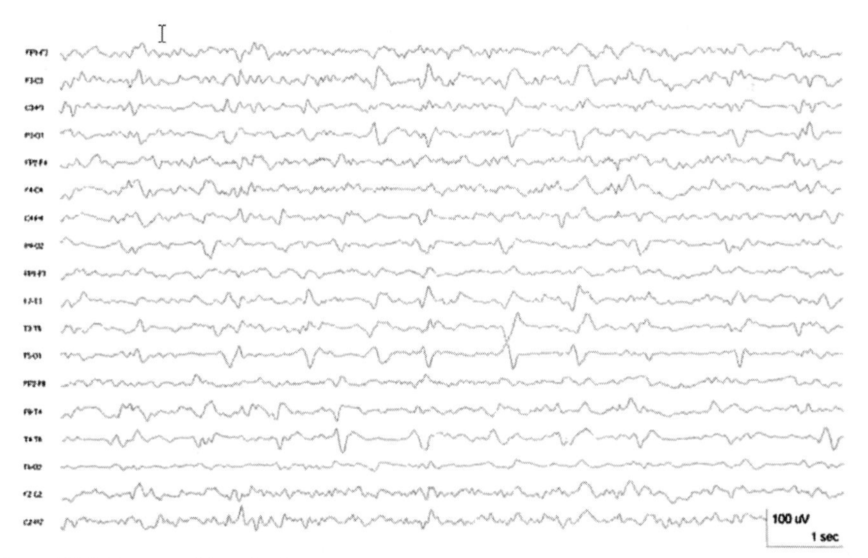


**Fig. 8.** BIPLEDs are evident in the EEG in a patient with prolonged hypoglycemia. Electrodes are placed in the 10–20 international electrode convention. The electrodes are arranged in a bipolar montage. The first and third set of 4 electrodes are on the left side of the head, and the second and fourth set of 4 electrodes are on the right side of the head. Within each set the electrodes are arranged anterior to posterior with the first and second sets representing midline electrodes, and the third and fourth sets representing lateral electrodes. The bottom 2 electrode pairs are $F_z$ to $C_z$, and $C_z$ to $P_z$. (*Reprinted from* Brenner RP. EEG in encephalopathy and coma. Am J Electroneurodiagn Technol 2003;43(3):164–84; with permission.)

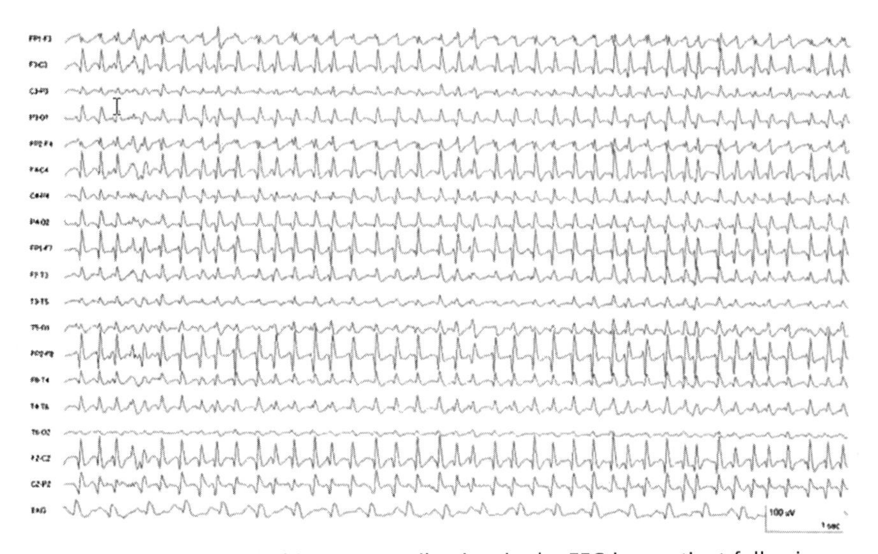

**Fig. 9.** Generalized nonconvulsive status epilepticus in the EEG in a patient following cerebral anoxia. Electrodes are placed in the 10–20 international electrode convention. The electrodes are arranged in a bipolar montage. The first and third set of 4 electrodes are on the left side of the head, and the second and fourth set of 4 electrodes are on the right side of the head. Within each set the electrodes are arranged anterior to posterior with the first and second sets representing midline electrodes, and the third and fourth sets representing lateral electrodes. The bottom 3 electrode pairs are $F_z$ to $C_z$, and $C_z$ to $P_z$ with the bottom trace the electrocardiogram (ECG). (*Reprinted from* Brenner RP. EEG in encephalopathy and coma. Am J Electroneurodiagn Technol 2003;43(3):164–84; with permission.)

### *Electrolytes*

Resting membrane potential, action potentials and their generation are controlled by both extra- and intracellular electrolyte concentrations. Many medications have effects on electrolyte concentrations. For example, diuretics are considered first-line medications for treatment of hypertension,[88–91] a common condition in the elderly. Chronic use of diuretics may lead to total body depletion of potassium. Because potassium is primarily an intracellular electrolyte, hypokalemia may be difficult to reverse acutely. Similarly divalent cations such as magnesium and manganese may have profound effects on the nervous system.

## WORKUP

The workup has to be targeted to the likely cause of delayed arousal. A thorough knowledge of the patient's medical history, medications and nature of the surgical procedure is essential. The timeline of the workup of delayed arousal is highly variable and depends on the clinical scenario in which we encounter the patient, and clinical judgment concerning the differential diagnosis. For example, in the patient who has undergone a carotid endarterectomy in which minimal medication was administered, the time threshold to explore a possible ischemic cause of delayed arousal is very short. In contrast, for the elderly patient with a prior history of organ dysfunction who has undergone a long procedure and has arrived at the recovery area at a low temperature after receiving a higher dose of medications, a longer time threshold is tolerated, as probable metabolic causes are considered.

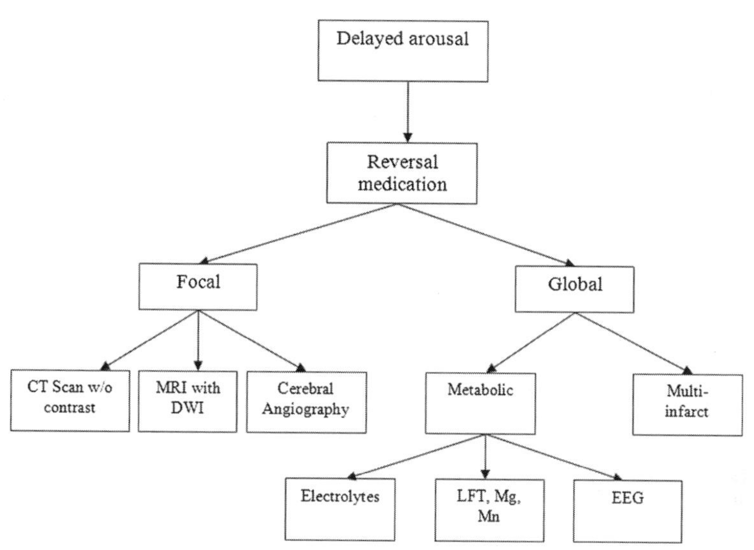


**Fig. 10.** An algorithm to work up a patient with delayed arousal. CT, computerized tomography; MRI, magnetic resonance imaging; DWI, diffusion-weighted imaging; LFT, liver function tests; Mg, magnesium levels; Mn, manganese levels; and EEG, electroencephalogram.

To the degree that it is possible, a neurologic examination should be performed immediately including the cranial nerves, and the motor and sensory pathways. Frequently, little information can be derived.

The most common cause of delayed arousal is overdose of a sedative-hypnotic medication. Several medications to reverse narcotic and benzodiazepine overdose are available and should be tried. However, should these fail, then a systematic review of other metabolic and structural possibilities needs to be carried out (**Fig. 10**).

Metabolic considerations can be immediately and easily determined by an electrolyte panel including sodium, potassium, carbon dioxide, chloride, blood urea nitrogen, and glucose. Other electrolyte tests may take longer to be reported such as magnesium, manganese, lactate, elevated liver function tests, and so forth.

Based on the procedures that the patient has undergone and the clinical differential diagnosis, an evaluation of structural causes should be looked into including MRI with DWI or CT scan. Based on the findings from this study, cerebral angiography may be necessary.

Because most of our anesthetics have context-sensitive half-times, elimination of medications may be significantly prolonged. This fact alone makes it difficult to provide an exact timeline of the steps to take at each exact point in time. Instead, we have provided an algorithm to focus on the workup of delayed arousal, with attention to the fact that the elderly population has a high variability for many different characteristics, including arousal.

## SUMMARY

Elderly patients have medical and psychological problems affecting all major organ systems. These problems may alter the pharmacokinetics and/or pharmacodynamics of medications, or expose previous neurologic deficits simply as a result of sedation. Delayed arousal, therefore, may arise from structural problems that are pre-existent or new, or metabolic or functional disorders such as convulsive or nonconvulsive seizures. Determining the cause of delayed arousal may require clinical, chemical, and structural tests. Structural problems that impair consciousness arise from a small number of focal lesions to specific areas of the central nervous system, or from pathology affecting the cerebrum. In general, focal or multifocal lesions can be identified by CT, or DWI. An algorithm is presented that outlines a workup for an elderly patient with delayed arousal.

## REFERENCES


1. Lazar RM, Fitzsimmons BF, Marshall RS, et al. Midazolam challenge reinduces neurological deficits after transient ischemic attack. Stroke 2003;34:794–6.
2. Saper CB, Scammell TE, Lu J. Hypothalamic regulation of sleep and circadian rhythms. Nature 2005;437(3):1257–63.
3. Moruzzi G, Magoun HW. Brain stem reticular formation and activation of the EEG. Electroencephalogr Clin Neurophysiol 1949;1(7063):455–73.
4. Saper CB, Chou TC, Scammell TE. The sleep switch: hypothalamic control of sleep and wakefulness. Trends Neurosci 2001;24(12):726–31.
5. Laureys S, Boly M, Maquet P. Tracking the recovery of consciousness from coma. J Clin Invest 2006;116(7):1823–5.
6. Alkire MT, Miller J. General anesthesia and the neural correlates of consciousness. Prog Brain Res 2005;150:229–44.
7. Hallanger AE, Levey AI, Lee HJ, et al. The origins of cholinergic and other subcortical afferents to the thalamus in the rat. J Comp Neurol 1987;262(1):105–24.
8. Strecker RE, Morairty S, Thakkar MM, et al. Adenosinergic modulation of basal forebrain and preoptic/anterior hypothalamic neuronal activity in the control of behavioral state. Behav Brain Res 2000;115(2):183–204.
9. Glenn LL, Steriade M. Discharge rate and excitability of cortically projecting intralaminar thalamic neurons during waking and sleep states. J Neurosci 1982;2(10): 1387–404.
10. Keifer JC, Baghdoyan HA, Lydic R. Pontine cholinergic mechanisms modulate the cortical electroencephalographic spindles of halothane anesthesia. Anesthesiology 1996;84(4):945–54.
11. Miller JW, Ferrendelli JA. Characterization of GABAergic seizure regulation in the midline thalamus. Neuropharmacology 1990;29(7):649–55.
12. Alkire MT, McReynolds JR, Hahn EL, et al. Thalamic microinjection of nicotine reverses sevoflurane-induced loss of righting reflex in the rat. Anesthesiology 2007;107(2):264–72.
13. Gerashchenko D, Blanco-Centurion C, Greco MA, et al. Effects of lateral hypothalamic lesion with the neurotoxin hypocretin-2-saporin on sleep in Long-Evans rats. Neuroscience 2003;116(1):223–35.
14. Lee MG, Hassani OK, Jones BE. Discharge of identified orexin/hypocretin neurons across the sleep-waking cycle. J Neurosci 2005;25(28):6716–20.
15. Verret L, Goutagny R, Fort P, et al. A role of melanin-concentrating hormone producing neurons in the central regulation of paradoxical sleep. BMC Neurosci 2003;4:19.
16. Lee MG, Hassani OK, Alonso A, et al. Cholinergic basal forebrain neurons burst with theta during waking and paradoxical sleep. J Neurosci 2005;25(17):4365–9.
17. Aston-Jones G, Bloom FE. Activity of norepinephrine-containing locus coeruleus neurons in behaving rats anticipates fluctuations in the sleep-waking cycle. J Neurosci 1981;1(8):876–86.

18. Fornal C, Auerbach S, Jacobs BL. Activity of serotonin-containing neurons in nucleus raphe magnus in freely moving cats. Exp Neurol 1985;88(3):590–608.
19. Steininger TL, Alam MN, Gong H, et al. Sleep-waking discharge of neurons in the posterior lateral hypothalamus of the albino rat. Brain Res 1999;840(1-2):138–47.
20. Estabrooke IV, McCarthy MT, Ko E, et al. Fos expression in orexin neurons varies with behavioral state. J Neurosci 2001;21(5):1656–62.
21. Mileykovskiy BY, Kiyashchenko LI, Siegel JM. Behavioral correlates of activity in identified hypocretin/orexin neurons. Neuron 2005;46(5):787–98.
22. Thannickal TC, Moore RY, Nienhuis R, et al. Reduced number of hypocretin neurons in human narcolepsy. Neuron 2000;27(3):469–74.
23. Peyron C, Faraco J, Rogers W, et al. A mutation in a case of early onset narcolepsy and a generalized absence of hypocretin peptides in human narcoleptic brains. Nat Med 2000;6(9):991–7.
24. Ripley B, Overeem S, Fujiki N, et al. CSF hypocretin/orexin levels in narcolepsy and other neurological conditions. Neurology 2001;57(12):2253–8.
25. Peyron C, Tighe DK, van den Pol AN, et al. Neurons containing hypocretin (orexin) project to multiple neuronal systems. J Neurosci 1998;18(23):9996–10015.
26. Sakurai T, Amemiya A, Ishii M, et al. Orexins and orexin receptors: a family of hypothalamic neuropeptides and G protein-coupled receptors that regulate feeding behavior. Cell 1998;92(4):573–85.
27. Yasuda Y, Takeda A, Fukuda S, et al. Orexin a elicits arousal electroencephalography without sympathetic cardiovascular activation in isoflurane-anesthetized rats. Anesth Analg 2003;97(6):1663–6.
28. Kushikata T, Hirota K, Yoshida H, et al. Orexinergic neurons and barbiturate anesthesia. Neuroscience 2003;121(4):855–63.
29. Kelz MB, Sun Y, Chen J, et al. An essential role for orexins in emergence from general anesthesia. Proc Natl Acad Sci U S A 2008;105(4):1309–14.
30. McGinty DJ, Sterman MB. Sleep suppression after basal forebrain lesions in the cat. Science 1968;160(833):1253–5.
31. Sherin JE, Shiromani PJ, McCarley RW, et al. Activation of ventrolateral preoptic neurons during sleep. Science 1996;271(5246):216–9.
32. Ko EM, Estabrooke IV, McCarthy M, et al. Wake-related activity of tuberomammillary neurons in rats. Brain Res 2003;992(2):220–6.
33. John J, Wu MF, Boehmer LN, et al. Cataplexy-active neurons in the hypothalamus: implications for the role of histamine in sleep and waking behavior. Neuron 2004;42(4):619–34.
34. Chou TC, Bjorkum AA, Gaus SE, et al. Afferents to the ventrolateral preoptic nucleus. J Neurosci 2002;22(3):977–90.
35. Gallopin T, Fort P, Eggermann E, et al. Identification of sleep-promoting neurons in vitro. Nature 2000;404(6781):992–5.
36. Martin-Schild S, Gerall AA, Kastin AJ, et al. Differential distribution of endomorphin 1- and endomorphin 2-like immunoreactivities in the CNS of the rodent. J Comp Neurol 1999;405(4):450–71.
37. Vincent SR, Hokfelt T, Wu JY. GABA neuron systems in hypothalamus and the pituitary gland. Immunohistochemical demonstration using antibodies against glutamate decarboxylase. Neuroendocrinology 1982;34(2):117–25.
38. Marcus JN, Aschkenasi CJ, Lee CE, et al. Differential expression of orexin receptors 1 and 2 in the rat brain. J Comp Neurol 2001;435(1):6–25.
39. Lukatch HS, MacIver MB. Synaptic mechanisms of thiopental-induced alterations in synchronized cortical activity. Anesthesiology 1996;84(6):1425–34.

40. Hentschke H, Schwarz C, Antkowiak B. Neocortex is the major target of sedative concentrations of volatile anaesthetics: strong depression of firing rates and increase of GABAA receptor-mediated inhibition. Eur J Neurosci 2005;21(1):93–102.
41. Velly LJ, Rey MF, Bruder NJ, et al. Differential dynamic of action on cortical and subcortical structures of anesthetic agents during induction of anesthesia. Anesthesiology 2007;107(2):202–12.
42. Antognini JF, Buonocore MH, Disbrow EA, et al. Isoflurane anesthesia blunts cerebral responses to noxious and innocuous stimuli: a fMRI study. Life Sci 1997;61(24):349–54.
43. Vahle-Hinz C, Detsch O, Siemers M, et al. Contributions of GABAergic and glutamatergic mechanisms to isoflurane-induced suppression of thalamic somatosensory information transfer. Exp Brain Res 2007;176(1):159–72.
44. Morrison JH, Hof PR. Selective vulnerability of corticocortical and hippocampal circuits in aging and Alzheimer's disease. Prog Brain Res 2002;136:467–86.
45. Page TL, Einstein M, Duan H, et al. Morphological alterations in neurons forming corticocortical projections in the neocortex of aged Patas monkeys. Neurosci Lett 2002;317(1):37–41.
46. Terry RD, Katzman R. Life span and synapses: will there be a primary senile dementia? Neurobiol Aging 2001;22(3):347–8.
47. Dickstein DL, Kabaso D, Rocher AB, et al. Changes in the structural complexity of the aged brain. Aging Cell 2007;6(3):275–84.
48. Terry RD, Masliah E, Salmon DP, et al. Physical basis of cognitive alterations in Alzheimer's disease: synapse loss is the major correlate of cognitive impairment. Ann Neurol 1991;30(4):572–80.
49. Downs JL, Dunn MR, Borok E, et al. Orexin neuronal changes in the locus coeruleus of the aging rhesus macaque. Neurobiol Aging 2007;28(8):1286–95.
50. Meltzer CC, Smith G, DeKosky ST, et al. Serotonin in aging, late-life depression, and Alzheimer's disease: the emerging role of functional imaging. Neuropsychopharmacology 1998;18(6):407–30.
51. Yanai K, Watanabe T, Meguro K, et al. Age-dependent decrease in histamine H1 receptor in human brains revealed by PET. Neuroreport 1992;3(5):433–6.
52. Yanai K, Tashiro M. The physiological and pathophysiological roles of neuronal histamine: an insight from human positron emission tomography studies. Pharmacol Ther 2007;113(1):1–15.
53. Azmitia EC, Whitaker-Azmitia PM. Awakening the sleeping giant: anatomy and plasticity of the brain serotonergic system. J Clin Psychiatry 1991;52(Suppl):4–16.
54. Arranz B, Eriksson A, Mellerup E, et al. Effect of aging in human cortical pre- and postsynaptic serotonin binding sites. Brain Res 1993;620(1):163–6.
55. Iyo M, Yamasaki T. The detection of age-related decrease of dopamine D1, D2 and serotonin 5-HT2 receptors in living human brain. Prog Neuropsychopharmacol Biol Psychiatry 1993;17(3):415–21.
56. Allen LS, Hines M, Shryne JE, et al. Two sexually dimorphic cell groups in the human brain. J Neurosci 1989;9(2):497–506.
57. Hofman MA, Swaab DF. The sexually dimorphic nucleus of the preoptic area in the human brain: a comparative morphometric study. J Anat 1989;164:55–72.
58. Senut MC, de Bilbao F, Lamour Y. Age-related loss of galanin-immunoreactive cells in the rat septal area. Neurosci Lett 1989;105(3):257–62.
59. Toescu EC, Xiong J. Metabolic substrates of neuronal aging. Ann N Y Acad Sci 2004;1019:19–23.
60. Thibault O, Landfield PW. Increase in single L-type calcium channels in hippocampal neurons during aging. Science 1996;272(5264):1017–20.

61. Mattson MP. Neuronal life-and-death signaling, apoptosis, and neurodegenerative disorders. Antioxid Redox Signal 2006;8(11–12):1997–2006.
62. Benet LZ, Hoener BA. Changes in plasma protein binding have little clinical relevance. Clin Pharmacol Ther 2002;71(3):115–21.
63. McLean AJ, Le Couteur DG. Aging biology and geriatric clinical pharmacology. Pharmacol Rev 2004;56(2):163–84.
64. Schmucker DL. Liver function and phase I drug metabolism in the elderly: a paradox. Drugs Aging 2001;18(11):837–51.
65. Matteo RS, Schwartz AE, Ornstein E, et al. Pharmacokinetics of sufentanil in the elderly surgical patient. Can J Anaesth 1990;37(8):852–6.
66. Hughes MA, Glass PS, Jacobs JR. Context-sensitive half-time in multicompartment pharmacokinetic models for intravenous anesthetic drugs. Anesthesiology 1992;76(3):334–41.
67. Schraag S, Mohl U, Hirsch M, et al. Recovery from opioid anesthesia: the clinical implication of context-sensitive half-times. Anesth Analg 1998;86(1):184–90.
68. Scott JC, Stanski DR. Decreased fentanyl and alfentanil dose requirements with age. A simultaneous pharmacokinetic and pharmacodynamic evaluation. J Pharmacol Exp Ther 1987;240(1):159–66.
69. Feely J, Coakley D. Altered pharmacodynamics in the elderly. Clin Geriatr Med 1990;6(2):269–83.
70. Turnheim K. When drug therapy gets old: pharmacokinetics and pharmacodynamics in the elderly. Exp Gerontol 2003;38(8):843–53.
71. Bailey JM. Technique for quantifying the duration of intravenous anesthetic effect. Anesthesiology 1995;83(5):1095–103.
72. Schnider TW, Minto CF, Shafer SL, et al. The influence of age on propofol pharmacodynamics. Anesthesiology 1999;90(6):1502–16.
73. Kreuer S, Schreiber JU, Bruhn J, et al. Impact of patient age on propofol consumption during propofol-remifentanil anaesthesia. Eur J Anaesthesiol 2005;22(2):123–8.
74. Bailey JM. Context-sensitive half-times: what are they and how valuable are they in anaesthesiology? Clin Pharmacokinet 2002;41(11):793–9.
75. Bailey JM. Context-sensitive half-times and other decrement times of inhaled anesthetics. Anesth Analg 1997;85(3):681–6.
76. Matsuura T, Oda Y, Tanaka K, et al. Advance of age decreases the minimum alveolar concentrations of isoflurane and sevoflurane for maintaining bispectral index below 50. Br J Anaesth 2009;102(3):331–5.
77. Eger EI 2nd. Age, minimum alveolar anesthetic concentration, and minimum alveolar anesthetic concentration-awake. Anesth Analg 2001;93(4):947–53.
78. Barber P, Darby D, Desmond P, et al. Identification of major ischemic change: diffusion-weighted imaging versus computed tomography. Stroke 1999;30:2059–65.
79. Fiebach JB, Schellinger PD, Jansen O, et al. CT and diffusion-weighted MR imaging in randomized order: diffusion-weighted imaging results in higher accuracy and lower interrater variability in the diagnosis of hyperacute ischemic stroke. Stroke 2002;33(9):2206–10.
80. Lansberg MG, Thijs VN, O'Brien MW, et al. Evolution of apparent diffusion coefficient, diffusion-weighted, and T2-weighted signal intensity of acute stroke. AJNR Am J Neuroradiol 2001;22(4):637–44.
81. Brenner RP. EEG in encephalopathy and coma. Am J Electroneurodiagn Technol 2003;43(3):164–84.
82. Kaplan PW. The EEG in metabolic encephalopathy and coma. J Clin Neurophysiol 2004;21(5):307–18.

83. Chatrian G-E. Coma, other states of altered responsiveness, and brain death. In: Daly DD, Pedley TA, editors. Current practice of clinical electroencephalography. 2nd edition. New York: Raven Press; 1990. p. 425–87.
84. Goudswaard AN, Stolk RP, Zuithoff P, et al. Patient characteristics do not predict poor glycaemic control in type 2 diabetes patients treated in primary care. Eur J Epidemiol 2004;19(6):541–5.
85. Hennis A, Corbin D, Fraser H. Focal seizures and non-ketotic hyperglycaemia. J Neurol Neurosurg Psychiatr 1992;55(3):195–7.
86. Maccario M, Messis CP, Vastola EF. Focal seizures as a manifestation of hyperglycemia without ketoacidosis. A report of seven cases with review of the literature. Neurology 1965;15:195–206.
87. Duckworth W, Abraira C, Moritz T, et al. Glucose control and vascular complications in veterans with type 2 diabetes. N Engl J Med 2009;360(2):129–39.
88. Psaty BM, Smith NL, Siscovick DS, et al. Health outcomes associated with antihypertensive therapies used as first-line agents. A systematic review and meta-analysis. JAMA 1997;277(9):739–45.
89. Beckett NS, Peters R, Fletcher AE, et al. Treatment of hypertension in patients 80 years of age or older. N Engl J Med 2008;358(18):1887–98.
90. Blumenstein M, Romaszko J, Calderon A, et al. Antihypertensive efficacy and tolerability of aliskiren/hydrochlorothiazide (HCT) single-pill combinations in patients who are non-responsive to HCT 25 mg alone. Curr Med Res Opin 2009;25(4):903–10.
91. Kaneshiro Y, Ichihara A, Sakoda M, et al. Add-on benefits of amlodipine and thiazide in nondiabetic chronic kidney disease stage 1/2 patients treated with valsartan. Kidney Blood Press Res 2009;32(1):51–8.

# Postoperative Delirium in the Elderly Surgical Patient

Frederick E. Sieber, MD[a,b,*]

**KEYWORDS**

- Delirium • Elderly • Aged cognition disorders
- Postoperative complications/diagnosis

## CASE PRESENTATION

A 72-year-old white woman presents to the emergency room with a right femoral neck fracture. The patient is American Society of Anesthesiologists physical status 3 with a history of hypertension, atrial fibrillation, severe chronic obstructive pulmonary disease (COPD) requiring home $O_2$, a stroke 10 years previously with residual mild left hemiparesis, and an anxiety disorder. Preoperative laboratory values include: white blood cell count $8950 \times 10^3/\mu L$; hematocrit 39.2; blood urea nitrogen 16 mg/dL; creatinine 0.8 mg/dL; sodium 141 mEq/L; potassium 4.4 mEq/L; and normal coagulation studies. Preoperative medications include: cardizem 120 mg daily, coumadin 2.5 mg daily, digoxin 0.125 mg daily, albuterol, and diazepam 5 mg twice daily. Before hip fracture the patient was living alone and functioning independently.

The patient underwent a bipolar hip replacement under spinal anesthesia with propofol sedation. Postoperatively the patient was admitted to the intensive care unit (ICU) secondary to her underlying pulmonary comorbidities. The patient was brought to the ICU awake and alert with an initial Patient At Risk score of 10. While in the ICU the patient resumed her previous medications, including diazepam. On the first night in the ICU, she suffered a bradycardic respiratory arrest following administration of hydromorphone for pain. This complication required intubation and short-term ventilator management. By the second postoperative day the patient was extubated and transferred to the floor. Over the next several days the patient developed a left lower lobe pneumonia, which was treated with antibiotics.

[a] Department of Anesthesiology, Johns Hopkins Bayview Medical Center, Johns Hopkins Medical Institutions, 4940 Eastern Avenue, A588, Baltimore, MD 21224, USA
[b] Anesthesiology and Critical Care Medicine, Johns Hopkins University School of Medicine, Baltimore, MD, USA
* Department of Anesthesiology, Johns Hopkins Bayview Medical Center, Johns Hopkins Medical Institutions, 4940 Eastern Avenue, A588, Baltimore, MD 21224.
*E-mail address:* fsieber1@jhmi.edu

Anesthesiology Clin 27 (2009) 451–464
doi:10.1016/j.anclin.2009.07.009
**anesthesiology.theclinics.com**

In addition to these complications, the patient sustained an episode of delirium beginning in the ICU and lasting for a total of 5 days. While intubated and ventilated, features of altered consciousness, inattention, and disorganized thinking were observed when a Confusion Assessment Method (CAM-ICU) evaluation for delirium was performed. Following extubation, in both the ICU and on the surgical floor, a positive CAM score was given during formal delirium testing because of fluctuations in mental status, inattention, and disorientation. The patient's altered mental status was slow to clear, interfering with her rehabilitation and leading to a prolonged hospital stay. Discharge to a rehabilitation facility occurred on postoperative day 14. At 30 days postoperatively, the patient was discharged home from the rehabilitation facility.

At 50 days postoperatively the patient was readmitted for an exacerbation of her COPD. At that time her chest radiograph was clear. On admission, the patient was delirious and judged incompetent to make her own medical decisions. After discussion with the family, the patient was made DNR/DNI (do not resuscitate/do not intubate). Intubation was deferred, and her respiratory failure was treated with bilevel positive airway pressure. She was discharged home 4 days later and died on the 64th postoperative day.

## INTRODUCTION

This issue deals with one of the common complications seen postoperatively in the elderly, delirium. The discussion is not meant to provide a comprehensive treatise on delirium management. Instead, the focus is on relevant issues in Anesthesia practice. Toward this end clinical aspects of management, directly under the control of the anesthesiologist, as determined by the case presentation, have been emphasized. This specific case presentation illustrates several points pertinent to clinical presentation and management of postoperative delirium in the elderly surgical patient.

## EPIDEMIOLOGY

Delirium is a common complication following surgery in the geriatric population. The incidence of postoperative delirium varies depending on the type of surgery (**Table 1**)[1] The reported incidence of delirium following cardiac surgery ranges from 13.5% to 21%.[2,3] In noncardiac procedures, surgery specific risk as defined by the American Heart Association[4] and risk of delirium generally mirror each other. Overall, the incidence of postoperative delirium is estimated at 10% in elderly patients following major elective noncardiac surgery.[5] Postoperative delirium usually presents around 24 hours

**Table 1**
**Surgical procedure and incidence of postoperative delirium**

| Surgical Procedure | Incidence of Postoperative Delirium (%) | References |
|---|---|---|
| Lung transplant | 73 | 1 |
| Cardiac | 13.5–21 | 2,3 |
| Urologic | 5.7 | 1 |
| Laparoscopic general surgery >4 h | 2 | 72 |
| Open general surgery | 17 | 73 |
| Elective abdominal aortic aneurysm | 33 | 74 |
| Elective hip replacement | 7.3–14.7 | 6,35,75 |
| Elective knee replacement | 11 | 76 |

postoperatively and resolves in most patients within 48 hours.[6] However, postoperative delirium may be persistent, with episodes lasting months.

Delirium incidence following orthopedic procedures is dependent on urgency of the procedure and underlying frailty of the patient population. With elective joint replacement, postoperative delirium does not seem to be a significant issue. Even though the incidence of postoperative delirium has been reported in the range of 3.6% to 28%,[7] the length of the episodes is usually only 1 day and does not seem to be a major postoperative problem.[8] On the other hand, semiurgent hip fracture repair in high-risk patients is associated with a 35% average incidence of postoperative delirium.[9] Delirium following hip fracture repair often can endure beyond the period of hospitalization. For instance, in hip fracture patients persistent delirium can be detected in 39%, 33%, and 6% of patients at hospital discharge, 1 month postoperatively, and 6 months postoperatively, respectively.[10]

Comment: The case presentation represents a patient at high risk for postoperative delirium as she is frail, undergoing a semiurgent orthopedic procedure, and has significant comorbidities. The delirium episode suffered by the patient was persistent in nature as it was slow to clear during initial hospitalization, and recurred with the second hospitalization.

## FINANCIAL IMPLICATIONS

Postoperative delirium is independently associated with an increased risk of remaining in the hospital, an increased risk of early and long-term mortality, increased physical dependence, and an increased rate of discharge to a nursing home.[11,12] Persistent delirium is associated with even poorer outcomes in terms of decline in activities of daily living, new nursing home placement, or death.[10]

Incident, but not prevalent, delirium is an important predictor of longer hospital stay and increased costs.[13] Overall, 2 to 3 million elderly patients per year sustain delirium during their hospital stay, involving more than 17.5 million inpatient days and accounting for over $4 billion in Medicare expenditure.[14] Milbrandt and colleagues[15] determined that delirium in mechanically ventilated medical ICU patients is associated with an incremental ICU cost of about $9000 per patient. Milbrandt and colleagues[15] project that the yearly costs associated with delirium in the medical ICU patient to be $6.5 to $20.4 billion. Others have estimated that the national burden of delirium on the health care system ranges from $38 billion to $152 billion each year.[16] Whether these estimates apply to surgical ICU patients is yet to be determined. In a study cohort of 500 elective surgical patients at the Cleveland Clinic, the incidence of postoperative delirium was 11.4%, and average costs per patient were increased by $908, $1400, and $400 for nursing, technical services, and professional consultative fees, respectively. This expense accounted for a greater than $2500 cost increase per surgical patient sustaining delirium.[17]

Comment: The postoperative complications that occurred in the case presented (delirium, pneumonia, respiratory arrest) were associated prolonged hospital stay, hospital readmission, and eventual death.

## DIAGNOSIS

Delirium is a syndrome characterized by acute onset of variable and fluctuating changes in level of consciousness accompanied by a range of other mental symptoms. By convention, the presence or absence of delirium is based on application of diagnostic criteria articulated in the fourth edition of the Diagnostic and Statistical Manual of Mental Disorders (DSM-IV), "The essential feature of delirium is a disturbance in consciousness that is accompanied by a change in cognition that cannot be better accounted for by a preexisting or evolving dementia" (**Box 1**).[18]

The diagnosis of delirium is challenging because it has variable presentations that include disturbance in one or more of the following domains: orientation, thought process, perception, memory, mood, and behavior with or without hyperactivity. Nevertheless, recent advances in clinical measurement have concluded that delirium can be diagnosed, and its severity quantified, with a high degree of reliability and validity using structured instruments applied by well-trained examiners.[19,20] There are advantages and disadvantages for each delirium instrument. In reviewing the orthopedic literature, the most widely used diagnostic assessment methods for delirium are the CAM, Mini-Mental State Examination (MMSE), and Organic Brain Syndrome Scale.[9]

The CAM[21] is a bedside rating scale developed to assist nonpsychiatrically trained clinicians in the rapid and accurate diagnosis of delirium in both clinical and research settings. The CAM follows DSM-III-R criteria for delirium but can be easily adapted to approximate DSM-IV criteria, which are similar. CAM is designed to be administered by any clinician, including physicians or nurses, and may also be administered by trained lay interviewers. Data suggest that geriatricians, nurses, and trained lay interviewers perform as well as psychiatrists in rating the CAM.[20] Interrater reliability of the CAM is high, with $\kappa = 1$ for diagnosis of presence or absence of delirium. The convergent validity of the CAM against other measures is also high: $\kappa = 0.64$ for the MMSE, $\kappa = 0.59$ for the story completion task, $\kappa = 0.82$ for the Visual Analog Scale for Confusion, and $\kappa = 0.66$ for the digit span test. The sensitivity of the CAM against the gold standard of psychiatric diagnosis is 94% to 100%, and specificity 90% to 95%.[21] The CAM has been adapted for use in ventilated ICU patients in the form of the CAM-ICU. The CAM-ICU has a demonstrated sensitivity of 93% to 100%, and high interrater reliability ($\kappa = 0.96$) in the detection of delirium.[22]

Delirium is commonly superimposed on a preexisting dementia. Several clinical features help to distinguish dementia from delirium (**Table 2**). Despite this challenge, the distinction of delirium from dementia, or the recognition of delirium in patients with preexisting dementia can usually be made because delirium symptoms tend to dominate the clinical picture.[23] However, evaluation of delirium in the context of underlying dementia may require use of several instruments in addition to the CAM. To assist in diagnostic accuracy, the MMSE may be used as a screening and diagnostic scale for cognitive impairment.[24] To assess attention, the MMSE's immediate repetition of three objects and a backward-spelled word ("d-l-r-o-w") items can be very useful.

**Box 1**
**DSM-IV diagnostic criteria for 293.0 delirium**

A. Disturbance of consciousness (ie, reduced clarity of awareness of the environment) with reduced ability to focus, sustain, or shift attention

B. A change in cognition (such as memory deficit, disorientation, language disturbance) or the development of a perceptual disturbance that is not better accounted for by a preexisting, established, or evolving dementia

C. The disturbance develops over a short period of time (usually hours to days) and tends to fluctuate during the course of the day

D. There is evidence from the history, physical examination, or laboratory findings that the disturbance is caused by the direct physiologic consequences of a general medical condition

*Reprinted with permission from* the Diagnostic and Statistical Manual of Mental Disorders, Text Revision, Fourth Edition, (Copyright 2000). American Psychiatric Association.

**Table 2**
**Distinguishing delirium from dementia**

| | Delirium | Dementia |
|---|---|---|
| Onset | Acute or subacute | Insidious |
| Course | Fluctuating, usually revolves over days to weeks | Progressive |
| Conscious level | Often impaired, can fluctuate rapidly | Clear until later stages |
| Cognitive defects | Poor short-term memory, poor attention span | Poor short-term memory, attention less affected until severe |
| Hallucinations | Common, especially visual | Often absent |
| Delusions | Fleeting, nonsystematized | Often absent |
| Psychomotor activity | Increased, reduced, or unpredictable | Can be normal |

*Data from* Brown TM, Boyle MF. Delirium. BMJ 2002;325:644–7.
*Data from* Ref.[77]

Digit span is another formal, widely used screening tool that is an assessment of working memory and attention. Corroboration can be sought in the digit span test, in which inability to repeat at least five numbers forward without errors indicates inattention.[25]

The CAM is not designed to measure symptom severity. Several methods have been developed to quantify delirium severity and to monitor its course.[20] The most widely used is the Delirium Rating Scale, revised (DRS-R-98).[26] The DRS-R-98 includes 13 symptom items as a severity scale and three diagnostic items, and is used as an adjunct to the DSM-IV criterion for delirium. The interrater reliability and internal consistency of DRS-R-98 is high (intraclass correlation coefficient of 0.98–0.99, Cronbach a coefficient of 0.87–0.90).[26]

Comment: In the case presentation, CAM and CAM-ICU were the instruments used to diagnose delirium.

## MECHANISM

Delirium may occur through a variety of potential pathophysiologic mechanisms,[27] and different mechanisms apply in different situations. Although the mechanism of delirium is not yet fully understood, the current basic science hypothesis is that delirium is produced by some combination of increased dopaminergic activity, decreased cholinergic activity, and decreased γ-aminobutyric acid (GABA)-ergic activity.[28] Because cholinergic[29] and GABAergic[30] tone decrease with aging, it is no surprise that aging is accompanied by an increased incidence of delirium. Although dopaminergic activity also declines with age, as indicated by the increased incidence of parkinsonism, patients with Parkinson's disease also take medications that increase dopaminergic activity in a manner that could increase the likelihood of delirium. One model of delirium[28] recognizes how increased dopaminergic tone, decreased cholinergic tone, and decreased GABAergic tone can lead to a considerable decrease in the inhibitory GABAergic input from the basal ganglia to the thalamus. Because the thalamus is the gateway for sensory input and also seems to mediate interaction between distinct regions of the neocortex, failure to modulate its activity could lead to the altered sensorium and confusion generally associated with delirium.

The current clinical hypothesis is that the onset of delirium involves an interaction between predisposing and precipitating risk factors for delirium.[31] The following paragraph summarizes current thinking in geriatrics concerning risk factors of delirium and their interplay in causing postoperative delirium. It is paraphrased from an article by Dr. Edward Marcantonio in the Annals of Long-Term Care.[32]

> *Delirium epitomizes an atypical presentation of disease[33] in which acute illness is manifested in the most vulnerable organ system or "the weakest link"—in this case, the brain. This theory holds that the normal aging process can be characterized as "homeostenosis," the progressive constriction of each organ system's ability to respond to stress. In addition, the aging brain is more likely to be affected by diseases and drugs that cloud the sensorium. The sum of these effects leads some elderly to be teetering on the brink of neurodysfunction. Add any precipitating factor for delirium or small stressor, and these individuals develop acute worsening of their mental status. Healthier elderly can also become delirious, but they would have to be sicker.*

This concept has been validated empirically in medical patients by Inouye and Charpentier,[34] who developed a risk model for delirium that demonstrated that the greater the number of preexisting vulnerability factors, the less acute are the stressors required to invoke delirium. The important preexisting vulnerability factors defined in the medical model of delirium are visual impairment, severe illness, cognitive impairment, and dehydration. Kalisvaart and colleagues[35] attempted to validate the medical risk factor model of delirium in elderly hip surgery patients. This study demonstrated the usefulness of the medical risk factor model in predicting postoperative delirium in surgery patients, and supports the concept that when more preexisting vulnerability factors are present, there is a higher risk for postoperative delirium.

Comment: In the case presentation, the two preexisting vulnerability risk factors identified from the medical model of delirium were dehydration (elevated blood urea nitrogen/creatinine) and severe medical illness (COPD). The occurrence of important precipitating events, such as respiratory arrest and development of pneumonia, led to the onset of delirium in this frail individual.

## TREATMENT ISSUES

The mainstay of delirium management is prevention. The approach involves control or elimination of modifiable risk factors. Many of these risk factors are under the control of the health care provider, both nurses and physicians. For the purposes of this discussion, the focus will be on those factors that are directly under the control of the anesthesiologist. For one, abnormal laboratory values (especially electrolytes and glucose)[36] and hemoglobin values less than 10 g%[37] have been associated with postoperative delirium.

Pain at rest is associated with postoperative delirium.[38] However, management of postoperative pain in the elderly can be complicated for several reasons. There seems to be an age-related increase in pain threshold[39] as well as a tendency for elders to underreport pain. Cognitive impairment can make pain assessment and treatment difficult. Side effects from medications, particularly the opioids, are more likely to occur in older patients. Given the above, a multimodal approach to pain management using nonsteroidal anti-inflammatory agents or other nonopioids allows lower doses of drugs to be used, thus helping to reduce potential side effects.[40] For pharmacologic guidance in multimodal therapy, the reader is referred to the three-step conceptual model developed by the World Health Organization.[41] When narcotics are used for pain management, there is no difference in cognitive outcome when comparing fentanyl, morphine, and hydromorphone.[42] Meperidine is the only narcotic that has been definitively associated with delirium.[43] When intravenous and epidural administration of narcotics is compared, there is no difference in cognitive outcome.[42] However, studies suggest that patients who receive oral opioids as their sole means of postoperative pain control are at less risk of developing delirium than those receiving intravenous patient-controlled analgesia.[44]

The patient's medication profile should be carefully assessed for any drugs that have been associated with delirium in the elderly. Among drugs commonly used in anesthetic practice, sevoflurane[45] and benzodiazepines[43] have been implicated in the development of delirium. Several reviews contain extensive lists of drugs known to provoke delirium.[46,47] Of note, the general consensus is that medications with anticholinergic effects should be avoided.[48] Simplification of the medication regimen is important to decrease polypharmacy as multiple drug interactions can compound central nervous system effects. The Beers criteria for potentially inappropriate medications in the elderly are a helpful guide in determining which medications to avoid or eliminate.[49]

The role of sedative and analgesic medications as iatrogenic risk factors for delirium has been described in ICU patients.[50] The use of opioids is strongly related to the development of ICU delirium.[51] Lorazepam has been shown to be an independent risk factor for the transitioning of ICU patients into delirium.[52] Based on the high incidence of delirium in sedated ICU patients, the Society of Critical Care Medicine's guidelines recommend that when managing ventilated patients with sedatives, ICU teams set clinically appropriate target sedation levels using a well-validated sedation scale, and periodically assess patient mental status.[53]

Dexmedetomidine may be the drug of choice for long-term sedation in the ICU, as several studies demonstrate that its use leads to a decreased incidence of ICU delirium as well as ventilator days.[54,55] Despite evidenced-based information concerning appropriate drug use for ICU sedation, at present it is unclear whether there is an optimal anesthetic agent for intraoperative use that leads to less postoperative delirium.

Despite the many possible approaches to delirium prevention, only two randomized trials have demonstrated that any intervention is useful in delirium prevention.[56] One proven intervention involves the use of structured clinical protocols to assist in preventing episodes of delirium. Specialist delirium units that focus on assessing for delirium risk factors with targeted risk factor modification may represent a best practice model.[57] As an alternative to the delirium unit, a combined geriatric-orthopedic approach using proactive geriatric consultation was found to decrease delirium incidence in hip fracture patients by more than one-third.[58]

Another area of delirium prevention focuses on prophylactic administration of drugs used in managing delirium. Drug studies using this strategy have concentrated on patients undergoing orthopedic procedures.[59] Low-dose haloperidol (1.5 mg/day) given prophylactically to elderly hip surgery patients does not reduce the incidence of postoperative delirium, but does decrease the severity and duration of the delirium episodes.[60] Donazepil, when given prophylactically, does not decrease delirium incidence in elderly patients undergoing total joint replacement.[8,61] Several trials are currently underway to determine whether prophylactic administration of the atypical antipsychotics is useful in preventing postoperative delirium.

Comment: Attention to any possible drug interactions is important before administration of any medications. In the case presentation, the combined respiratory depressant effects of benzodiazepines and opioids caused a respiratory arrest in a patient with severe COPD. Multimodal pain therapy may have been a better option given the underlying comorbidities. In patients at high risk for respiratory failure, postoperative regional techniques or nonopioid analgesics should be considered.

## ROLE OF ANESTHESIA

Recent reviews have examined whether general or regional anesthesia is associated with a greater risk of postoperative delirium.[62] Most studies examining **elective** surgery suggest no difference in postoperative delirium when regional and general anesthesia are compared. Yet there are data following total hip replacement in elderly patients suggesting that persistent mental status changes are greater after general than after epidural anesthesia (7/31 vs 0/29, respectively, $P<.01$).[63] In contrast to elective procedures, evidence suggests that type of anesthesia influences delirium with the **urgent** surgery of hip fracture repair. A Cochrane review compared outcome differences in hip fracture patients who received regional and general anesthesia.[64] Based on 5 randomized controlled trials meeting the inclusion criteria, the number of patients who experienced postoperative confusional state was 11 of 117 (9.4%) in the regional anesthesia group and 23 of 120 (19.2%) in the general anesthesia group (risk ratio 0.50, 95% confidence interval 0.26–0.95; overall effect $z = 2.12$, $P = .03$). The investigators conclude that with hip fracture surgery, regional anesthesia, compared with general anesthesia, is associated with a 2-fold reduced risk of acute postoperative confusion.

Much of the controversy surrounding the issue of postoperative delirium in regional versus general anesthesia can be attributed to issues with study design. The important study design problems that have been identified are: sedation during regional anesthesia in many of the previous studies was uncontrolled; postoperative pain management was uncontrolled; and patients at highest risk for postoperative delirium were excluded. **Table 3** outlines some of the methodological flaws of the important studies to date.

Control of the level of sedation is extremely important in any study looking at regional versus general differences. Sedative medications are iatrogenic risk factors for delirium.[50] More important, evidence suggests that in routine anesthesia practice, sedation levels consistent with general anesthesia commonly occur. Thus, if sedation is not controlled, the anesthetic level seen by the brain may be similar regardless of

**Table 3**
**Design flaws in studies that examined incidence of delirium in regional versus general anesthesia**

| Study | Sedation During Regional Anesthesia Controlled (Yes or No) | Postoperative Pain Management Controlled (Yes or No) | Patients with Dementia Included? (Yes or No) |
|---|---|---|---|
| Williams-Russo et al[76] | No | No | No |
| Chung et al, 1987[69] | No[a] | Yes (meperidine used) | No |
| Chung et al, 1989[70] | No | Yes (meperidine used) | No |
| Berggren et al[78] | Yes (meperidine premedication) | No comment | No |
| Crul et al[79] | Yes (atropine, nicomorphine, droperidol premedication) | No comment | No |
| Campbell et al[80] | Yes (no sedation) | No | No |
| Bigler et al[81] | No | No comment | No |
| Cook et al[82] | No | No comment | No |

[a] Attempted verbal reassurance only; anxiety treated with droperidol and fentanyl.

regional or general anesthesia. This similarity would tend to negate any possible differences in cognitive outcome between the 2 anesthetic techniques. For instance, closed claims analysis suggests that excessive sedation is an important predisposing factor for cardiac arrest during spinal anesthesia.[65] In closed claims analysis of monitored anesthetic care, excessive sedation leading to respiratory depression has been identified as an important mechanism of patient injury.[66] Recent studies examining the level of sedation during surgical procedures requiring light to moderate sedation demonstrate that 24.5% of the time patients' level of sedation is consistent with general anesthesia by clinical assessment.[67] Only one study in **Table 3**, by Campbell and colleagues, properly controlled sedation in the local/regional group. This study involved cataract surgery whereby the local anesthesia group received no sedation. However, the study is underpowered to make any conclusions about anesthetic effects. Current studies report a 4% delirium incidence following cataract surgery,[68] and power analysis shows that greater than 500 cataract patients would be required to show a difference in regional versus general groups (n = 169 for the study by Campbell and colleagues). The other studies that attempted to control sedation in the regional group premedicated patients with drugs known to be associated with delirium.[47]

The importance of controlling intraoperative sedation is emphasized by the two studies by Chung and colleagues in **Table 3**. In 1987, Chung and colleagues compared 44 elderly patients randomized to either spinal or general anesthesia.[69] In the spinal anesthesia group the goal was for intraoperative sedation to consist primarily of verbal reassurance by the anesthetist. Out of 20 patients in the spinal anesthesia group, 15 required no sedation and 5 required administration of fentanyl (mean dose = 80 μg) and droperidol (mean dose = 0.9 mg). Using this paradigm, there was a 12.5% incidence of postoperative delirium by day three in the general anesthesia group versus 0% in the spinal anesthesia group. In 1989, Chung and colleagues randomized 44 elderly patients to receive spinal anesthesia with sedation or general anesthesia.[70] However, the type and level of sedation was not controlled. There was no difference in postoperative delirium between the general and spinal anesthetic groups. These two studies suggest collectively that minimal sedation during regional anesthesia may have less of an effect on incidence of postoperative delirium than general anesthesia or uncontrolled sedation during regional anesthesia.

Control of postoperative pain is important in any study looking at regional versus general differences. Evidence suggests that in patients undergoing noncardiac surgery, higher pain scores at rest during the first three postoperative days are associated with postoperative delirium.[38] In fact, increased levels of both preoperative and postoperative pain are risk factors for development of postoperative delirium.[44] In the hip fracture population, Morrison and colleagues[71] found that cognitively intact individuals with poorly controlled pain were nine times more likely to become delirious. In **Table 3**, the two studies that controlled postoperative pain management used drugs that have a known association with delirium.[43]

Including patients with preexisting vulnerability factors and at high risk for postoperative delirium is important in any study looking at regional versus general differences. This patient population is precisely that in which therapeutic interventions could have the greatest effect! No study in **Table 3** systematically included and studied patients with the important vulnerability risk factors of visual impairment, severe illness, cognitive impairment, and dehydration.[34] In particular, high-risk patients such as those with dementia were excluded.

Comment: Type of anesthesia did not precipitate the episode of delirium in the case presentation. The patient received spinal anesthesia. Evidence suggests that this type of anesthetic in hip fracture repair is associated with a decreased incidence of postoperative delirium. On the other hand, the means of pain management played a key role in the patient's postoperative course. Administration of narcotics in the setting of severe underlying COPD precipitated a respiratory arrest and a host of other ensuing complications. Whereas the goal of obtaining adequate postoperative pain relief is laudable, the means by which this is obtained must take into account underlying comorbidities.

## REFERENCES

1. Dyer CB, Ashton CM, Teasdale TA. Postoperative delirium. A review of 80 primary data-collection studies. Arch Intern Med 1995;155:461–5.
2. van der Mast RC, van den Broek WW, Fekkes D, et al. Incidence of and preoperative predictors for delirium after cardiac surgery. J Psychosom Res 1999;46:479–83.
3. Koster S, Oosterveld FG, Hensens AG, et al. Delirium after cardiac surgery and predictive validity of a risk checklist. Ann Thorac Surg 2008;86:1883–7.
4. Eagle KA, Berger PB, Calkins H, et al. ACC/AHA guideline update for perioperative cardiovascular evaluation for noncardiac surgery—executive summary. A report of the American College of Cardiology/American heart association task force on practice guidelines (committee to update the 1996 guidelines on perioperative cardiovascular evaluation for noncardiac surgery). Anesth Analg 2002;94:1052–64.
5. Rasmussen LS, Jt M. Central nervous system dysfunction after anesthesia in the geriatric patient. Anesthesiol Clin North America 2000;18:59–70.
6. Duppils GS, Wikblad K. Acute confusional states in patients undergoing hip surgery, a prospective observation study. Gerontology 2000;46:36–43.
7. Bruce AJ, Ritchie CW, Blizard R, et al. The incidence of delirium associated with orthopedic surgery: a meta-analytic review. Int Psychogeriatr 2007;19:197–214.
8. Liptzin B, Laki A, Garb JL, et al. Donepezil in the prevention and treatment of post-surgical delirium. Am J Geriatr Psychiatry 2005;13:1100–6.
9. Bitsch M, Foss N, Kristensen B, et al. Pathogenesis of and management strategies for postoperative delirium after hip fracture: a review. Acta Orthop Scand 2004;75:378–89.
10. Marcantonio ER, Flacker JM, Michaels M, et al. Delirium is independently associated with poor functional recovery after hip fracture. J Am Geriatr Soc 2000;48:618–24.
11. Holmes J, House A. Psychiatric illness predicts poor outcome after surgery for hip fracture: a prospective cohort study. Psychol Med 2000;30:921–9.
12. Nightingale S, Holmes J, Mason J, et al. Psychiatric illness and mortality after hip fracture. Lancet 2001;357:1264–5.
13. McCusker J, Cole MG, Dendukuri N, et al. Does delirium increase hospital stay? J Am Geriatr Soc 2003;51:1539–46.
14. Pandharipande P, Jackson J, Ely EW. Delirium: acute cognitive dysfunction in the critically ill. Curr Opin Crit Care 2005;11:360–8.
15. Milbrandt EB, Deppen S, Harrison PL, et al. Costs associated with delirium in mechanically ventilated patients. Crit Care Med 2004;32:955–62.
16. Leslie DL, Marcantonio ER, Zhang Y, et al. One-year health care costs associated with delirium in the elderly population. Arch Intern Med 2008;168:27–32.
17. Franco K, Litaker D, Locala J, et al. The cost of delirium in the surgical patient. Psychosomatics 2001;42:68–73.

18. Diagnostic and statistical manual of mental disorders, fourth edition text revision (DSM-IV-TR). 4th edition. Washington, DC: American Psychiatric Publishing, Inc.; 2000.
19. Lyketsos CG, Steinberg M. Behavioral measures for cognitive disorders. In: Rush AJ, First MB, Blacker D, editors. Handbook of psychiatric measures. Washington, DC: American Psychiatric Association; 2000. p. 393–416.
20. Steinberg M, Lyketsos CG. Measures for the non-cognitive neuropsychiatric symptoms of the cognitive disorders. In: Rush AJ, First MB, Blacker D, editors. Handbook of psychiatric measures. 2nd edition. Washington, DC: American Psychiatric Association; 2007.
21. Inouye SK, van Dyck CH, Alessi CA, et al. Clarifying confusion: the confusion assessment method. A new method for detection of delirium. Ann Intern Med 1990;113:941–8.
22. Ely EW, Inouye SK, Bernard GR, et al. Delirium in mechanically ventilated patients: validity and reliability of the confusion assessment method for the intensive care unit (CAM-ICU). JAMA 2001;286:2703–10.
23. Trzepacz PT, Mulsant BH, Amanda Dew M, et al. Is delirium different when it occurs in dementia? A study using the delirium rating scale. J Neuropsychiatry Clin Neurosci 1998;10:199–204.
24. Folstein MFFS, McHugh PR. "Mini-mental state". A practical method for grading the cognitive state of patients for the clinician. J Psychiatr Res 1975;12:189–98.
25. Pompei P, Foreman M, Cassel CK, et al. Detecting delirium among hospitalized older patients. Arch Intern Med 1995;155:301–7.
26. Trzepacz PT, Mittal D, Torres R, et al. Validation of the delirium rating scale-revised-98: comparison with the delirium rating scale and the cognitive test for delirium. J Neuropsychiatry Clin Neurosci 2001;13:229–42.
27. Flacker JM, La L. Neural mechanisms of delirium: current hypotheses and evolving concepts. J Gerontol A Biol Sci Med Sci 1999;54:B239–46.
28. Gaudreau JD, Gagnon P. Psychotogenic drugs and delirium pathogenesis: the central role of the thalamus. Med Hypotheses 2005;64:471–5.
29. White P, Hiley CR, Goodhardt MJ, et al. Neocortical cholinergic neurons in elderly people. Lancet 1977;1:668–71.
30. Leventhal AG, Wang Y, Pu M, et al. GABA and its agonists improved visual cortical function in senescent monkeys. Science 2003;300:812–5.
31. Inouye SK. Delirium in older persons. N Engl J Med 2006;354:1157–65.
32. Marcantonio E.R. Ask the expert question and answer how can a urinary tract infection precipitate delirium in an older patient? 2002;10:56.
33. Resnick NM, Marcantonio ER. How should clinical care of the aged differ? Lancet 1997;350:1157–8.
34. Inouye SK, Charpentier PA. Precipitating factors for delirium in hospitalized elderly persons, predictive model and interrelationship with baseline vulnerability. JAMA 1996;275:852–7.
35. Kalisvaart KJ, Vreeswijk R, de Jonghe JF, et al. Risk factors and prediction of postoperative delirium in elderly hip-surgery patients: implementation and validation of a medical risk factor model. J Am Geriatr Soc 2006;54:817–22.
36. Marcantonio ER, Goldman L, Mangione CM, et al. A clinical prediction rule for delirium after elective noncardiac surgery. JAMA 1994;271:134–9.
37. Marcantonio ER, Goldman L, Orav EJ, et al. The association of intraoperative factors with the development of postoperative delirium. Am J Med 1998;105: 380–4.

38. Lynch EP, Lazor MA, Gellis JE, et al. The impact of postoperative pain on the development of postoperative delirium. Anesth Analg 1998;86:781–5.
39. Gibson SJ, Helme RD. Age-related differences in pain perception and report. Clin Geriatr Med 2001;17:433–56.
40. Aubrun F, Marmion F. The elderly patient and postoperative pain treatment. Best Pract Res Clin Anaesthesiol 2007;21:109–27.
41. Karani R, Meier DE. Systemic pharmacologic postoperative pain management in the geriatric orthopaedic patient. Clin Orthop 2004;26–34.
42. Fong HK, Sands LP, Leung JM. The role of postoperative analgesia in delirium and cognitive decline in elderly patients: a systematic review. Anesth Analg 2006;102:1255–66.
43. Marcantonio ER, Juarez G, Goldman L, et al. The relationship of postoperative delirium with psychoactive medications. JAMA 1994;272:1518–22.
44. Vaurio LE, Sands LP, Wang Y, et al. Postoperative delirium: the importance of pain and pain management. Anesth Analg 2006;102:1267–73.
45. Aono J, Ueda W, Mamiya K, et al. Greater incidence of delirium during recovery from sevoflurane anesthesia in preschool boys. Anesthesiology 1997;87:1298–300.
46. Alagiakrishnan K, Wiens CA. An approach to drug induced delirium in the elderly. Postgrad Med J 2004;80:388–93.
47. Brown T. Drug-induced delirium. Semin Clin Neuropsychiatry 2000;5:113–24.
48. Pratico C, Quattrone D, Lucanto T, et al. Drugs of anesthesia acting on central cholinergic system may cause post-operative cognitive dysfunction and delirium. Med Hypotheses 2005;65:972–82.
49. Fick DM, Cooper JW, Wade WE, et al. Updating the beers criteria for potentially inappropriate medication use in older adults: results of a US consensus panel of experts. Arch Intern Med 2003;163:2716–24.
50. Pandharipande P, Ely EW. Sedative and analgesic medications: risk factors for delirium and sleep disturbances in the critically ill. Crit Care Clin 2006;22:313–27, vii.
51. Dubois MJ, Bergeron N, Dumont M, et al. Delirium in an intensive care unit: a study of risk factors. Intensive Care Med 2001;27:1297–304.
52. Pandharipande P, Shintani A, Peterson J, et al. Lorazepam is an independent risk factor for transitioning to delirium in intensive care unit patients. Anesthesiology 2006;104:21–6.
53. Jacobi J, Fraser GL, Coursin DB, et al. Clinical practice guidelines for the sustained use of sedatives and analgesics in the critically ill adult. Crit Care Med 2002;30:119–41.
54. Pandharipande PP, Pun BT, Herr DL, et al. Effect of sedation with dexmedetomidine vs lorazepam on acute brain dysfunction in mechanically ventilated patients: the MENDS randomized controlled trial. JAMA 2007;298:2644–53.
55. Riker RR, Shehabi Y, Bokesch PM, et al. Dexmedetomidine vs midazolam for sedation of critically ill patients: a randomized trial. JAMA 2009;301:489–99.
56. Siddiqi N, Stockdale R, Britton AM, et al. Interventions for preventing delirium in hospitalised patients. Cochrane Database Syst Rev 2007;(2):CD005563.
57. Inouye SK, Bogardus ST Jr, Charpentier PA, et al. A multicomponent intervention to prevent delirium in hospitalized older patients. N Engl J Med 1999;340:669–76.
58. Marcantonio ER, Flacker JM, Wright RJ, et al. Reducing delirium after hip fracture: a randomized trial. J Am Geriatr Soc 2001;49:516–22.
59. Bourne RS, Tahir TA, Borthwick M, et al. Drug treatment of delirium: past, present and future. J Psychosom Res 2008;65:273–82.

60. Kalisvaart KJ, de Jonghe JF, Bogaards MJ, et al. Haloperidol prophylaxis for elderly hip-surgery patients at risk for delirium: a randomized placebo-controlled study. J Am Geriatr Soc 2005;53:1658–66.
61. Sampson EL, Raven PR, Ndhlovu PN, et al. A randomized, double-blind, placebo-controlled trial of donepezil hydrochloride (Aricept) for reducing the incidence of postoperative delirium after elective total hip replacement. Int J Geriatr Psychiatry 2007;22:343–9.
62. Bryson GL, Wyand A. Evidence-based clinical update: general anesthesia and the risk of delirium and postoperative cognitive dysfunction. Can J Anaesth 2006;53:669–77.
63. Hole A, Terjesen T, Breivik H. Epidural versus general anaesthesia for total hip arthroplasty in elderly patients. Acta Anaesthesiol Scand 1980;24:279–87.
64. Parker MJ, Handoll HH, Griffiths R. Anaesthesia for hip fracture surgery in adults. Cochrane Database Syst Rev. 2004;(4):CD000521.
65. Caplan RA, Ward RJ, Posner K, et al. Unexpected cardiac arrest during spinal anesthesia: a closed claims analysis of predisposing factors. Anesthesiology 1988;68:5–11.
66. Bhananker SM, Posner KL, Cheney FW, et al. Injury and liability associated with monitored anesthesia care: a closed claims analysis. Anesthesiology 2006;104:228–34.
67. Chisholm CJ, Zurica J, Mironov D, et al. Comparison of electrophysiologic monitors with clinical assessment of level of sedation. Mayo Clin Proc 2006;81:46–52.
68. Milstein A, Pollack A, Kleinman G, et al. Confusion/delirium following cataract surgery: an incidence study of 1-year duration. Int Psychogeriatr 2002;14:301–6.
69. Chung F, Meier R, Lautenschlager E, et al. General or spinal anesthesia: which is better in the elderly? Anesthesiology 1987;67:422–7.
70. Chung FF, Chung A, Meier RH, et al. Comparison of perioperative mental function after general anaesthesia and spinal anaesthesia with intravenous sedation. Can J Anaesth 1989;36:382–7.
71. Morrison RS, Magaziner J, Gilbert M, et al. Relationship between pain and opioid analgesics on the development of delirium following hip fracture. J Gerontol A Biol Sci Med Sci 2003;58:76–81.
72. Nishikawa K, Nakayama M, Omote K, et al. Recovery characteristics and postoperative delirium after long-duration laparoscope-assisted surgery in elderly patients: propofol-based vs. sevoflurane-based anesthesia. Acta Anaesthesiol Scand 2004;48:162–8.
73. Kaneko T, Takahashi S, Naka T, et al. Postoperative delirium following gastrointestinal surgery in elderly patients. Surg Today 1997;27:107–11.
74. Benoit AG, Campbell BI, Tanner JR, et al. Risk factors and prevalence of perioperative cognitive dysfunction in abdominal aneurysm patients. J Vasc Surg 2005;42:884–90.
75. Galanakis P, Bickel H, Gradinger R, et al. Acute confusional state in the elderly following hip surgery: incidence, risk factors and complications. Int J Geriatr Psychiatry 2001;16:349–55.
76. Williams-Russo P, Sharrock NE, Mattis S, et al. Cognitive effects after epidural vs general anesthesia in older adults. A randomized trial. JAMA 1995;274:44–50.
77. Brown TM, Boyle MF. Delirium. BMJ 2002;325:644–7.
78. Berggren D, Gustafson Y, Eriksson B, et al. Postoperative confusion after anesthesia in elderly patients with femoral neck fractures. Anesth Analg 1987;66:497–504.

79. Crul BJ, Hulstijn W, Burger IC. Influence of the type of anaesthesia on post-operative subjective physical well-being and mental function in elderly patients. Acta Anaesthesiol Scand 1992;36:615–20.
80. Campbell DN, Lim M, Muir MK, et al. A prospective randomised study of local versus general anaesthesia for cataract surgery. Anaesthesia 1993;48:422–8.
81. Bigler D, Adelhoj B, Petring OU, et al. Mental function and morbidity after acute hip surgery during spinal and general anaesthesia. Anaesthesia 1985;40:672–6.
82. Cook PT, Davies MJ, Cronin KD, et al. A prospective randomised trial comparing spinal anaesthesia using hyperbaric cinchocaine with general anaesthesia for lower limb vascular surgery. Anaesth Intensive Care 1986;14:373–80.

# Postoperative Urinary Retention

Daniela M. Darrah, MD[a], Tomas L. Griebling, MD, MPH[b,c], Jeffrey H. Silverstein, MD[d,e,*]

**KEYWORDS**

- Urinary retention • Postoperative complications
- Postoperative care • Geriatrics • Voiding dysfunction

An 82-year-old male with a history of non–insulin-dependent diabetes and hypertension, both well controlled with medication, is admitted to the post anesthesia care unit (PACU) following a right inguinal herniorrhaphy. The procedure was accomplished under spinal anesthesia using 1.2 mL 0.5% bupivacaine. Blood loss was minimal and he received 1200 mL of balanced salt solution during the procedure. On admission to the PACU he is mildly sedated but arousable and reports no pain. He has some movement in his toes, but his lower extremity is still weak. Within 2 hours of his arrival, the spinal has regressed and he complains of only moderate pain. The facility requires that patients following a herniorrhaphy void before discharge, but the patient cannot urinate. One hour later he still cannot urinate and informs the nurse that he has had some prostate issues in the past.

Should you:
1) perform an in-out catheterization and discharge the patient?
2) discharge the patient with an indwelling catheter?
3) be patient and allow the patient more time to void?
4) perform an ultrasound exam of the bladder?
5) administer a small dose of naloxone?

---

JH Silverstein is partially funded by the National Institute on Aging Grants R01 AG029656 and R01 AG030141.

[a] Department of Anesthesiology, Mount Sinai School of Medicine, 1 Gustave L. Levy Place, Box 1010, New York, NY 10029-6500, USA
[b] Department of Urology, University of Kansas School of Medicine, Mailstop 301, 3901 Rainbow Boulevard, Kansas City, KS 66160, USA
[c] The Landon Center on Aging, University of Kansas School of Medicine, Mailstop 301, 3901 Rainbow Boulevard, Kansas City, KS 66160, USA
[d] Departments of Anesthesiology, Surgery, and Geriatrics and Adult Development, Mount Sinai School of Medicine, 1 Gustave L. Levy Place, Box 1010, New York, NY 10029-6574, USA
[e] Program for the Protection of Human Subjects, Mount Sinai School of Medicine, Box 1010, 1 Gustave L. Levy Place, New York, NY 10029-6574, USA
* Corresponding author.
*E-mail address:* jeff.silverstein@mssm.edu (J.H. Silverstein).

Anesthesiology Clin 27 (2009) 465–484
doi:10.1016/j.anclin.2009.07.010
anesthesiology.theclinics.com
1932-2275/09/$ – see front matter 

Postoperative urinary retention (PUR) can complicate any surgical procedure and is not limited to patients with preexisting urinary symptoms. Although often regarded by clinicians as a trivial or minor complication, urinary retention can be a significant source of patient anxiety and discomfort. Retention prolongs hospital stay, increases costs, and may result in significant morbidity.[1,2] In elderly patients, urinary retention can be associated with restlessness, confusion, and potential development of delirium. Urethral catheterization to treat postoperative retention conveys the risk of urinary tract infection, which increases every day a catheter remains in place.[3,4] Catheterization can result in urethral strictures, the need for additional surgery, and may be associated with a higher hospital mortality rate in vulnerable patient populations.[5] Even a single episode of bladder overdistention may lead to the deposition of collagen between the smooth muscle fibers of the detrusor, reducing their contractile function and leading to chronic impairment of bladder emptying or atony.[6] Irreversible damage to bladder nerves and postjunctional membranes has also been described.[7]

## PHYSIOLOGY OF MICTURITION

The control of micturition is a complex process involving multiple afferent and efferent neural pathways, reflexes, and central and peripheral neurotransmitters. The perioperative period includes myriad insults that may interrupt this process and promote the development of urinary retention.

The bladder is under sympathetic, parasympathetic, and somatic neural control via the hypogastric, pelvic, and pudendal nerves, respectively. Lower motor neurons are under the control of upper motor neurons located in the pons, midbrain, and cerebral cortex. The storage phase of the micturition reflex is mediated by sympathetic stimulation. $\beta_3$-adrenergic receptors are found throughout the detrusor; stimulation by norepinephrine or epinephrine results in smooth muscle relaxation and permits bladder filling. Alpha-adrenergic receptors predominate in the internal urethral sphincter in both men and women, where sympathetic activation maintains contraction. Alpha receptors are also densely found throughout the bladder neck, prostate, and prostatic capsule.[8] The external urethral sphincter is a striated muscle under voluntary control. Sphincter muscle neurons located in Onuf's nucleus, in the S2-S4 segments of the spinal cord, send axons into the pudendal nerve.[9] Acetylcholine released from these axons binds to postjunctional nicotinic receptors and causes constriction of the external urethral sphincter.

When the bladder volume exceeds approximately 300 mL, impulses from stretch receptors in the bladder wall reach the sensory cortex via the pelvic splanchnic nerves; the voiding reflex can then be facilitated by centers in the pons or inhibited by midbrain centers. Central control of micturition involves multiple neurotransmitters including dopamine and serotonin. Normal bladder capacity ranges from 400 to 600 mL.[10]

The efferent limb of the micturition reflex, via parasympathetic motor nerve fibers, runs with spinal nerves from the S2 and S3 levels. These fibers terminate in ganglia within the bladder wall; short, postganglionic fibers innervate the detrusor and internal sphincter. For voiding to take place, tonic inhibition from the motor cortex must be interrupted, allowing the efferent parasympathetics to produce electrical silencing and relaxation of the external sphincter followed by detrusor contraction. Finally, the pelvic floor relaxes and the levator ani descends, allowing micturition to occur.[11]

Multiple facets of surgery, anesthesia, and the perioperative experience may interrupt the micturition reflex. Anesthesia, sedation, and analgesics interfere with the afferent limb by dulling the sensation and perception of bladder fullness, allowing painless urinary retention to develop; 61% of postoperative patients fail to experience discomfort or a strong urge to void even as their bladder volume, as determined by ultrasound bladder scanning, exceeds 600 mL.[12] Normal functioning of the micturition reflex depends on a precise balance between sympathetic and parasympathetic tone, which is frequently disrupted during the perioperative period. Systemic sympathetic discharge and catecholamine release inhibit detrusor contraction and cause functional bladder outlet obstruction via an alpha-mediated increase in bladder outlet and proximal urethral tone. Distention of the bladder itself also leads to an increase in sympathetic motor activity.[8] Detrusor contraction can also be inhibited by a reflex involving afferent fibers of the pudendal nerve, the sacral spinal cord, and efferent pelvic parasympathetic nerves. This reflex can be triggered by peri-anal pain, dilation of the anal canal, and bladder overdistention.[13] Perineal or lower abdominal pain also inhibits the perineal relaxation that is necessary for voiding. Immobilization from intravenous lines, tubes, or drains and the need to void in the supine position can contribute to postoperative voiding dysfunction. One study found that postoperative urinary retention developed in 100% of male patients undergoing hip arthroplasty who were unable to void into a bottle while supine before surgery.[14] Some patients may also be hindered by stress, anxiety, and lack of privacy.

## DIAGNOSIS OF POSTOPERATIVE URINARY RETENTION

Many studies examining the etiology of postoperative urinary retention have come to contradictory conclusions. Reconciling conflicting results is complicated by variation in how urinary retention is defined. In the past, diagnosis relied on patient discomfort or the presence of a palpable bladder.[1,13,15] The accuracy of this method is questionable, as most postoperative urinary retention is painless and physical examination unreliable. Using ultrasound monitoring, Lamonerie and colleagues[16] found that only 46% of patients with a bladder volume exceeding 500 mL appreciated that their bladders were full and felt an urge to void. The diagnosis of bladder distention by nurses has been shown to agree with ultrasound in only 54% of cases.[17] The advent of ultrasound bladder scanning, which allows rapid and accurate assessment of bladder volume, has aided in the diagnosis of postoperative urinary retention for both clinical and research purposes and is becoming available in more patient care settings.[17,18] However, variation continues to exist in the time allowed for spontaneous voiding and in the bladder volume prompting catheterization.

## PERIOPERATIVE FACTORS INFLUENCING THE DEVELOPMENT OF URINARY RETENTION

### *Surgical Procedure*

Rates of postoperative urinary retention reported in the literature vary widely. Although some variation likely reflects differing methodologies and diagnostic thresholds, trends have emerged regarding which types of surgery are likely to be complicated by urinary retention (**Table 1**).

Reported rates of urinary retention among the mixed surgical populations of large hospitals vary from 4% to 29%.[19–21] Two groups recently demonstrated that from 16% to 24% of nonambulatory patients have urinary retention upon PACU discharge, as defined by failure to void with a sonographically demonstrated bladder volume of 600 or 500 mL, respectively.[16,22] The incidence of urinary retention following outpatient surgery has been shown to be procedure-dependent. Patients undergoing hernia or anal surgery, with a combined incidence of 17%, are considered high risk for the development of urinary retention.[17] When these high-risk surgeries are excluded, urinary retention has been found to complicate only 0.0% to 0.8% of ambulatory cases.[12,17]

**Table 1**
**Selected rates of postoperative urinary retention**

| Type of Surgery | Incidence of PUR | References |
| --- | --- | --- |
| Low-risk ambulatory surgery | 0.50% | 12 |
| Gynecological surgery | 0.00% | 12 |
| High-risk ambulatory surgery | 5.00% | 12 |
| Herniorrhaphy | | |
| Local anesthesia with sedation | 0.37% | 59 |
| Regional anesthesia | 2.42% | 59 |
| General anesthesia | 3.00% | 59 |
| Endoscopic hernia repair | 4.00%–22.20% | 19,24 |
| Anorectal surgery | 16.00%–20.00% | 12,13,28 |
| Mixed nonambulatory surgical | | |
| On PACU entry | 28.70% | 21 |
| On PACU discharge | 16.00%–23.70% | 16,22 |
| Gynecological surgery | 9.20% | 34 |
| Orthopedic | | |
| Total knee arthroplasty | 19.70% | 29 |
| Lower-limb joint replacement | 18.10% | 76 |

Patients undergoing inguinal hernia repair are particularly susceptible to postoperative urinary retention. Reported rates of retention after open inguinal or femoral herniorrhaphy vary from 5% to 26%.[12,15,23] Although some authors have found a decreased incidence with laparoscopic techniques, reports range from 4% to 22%.[24,25] Velasco and colleagues[26] reported results of a study examining postoperative complications from laparoscopic herniorrhaphy in 110 patients older than 65. The observed complication rate was 15%; however, 71% of these patients experienced acute PUR. Overall, 59% of patients were discharged on the day of surgery, and 33% were discharged on the next postoperative day.

Acute urinary retention is the most common complication after surgery for benign anorectal disease. While some series have reported incidences as low as 0.53%, the reported mean is around 15.00%.[27,28] Patients who experience an initial episode of urinary retention after anorectal surgery also appear to be prone to recurrent retention, with 50% requiring at least one additional catheterization in one study.[12]

Orthopedic patients have an elevated risk of postoperative urinary retention. Retention complicates 21% to 55% of knee arthroplasties and 11% to 48% of hip arthroplasties.[14,18,29–31] In addition to prolonging length of stay and impairing rehabilitation, urinary retention in this patient population poses a special concern, as transient bacteremia or urinary tract infection resulting from catheterization can cause deep infection in the prosthesis requiring its removal.[32] Deep joint sepsis has been reported in 0.5% to 6.2% of patients who develop urinary retention after total hip replacement.[33]

Postoperative urinary retention, diagnosed as a bladder volume in excess of preoperative bladder capacity, has been found to complicate 9.2% of elective gynecologic surgeries.[34] Although ambulatory gynecologic patients are frequently slow to void after surgery, they have been found to be at minimal risk for urinary retention, likely because of a high incidence of intraoperative catheterization resulting in decreased bladder volumes in the PACU.[17] One recent study suggests that up to 39% of women presenting for urogynecologic assessment experience an underlying degree of significant voiding difficulty before surgery.[35]

The incidence of urinary retention after cholecystectomy reported in the literature ranges from less than 1% to 30%.[1] However, the incidence encountered in current clinical practice likely reflects the lower range of this spectrum, as the incidence has dropped with widespread adoption of laparoscopy. A meta-analysis found a retention rate of only 1.4% in patients undergoing laparoscopic cholecystectomy; the overall rate for elective cholecystectomy in modern series varies from 0.7% to 6.5% with an open approach increasing the risk of urinary retention.[1,36,37]

Prolonged postoperative urinary retention is often seen in patients undergoing complex pelvic surgery for treatment of cancers. Radical hysterectomy for treatment of cervical or endometrial cancer can lead to urinary retention, usually secondary to disruption of the sympathetic innervation from the hypogastric plexus during inferolateral dissection of the cervix. The reported rate of urinary retention requiring catheter drainage for more than 1 month after radical hysterectomy is approximately 14%.[38] Normal voiding returned within 1 month in 85.5% of patients. Another group has shown similar results with approximately 14% of women undergoing either laparoscopic or open radical hysterectomy experiencing prolonged postoperative urinary retention.[39] Another study revealed that up to 30% of women reported a feeling of incomplete bladder emptying based on self-assessment, although this was not corroborated with actual measurements of postvoid residual urine volumes.[40]

Abdominal perineal resection (APR) for the treatment of colorectal cancer is also frequently associated with prolonged urinary retention. This is most often caused by disruption of innervation from the pudendal nerve associated with the anal dissection. Reported rates of urinary retention after APR range from 15% to more than 35% and 41% for women and men respectively.[41–43] A recent prospective study of 295 women who underwent surgery for rectal cancer compared results for anterior resection and abdominal perineal resection in terms of urinary and sexual outcomes.[44] In this series, APR was associated with a significantly higher rate of urinary retention compared with anterior resection (Odds Ratio 11.7; 95% confidence interval [CI] 4.15–32.9; $P < .001$).

## *Anesthetic Technique*

The evidence suggests that anesthetic technique affects the incidence of postoperative urinary retention. General anesthetics cause bladder atony by acting as smooth muscle relaxants and by interfering with autonomic regulation of detrusor tone. Some anesthetic agents have been shown to dramatically increase bladder capacity.[45] In vitro work with isolated human bladder strips has also demonstrated that clinical doses of halothane and thiopentone decrease bladder response to stimulation.[45] Sedative-hypnotics and volatile anesthetics inhibit the pontine micturition center and voluntary cortical control of the bladder, suppressing detrusor contraction and the micturition reflex.[46,47] Petros and colleagues[15] found that patients who underwent inguinal herniorrhaphy under general anesthesia with halothane, a potent smooth muscle relaxant, experienced a significantly higher rate of retention than cases performed with a lidocaine spinal anesthetic. The urodynamic effects of volatile anesthetics and sedative-hypnotics may be augmented by other agents commonly administered during a general anesthetic. Anticholinergic agents once commonly used for premedication and currently used in the management of the reversal of neuromuscular blockade may impair detrusor contractility and facilitate passive overfilling of the bladder by acting at cholinergic receptor sites in the smooth muscle of the bladder and urethra. However, despite the differences in their duration of action, the selection of glycopyrrolate or atropine for preventing the bradycardia associated with reversal agents has not been found to affect the incidence of urinary retention.[48] The use of sympathomimetic agents to treat intraoperative hypotension can also promote retention, via their effects on β receptors in the bladder and α receptors in the bladder neck and proximal urethra. Indeed, a statistically significant increase in retention, to 43.8%, has been shown in patients treated with ephedrine.[21]

Intrathecal local anesthetics interrupt the micturition reflex by blocking transmission of action potentials in the sacral spinal cord. Blockade of afferent nerves results in bladder analgesia, while lack of transmission in efferent fibers causes a detrusor blockade that outlasts motor blockade by as much as several hours. Most patients will be incapable of spontaneous voiding until the sensory level has regressed to the S3 level.[49] After spinal injection of isobaric bupivacaine (20 mg), hyperbaric bupivacaine (21.5 mg), or hyperbaric tetracaine (7.5 mg), sensory block takes 7 to 8 hours to regress to the S3 level.[50] With the use of longer-acting local anesthetics, the duration of detrusor blockade allows the bladder volume to significantly exceed preoperative bladder capacity.[49] Once the bladder is sufficiently overdistended, voiding remains impaired after return of function and urinary retention develops. Many authors have substantiated the association between spinal anesthesia with long-acting local anesthetics and postoperative urinary retention.[16,17,19,21,51,52] However, recovery of bladder function after spinal injection of low-dose, shorter-acting local anesthetics occurs early enough to prevent bladder overdistention and resulting retention in most cases. Ryan and colleagues[53] demonstrated a decrease in catheterization among patients undergoing herniorrhaphy with lidocaine spinal anesthesia to 6%, compared with 30% when bupivacaine or tetracaine were used. Mulroy and collegues[54] reported that retention developed in only 2 of 201 ambulatory patients receiving short-acting epidural or spinal anesthesia. In male patients undergoing inguinal herniorrhaphy, the risk of PUR was found to be greater after spinal anesthesia than epidural anesthesia.[55]

The risk of urinary retention after neuraxial anesthesia may be modulated by other factors in addition to local anesthetic dose and duration of action. A prospective, randomized trial demonstrated that the use of epidural anesthesia did not increase the incidence of retention after hemorrhoidectomy when intraoperative intravenous fluids were limited to 200 mL ± 2 mL/kg/h of Ringer's lactate solution.[56] Lumbar spinal surgery patients experience increased rates of PUR when intrathecal local anesthetics are administered with opioids.[57,58] The addition of fentanyl to spinal anesthesia and the choice of spinal over epidural anesthesia were found to significantly increase time to discharge of ambulatory surgical patients.[54]

Local anesthesia has no negative effects on bladder function and has been found to be associated with a lower incidence of postoperative urinary retention than neuraxial or general anesthesia. A review of 72 studies found that urinary retention occurred in only 0.37% of patients undergoing hernia repair when local anesthesia with sedation was used, as opposed to an incidence of 2.42% with regional anesthesia and 3.00% with general anesthesia.[59] Very low rates of retention after herniorrhaphy under local anesthesia with sedation may reflect improved postoperative pain control resulting from local anesthetic infiltration. Urinary retention after painful groin and pelvic operations is thought to be mediated in part by reflex inhibition of detrusor contraction in response to incisional or perineal pain and edema. Perineal or lower abdominal pain also impairs relaxation of the perineal musculature, which is necessary for voiding to occur. The use of paravertebral nerve block, which also provides good postoperative analgesia, has similarly been associated with minimal risk of urinary retention after herniorrhaphy.[60]

Some studies have found an association between operative time and the development of urinary retention.[1,16,21,51] Time to void after ambulatory surgery with short-acting spinal or epidural anesthesia has been shown to correlate with total anesthetic duration.[54] Longer operations may promote retention because of the administration of greater volumes of intravenous fluids or higher total doses of opioids and anesthetic agents; however, an association between longer procedures and urinary retention has not been confirmed in all studies.[61] Some authors have also concluded that anesthetic technique does not influence the incidence of retention.[20,34,61]

Irrespective of anesthetic modality, most patients are exposed to multiple medications throughout the perioperative period that could theoretically contribute to the development of urinary retention after surgery. By blocking the relaxing effect of beta receptors present in the bladder neck and proximal urethra, β-blockers may lead to alpha-sympathetic dominance and enhance bladder outflow resistance.[20] In neurosurgical patients, the use of β-blockers was associated with an increased risk of retention[62]; however, some studies have found that β-blockers do not influence the rate of retention.[51] Urinary retention has also been reported in association with the benzodiazepines clonazepam and diazepam and is thought to be caused by muscle relaxation.[63] The longer acting, more lipophilic benzodiazepines may be associated with higher rates of urinary retention owing to the more prolonged metabolic clearance of these agents after surgery.[63]

### *Intravenous Fluids*

Several studies have reported that the risk of postoperative urinary retention correlates with the volume of fluids administered during the perioperative period.[22,51,61] High fluid volumes are thought to cause retention via overdistention of the bladder wall. As the bladder fills with urine, the contractility of the detrusor increases. Optimum bladder emptying occurs at an approximate volume of 300 mL, after which detrusor contractility declines.[64] Once significantly overdistended, the bladder can no longer generate sufficient contractile force to empty and retention develops.[13]

Although aggressive fluid administration has been implicated in retention occurring after a variety of procedures, its role has been most conclusively supported in patients undergoing anorectal surgery. Several early articles reported the benefits of very tight fluid restriction. Campbell[65] reported that zero anorectal patients in a series of 100 experienced urinary retention when perioperative fluids were limited to 75 mL. Bailey and Ferguson[66] found that limiting perioperative fluids to 250 mL decreased the incidence to 4% from 15% in patients receiving fluids ad libitum. Several retrospective studies have advocated more moderate fluid restriction, linking the administration of intravenous fluids in excess of 1000 mL to an increased risk of retention after anorectal surgery.[13,52] One group found that increased perioperative fluid administration increases the risk of retention in patients undergoing surgery for benign anorectal disease, but not patients having hemorrhoidectomy.[28] The American Society of Colon and Rectal Surgeons currently recommends that perioperative fluids be limited to lower the incidence of urinary retention after ambulatory anorectal surgery.[67]

Several retrospective studies in herniorrhaphy patients have found a positive correlation between the volume of perioperative intravenous fluids (IVF) administered and the incidence of postoperative urinary retention. Petros and colleagues[15] found that the risk of PUR increased after 1200 mL of intraoperative fluid. Koch and colleagues[24] found that exceeding 500 mL postoperatively conferred increased risk, whereas the volume administered intraoperatively did not affect the incidence of retention. However, in a randomized prospective trial, restricting fluids to 500 mL failed to significantly decrease the incidence of urinary retention after hernia repair.[68]

The role that intravenous fluids play in the development of urinary retention after lower risk procedures remains unclear. Many authors have failed to find a relationship between volumes of IVF administered and the incidence of retention.[20,21,53,55,69–71]

Pavlin and colleagues[12] found that the incidence of retention in low-risk ambulatory surgery patients was unaffected by randomization to the administration of high or low intraoperative fluid volumes.

### *Postoperative Pain and Analgesia*

Postoperative pain may promote the development of urinary retention by increasing sympathetic activity, which inhibits detrusor contraction and increases outflow resistance. Perineal, lower abdominal, or pelvic pain can also directly inhibit initiation of the micturition reflex; this mechanism likely contributes to the elevated incidence of retention after hernia repair or anorectal surgery. The risk of urinary retention after hemorrhoidectomy has been found to correlate with disease severity and the amount of resection required. Distention and pain within the anal canal directly inhibit detrusor activity. More extensive dissection, resulting in increased postoperative pain and local edema, causes detrusor inhibition that promotes the development of urinary retention.[28] The risk of retention after anorectal surgery has been shown to increase with total analgesic requirement and decreases if opiates are used for pain control or if prophylactic analgesia is given with an indomethacin suppository.[13,28] The administration of local anesthetic into the operative site after hernia repair has been shown to decrease the time to voiding after surgery.[55] In neurosurgical patients, preoperative use of anti-inflammatory medications and narcotic analgesics has been found to decrease the risk of urinary retention.[62]

### *Opioids*

Although controlling postoperative pain may reduce the contribution of increased sympathetic tone and local pain reflexes to postoperative urinary retention, opioids interrupt the micturition reflex by several mechanisms. In vitro work with isolated strips of detrusor muscle has demonstrated that encephalins act as presynaptic inhibitors of acetylcholine release from postganglionic neurons.[72] Thus, opioid analgesics reduce parasympathetic tone within the bladder, decreasing detrusor tone and permitting passive filling. They also impair perception of bladder fullness and the urge to void, decrease activity in the pelvic nerves by depressing preganglionic neurons in the sacral parasympathetic nucleus, and cause detrusor-sphincter dyssynergy secondary to failure of sphincter relaxation.[73] Many studies have found that narcotic analgesia plays a significant role in the development of postoperative urinary retention and that the risk increases with escalating doses.[1,24,29,69] Opioid-mediated depression of bladder motility is largely secondary to action at the $\mu$-opioid receptor, and can be reversed by intravenous naloxone, which promotes detrusor contraction and sphincter relaxation. Small doses of IV naloxone (0.1 mg) have been shown to decrease bladder distention without reversing analgesia.[74]

Evidence suggests that some opioid analgesics have a greater impact on urinary function than others. One study found that meperidine use was an independent predictor of difficulty voiding after elective cholecystectomy.[36] It is also generally recommended that meperidine use be avoided in elderly patients owing to prolonged drug clearance, which can increase the risk for developing delirium. After orthopedic surgery, patients who received fentanyl for postoperative analgesia experienced significantly less urinary retention than those given morphine.[61,75]

Opioid-mediated urinary retention also appears to be influenced by route of administration. Several authors have demonstrated that risk is increased in patients using patient-controlled analgesia compared with those receiving intermittent intravenous or intramuscular opioids.[1,69] Although more effective pain control provided by patient-controlled analgesia (PCA) may lead to increased narcotic doses, some authors have found that the additional risk conferred by PCA use cannot be attributed solely to increased total opioid dose.[76] Steadier opioid plasma concentrations achieved by PCA may enhance their impact on urinary function. Intermittent low-dose (0.1 mg IV) naloxone has been shown to increase voiding frequency, decrease bladder scan residuals, and reduce the catheterization rate in orthopedic surgery patients receiving PCA morphine without affecting pain control.[75] However, the addition of ultra–low-dose naloxone (0.006 μg/kg/h to 0.05 μg/kg/h) to PCA morphine was not found to affect rates of postoperative urinary retention.[77]

### *Epidural Analgesia*

The highest rates of opioid-mediated urinary retention have generally been associated with epidural administration. A meta-analysis including 12,513 patients found that the use of epidural analgesia (EA) for postoperative pain control was associated with urinary retention in 23% of patients, a significant increase over the rate found in patients receiving intramuscular or PCA analgesia.[78] A meta-analysis of patients undergoing colorectal surgery found that the incidence of urinary retention increased from 1% to 10% when patients received EA instead of parenteral opioids.[79]

The effect of neuraxial opioids on voiding function may reflect peripheral, spinal, or supraspinal activity. Healthy volunteers given intrathecal morphine or sufentanil demonstrate impaired bladder contraction within 15 to 60 minutes.[80,81] Such rapid onset suggests that intrathecal opioids affect micturition primarily by inhibiting the spinal reflex responsible for detrusor contraction. A primary lumbar-spinal site of action is also supported by the increased incidence of urinary retention associated with lumbar compared with thoracic epidurals.[82] Intrathecal opioids depress preganglionic neurons in the sacral parasympathetic nucleus, decreasing pelvic nerve activity. They also activate μ and δ receptors in the dorsal horn of the spinal cord, inhibiting bladder afferents and attenuating perception of bladder sensation. Consequently, bladder capacity and compliance are increased and initiation of the micturition reflex is delayed.[83]

The extent to which epidural opioid administration negatively affects bladder motility varies with both duration of action and affinity for the μ and δ opioid receptors. Epidural morphine has been associated with rates of postoperative urinary retention as high as 10% to 15%.[84] In patients undergoing hip arthroplasty, use of epidural morphine was found to increase the incidence of bladder catheterization from 24% to 62%.[31] Healthy male volunteers given epidural morphine uniformly develop urinary retention characterized by detrusor relaxation and increased bladder capacity, which lasts an average of 14 to 16 hours.[80]

More lipophilic opioids impair bladder functioning to a lesser degree than hydrophilic morphine, as enhanced systemic uptake limits their activity at the sacral levels affecting urodynamics.[10] Recovery of normal lower urinary tract function is substantially quicker after intrathecal sufentanil than morphine.[81] A prospective, double-blind, randomized-controlled trial found that epidural anesthesia with sufentanil led to a lower incidence of micturition difficulties and bladder catheterization than morphine EA.[85] Epidural fentanyl has also been associated with a decreased incidence of urinary retention relative to morphine. One author reported that no cases of urinary retention requiring catheterization occurred in more than 3000 cases of postoperative analgesia with epidural fentanyl.[84] Animal studies have found that intrathecal fentanyl decreases mean peak urethral pressure along with bladder pressure, which may contribute to the decreased risk of bladder distention with fentanyl use.[73] A small study found that epidural tramadol, a weak μ-agonist and inhibitor of serotonin and norepinephrine uptake, increased bladder capacity and compliance without affecting voiding function.[86] Studies offer conflicting results on the dose-dependency of urinary retention after epidural opioids.[80,81]

### *Nonsteroidal Anti-inflammatory Drugs and Nonopioid Analgesics*

Concomitant administration of nonsteroidal anti-inflammatory drugs (NSAIDs) reduces postoperative opioid analgesic requirements and has been shown to decrease the incidence of postoperative nausea/vomiting and sedation, but not urinary retention.[87,88] The combination of propacetamol and ketoprofen was not found to decrease the incidence of retention in patients using morphine PCA after spinal surgery.[89] NSAIDS may actually facilitate urinary retention by inhibiting cyclooxygenase 2 (COX-2) and decreasing intravesical prostaglandin $E_2$ ($PGE_2$) levels. $PGE_2$ releases tachykinins, which stimulate detrusor smooth muscle and afferent nerve receptors, and has also been shown to relax urethral smooth muscle.[90] NSAID users have been found to experience a twofold increased risk of acute urinary retention.[63] The opioid-sparing effects of ketamine, when administered with morphine PCA after spinal surgery, were found to decrease the incidence of PUR in a small study.[91]

## DEMOGRAPHIC RISK FACTORS FOR POSTOPERATIVE URINARY RETENTION

### *Age and Gender*

Both gender and advancing age appear to modulate the risk of postoperative urinary retention. Multiple studies have concluded that older patients of both genders are at increased risk of retention.[16,19–22,28,61,69,76] The aging process includes multifactorial changes that alter voiding function and may promote the development of urinary retention after surgery.

Detrusor function deteriorates progressively with advancing age; changes may be myogenic or neurogenic in origin and include diminished detrusor contractility and pressure.[92,93] Even healthy older adults with normal urodynamic profiles exhibit evidence of impaired detrusor contractility.[92,93] In some it progresses to detrusor underactivity, characterized by contractions of decreased strength or duration that result in prolonged bladder emptying or failure to empty the bladder within a normal period.[94] Although the true incidence of overt detrusor underactivity remains unclear, the condition is particularly prevalent in frail elderly women, a population prone to PUR after orthopedic surgery. One study demonstrated that 79% of women with proximal hip fractures had bladder volumes greater than 300 mL on admission. Bladder overdistention was also present in 37% of patients before surgery and developed in 56% within the first 24 hours after surgery.[5]

Impaired bladder emptying is reported in 10.8% of women and 22.1% of men older than 60.[95] More than half of men older than 50 have lower urinary tract symptomatology.[96] Bladder outlet obstruction secondary to benign prostatic hyperplasia (BPH) is the primary source of bladder morbidity in elderly men, although some may experience comorbid detrusor decompensation, which can develop independently or in response to untreated BPH.[94] Several studies have confirmed that older males are at an increased risk for the development of PUR.[15,18,51]

Bladder sensation declines with advancing age and is manifested by an increase in the bladder volume prompting the urge to void.[92] Diabetes mellitus, one of the most common comorbid diseases in older adults, is often associated with impairment in bladder sensation, increased bladder capacity, and decreased contractility.[97] Some authors have found that patients with diabetes are prone to the development of postoperative urinary retention.[21,98] Impaired baseline bladder sensation may augment the contribution that decreased afferent activity secondary to anesthetics, sedative-hypnotics, and analgesics makes to the development of retention. The aged may also be more susceptible to the negative urodynamic effects of analgesic and anesthetic agents because many of these drugs have a prolonged duration of action in the elderly.

The impact that gender has on PUR in younger patients remains unclear. Some authors have found no link between gender and the risk of PUR.[21,29,52] Others have reported that females are at greater risk or that women between the ages of 21 and 40 are predisposed to retention.[13,20]

### *Abnormal Voiding History*

Whether patients with preoperative signs and symptoms of bladder outlet obstruction or other voiding dysfunction are predisposed to PUR remains unclear, but has been supported in some studies.[13,51] Tammela and colleagues[20] found that 80% of patients who developed postoperative urinary retention had abnormal voiding histories such as a history of retention after surgery or symptoms of bladder irritation or obstruction. One study of male herniorrhaphy patients found that postoperative urinary retention developed exclusively in patients with abnormal preoperative postvoiding residuals.[23] A previous history of urinary retention was found to be a predictor of PUR after knee arthroplasty.[29] One study found that whereas neither physical exam nor a detailed urological history could distinguish male hip arthroplasty patients at increased risk for retention, diminished preoperative peak urinary flow rate was a significant predictor of increased risk.[30]

However, many studies have refuted the claim that preoperative voiding dysfunction predisposes to the development of retention after surgery. Patients with preoperative signs and symptoms of bladder outlet obstruction undergoing surgery for benign anorectal disease were not found to be at increased risk of PUR.[28] Multiple studies of orthopedic surgery patients have concluded that a history of urological problems cannot predict those who will go on to develop urinary retention.[18,61,99] One recent prospective study examined 102 men undergoing either total knee or hip arthroplasty to determine if a history of voiding dysfunction measured by a standardized rating scale was predictive of PUR.[100] Although 30.4% of the men in this study developed PUR, only age older than 70 years was identified as a significant predictor variable. A case-control study of patients undergoing laparoscopic hernia repair found that those with a history of urinary retention, BPH, or prostate cancer were not at increased risk of PUR.[24]

## MANAGEMENT OF POSTOPERATIVE URINARY RETENTION

### *Preoperative Consultation*

The benefits of taking a more complete urological history as part of routine preoperative evaluation of surgical patients remains unclear, as baseline voiding dysfunction has not been consistently demonstrated to predict patients at increased risk of developing PUR. Ambulatory patients being considered for accelerated pathways permitting discharge without voiding may require screening for preoperative voiding dysfunction or a history of retention, as studies validating the safety of early discharge have excluded this patient population.[12,54]

### *Intraoperative Considerations*

High-risk patients may benefit from efforts to minimize the risk of bladder overdistention. Patients managed without indwelling urethral catheterization should be required to void immediately before surgery. One study found that 14% of patients undergoing common orthopedic and general surgery procedures had a sonographic bladder volume greater than 300 mL immediately before the induction of anesthesia.[64] Further research is required to determine optimum management of IV fluids; although lower fluid volumes may decrease retention rates in some patient populations, this effect must be balanced against the need to support the circulation when spinal or epidural anesthesia is used and the beneficial affect of adequate hydration on decreasing postoperative nausea and vomiting.

## *Diagnosis of Postoperative Urinary Retention*

Postoperative urinary retention is best diagnosed noninvasively with a portable ultrasound bladder scanner, which permits rapid and accurate measurement of bladder volume.[101] This approach has been shown to be superior to diagnosis dependent on physical exam or patient symptoms and avoids unnecessary catheterization of patients with minimal bladder volumes who have failed to void secondary to underresuscitation. The ideal bladder volume at which patients should be catheterized is unclear. The benefits of earlier intervention in preventing detrusor damage and possible persistent voiding dysfunction resulting from bladder overdistention must be weighed against exposing patients to the discomfort and infectious risks associated with catheterization. As normal adult bladder capacity ranges from 400 to 600 mL; a threshold of 600 mL has been recommended.[10,17] Several studies have demonstrated that elevated bladder volumes on PACU entry increase the subsequent risk of developing urinary retention and that the incidence of bladder overdistention on PACU discharge may be high.[16,22,71] Further investigation is warranted to determine the role of more widespread use of portable ultrasound bladder monitoring in the PACU.

## *Duration of Bladder Catheterization*

Urinary retention after ambulatory surgery is commonly managed with in-out urethral catheterization. However, the choice of indwelling or clean intermittent urethral catheterization for postoperative urinary retention in inpatients remains controversial. Animal studies have demonstrated that retention results in detrusor damage secondary to collagen infiltration and impaired contractility.[102,103] Many of these changes are reversible if the obstruction is relieved, and it has been suggested that bladder decompression facilitates normalization of detrusor contractility.[103] Consequently, some clinicians favor prolonged bladder decompression after an episode of acute urinary retention. A randomized study in patients undergoing total hip or knee replacement found that the use of indwelling catheters removed the morning after surgery decreased the risk of bladder distention, urinary retention, and the need for long-term catheterization compared with intermittent catheterization, without increasing the risk of urinary tract infection.[99] However, another randomized trial found that hip fracture patients who were intermittently catheterized on a regular schedule that prevented bladder overdistention experienced a quicker return to normal voiding than those managed with a preoperative indwelling catheter removed 48 hours after surgery.[104] Certain patients may be at increased risk for persistent voiding dysfunction and recurrent retention and therefore benefit from longer-term indwelling catheterization. Most rectal surgery patients require only 1 day of urinary drainage, but those with low-rectal cancers and metastatic lymph nodes are at increased risk of retention and best managed by transurethral catheterization for 5 days.[105] Further study is needed to clarify which patients benefit from indwelling catheterization as well as the optimal duration of bladder catheterization.

### *Pharmacological Therapy*

Several drugs, primarily alpha-blockers and parasympathomimetics, have been investigated for their potential to prevent or treat postoperative urinary retention. The noncompetitive, long-acting alpha-blocker phenoxybenzamine facilitates micturition by decreasing urethral outflow resistance and enhancing intravesical pressure. Several studies found that prophylactic treatment with phenoxybenzamine successfully decreased the incidence of postoperative urinary retention. This effect was demonstrated in small studies of patients undergoing abdominal or vaginal hysterectomy, hemorrhoidectomy, colorectal surgery, genital prolapse repair, and inguinal herniorrhaphy.[23,106,107] Phenoxybenzamine was found to decrease rates of postoperative urinary retention among patients receiving regional anesthesia with concomitant administration of large volumes of intravenous fluids to maintain blood pressure.[8] It was also found to decrease the incidence of retention, need for catheterization, and urinary tract infection in women undergoing elective caesarian section under epidural anesthesia and receiving epidural morphine for postoperative pain control.[108] However, most studies examining prophylactic alpha blockade to prevent postoperative urinary retention were conducted at a time when routine surgeries were followed by extended hospital stays that permitted monitoring for side effects. Phenoxybenzamine is rarely used clinically now because of the potential carcinogenic risk associated with this medication. Modern alpha-blockers such as tamsulosin, alfuzosin, or long-acting doxazosin also offer the advantage of initial administration at therapeutic doses without the need for titration. One study demonstrated that administration of prazosin around the time of hernia repair significantly reduced the incidence of urinary retention compared with placebo (10.8% versus 25.0%).[109] Catheterization rates were significantly reduced as well (3.5% versus 13.8%). Although enthusiasm for preoperative administration of alpha-blockers has waned in the era of ambulatory surgery and fast-track discharge, they are still frequently used in the postoperative treatment of urinary retention, particularly in men.

Interestingly, several benzodiazepines have also been considered for the prevention or treatment of urinary retention after surgery. A randomized controlled trial found that lorazepam administered 1 hour after operation in patients undergoing ambulatory gynecological surgery had no affect on the time to void after surgery.[70] Another study found that midazolam was an ineffective treatment for postoperative urinary retention.[110]

Parasympathomimetic agents such as bethanechol and urecholine theoretically act to increase bladder detrusor contractility. However, although a pharmacologic effect can be demonstrated, their clinical utility is limited owing to poor efficacy and unfavorable side-effect profiles. Hindley and colleagues[111] showed limited clinical improvement in voiding outcomes using a combination of $PGE_2$ and bethanechol compared with placebo. In a series of women undergoing radical hysterectomy, Madeiro and colleagues[112] demonstrated that although administration of bethanechol appeared to improve bladder emptying, it was associated with an increase in detrusor instability and urinary urgency symptoms.

Many patients presenting for surgery, particularly the elderly, take medications that affect voiding function. Optimal perioperative management of these patients remains unclear.

### *Discharge Criteria for Ambulatory Surgery Patients*

Traditionally, patients presenting for ambulatory surgery have been required to void before discharge; however, evidence suggests that this prerequisite may not be necessary for all patients. Fewer than 1% of patients undergoing nonpelvic surgery under general anesthesia, peripheral nerve block, or local anesthesia with sedation will develop urinary retention, defined as the inability to void at a bladder volume of 600 mL detected by bladder ultrasound. Most of these patients will void within 3 hours of their procedure. Requiring this low-risk population to void before discharge will delay 5% to 6% of discharges.[17] Pavlin and colleagues[12] found that low-risk patients could be safely discharged with instructions to return to hospital if voiding had not occurred within 6 to 8 hours of discharge. High-risk patients, those undergoing hernia or anorectal surgery or a procedure under spinal or epidural anesthesia, were monitored with bladder ultrasound and catheterized at a bladder volume of 600 mL. Catheterized patients had an elevated risk of reretention (25%).

The risk of urinary retention in low-risk patients undergoing spinal or epidural anesthesia with short-acting agents may also be sufficiently minimal to permit discharge before voiding.[54] Mulroy and colleagues[54] evaluated an accelerated discharge pathway for ambulatory patients undergoing procaine, lidocaine, or bupivacaine (6 mg or less) spinal anesthesia or epidural anesthesia with 2-chloroprocaine or lidocaine. Patients having hernia, rectal, or urologic surgery, those older than 70, and those with a prior history of voiding difficulty were excluded. Accelerated pathway patients who failed to void spontaneously were discharged if bladder ultrasound demonstrated a bladder volume less than 400 mL. Twenty-three percent of accelerated pathway patients were successfully discharged before voiding; none suffered voiding difficulty or had to return to hospital because of retention. The accelerated discharge protocol shortened discharge time by a mean of 22 minutes.[54]

## REFERENCES

1. Petros JG, Rimm EB, Robillard RJ. Factors influencing urinary tract retention after elective open cholecystectomy. Surg Gynecol Obstet 1992;174(6):497–500.
2. Williams MP, Wallhagen M, Dowling G. Urinary retention in hospitalized elderly women. J Gerontol Nurs 1993;19(2):7–14.
3. Getliffe K. Care of urinary catheters. Nurs Stand 1996;11(11):47–50.
4. Schaeffer AJ. Catheter-associated bacteriuria. Urol Clin North Am 1986;13(4):735–47.
5. Smith NK, Albazzaz MK. A prospective study of urinary retention and risk of death after proximal femoral fracture. Age Ageing 1996;25(2):150–4.
6. Hinman F. Editorial: postoperative over-distention of the bladder. Surg Gynecol Obstet 1976;142(6):901–2.
7. Tammela T, Kontturi M, Lukkarinen O. Postoperative urinary retention. II. Micturition problems after the first catheterization. Scand J Urol Nephrol 1986;20(4):257–60.
8. Leventhal A, Pfau A. Pharmacologic management of postoperative over-distention of the bladder. Surg Gynecol Obstet 1978;146(3):347–8.
9. de Groat WC. Integrative control of the lower urinary tract: preclinical perspective. Br J Pharmacol 2006;147(Suppl 2):S25–40.
10. Baldini G, Bagry H, Aprikian A, et al. Postoperative urinary retention: anesthetic and perioperative considerations. Anesthesiology 2009;110(5):1139–57.
11. Stallard S, Prescott S. Postoperative urinary retention in general surgical patients. Br J Surg 1988;75(11):1141–3.
12. Pavlin DJ, Pavlin EG, Fitzgibbon DR, et al. Management of bladder function after outpatient surgery. Anesthesiology 1999;91(1):42–50.

13. Toyonaga T, Matsushima M, Sogawa N, et al. Postoperative urinary retention after surgery for benign anorectal disease: potential risk factors and strategy for prevention. Int J Colorectal Dis 2006;21(7):676–82.
14. Waterhouse N, Beaumont AR, Murray K, et al. Urinary retention after total hip replacement. A prospective study. J Bone Joint Surg Br 1987;69(1):64–6.
15. Petros JG, Rimm EB, Robillard RJ, et al. Factors influencing postoperative urinary retention in patients undergoing elective inguinal herniorrhaphy. Am J Surg 1991;161(4):431–3 [discussion: 434].
16. Lamonerie L, Marret E, Deleuze A, et al. Prevalence of postoperative bladder distension and urinary retention detected by ultrasound measurement. Br J Anaesth 2004;92(4):544–6.
17. Pavlin DJ, Pavlin EG, Gunn HC, et al. Voiding in patients managed with or without ultrasound monitoring of bladder volume after outpatient surgery. Anesth Analg 1999;89(1):90–7.
18. Sarasin SM, Walton MJ, Singh HP, et al. Can a urinary tract symptom score predict the development of postoperative urinary retention in patients undergoing lower limb arthroplasty under spinal anaesthesia? A prospective study. Ann R Coll Surg Engl 2006;88(4):394–8.
19. Lau H, Lam B. Management of postoperative urinary retention: a randomized trial of in-out versus overnight catheterization. ANZ J Surg 2004;74(8):658–61.
20. Tammela T, Kontturi M, Lukkarinen O. Postoperative urinary retention. I. Incidence and predisposing factors. Scand J Urol Nephrol 1986;20(3):197–201.
21. Olsen S, Nielsen J. A study into postoperative urine retention in the recovery ward. British Journal of Anaesthetic & Recovery Nursing 2007;8(4):91–5.
22. Keita H, Diouf E, Tubach F, et al. Predictive factors of early postoperative urinary retention in the postanesthesia care unit. Anesth Analg 2005;101(2):592–6.
23. Goldman G, Leviav A, Mazor A, et al. Alpha-adrenergic blocker for posthernioplasty urinary retention. Prevention and treatment. Arch Surg 1988;123(1):35–6.
24. Koch CA, Grinberg GG, Farley DR. Incidence and risk factors for urinary retention after endoscopic hernia repair. Am J Surg 2006;191(3):381–5.
25. Lau H, Patil NG, Yuen WK, et al. Urinary retention following endoscopic totally extraperitoneal inguinal hernioplasty. Surg Endosc 2002;16(11):1547–50.
26. Velasco JM, Vallina VL, Esposito DJ, et al. Laparoscopic herniorrhaphy in the geriatric population. Am Surg 1998;64(7):633–7.
27. Hoff SD, Bailey HR, Butts DR, et al. Ambulatory surgical hemorrhoidectomy—a solution to postoperative urinary retention? Dis Colon Rectum 1994;37(12):1242–4.
28. Zaheer S, Reilly WT, Pemberton JH, et al. Urinary retention after operations for benign anorectal diseases. Dis Colon Rectum 1998;41(6):696–704.
29. Kumar P, Mannan K, Chowdhury AM, et al. Urinary retention and the role of indwelling catheterization following total knee arthroplasty. Int Braz J Urol 2006;32(1):31–4.
30. Redfern TR, Machin DG, Parsons KF, et al. Urinary retention in men after total hip arthroplasty. J Bone Joint Surg Am 1986;68(9):1435–8.
31. Walts LF, Kaufman RD, Moreland JR, et al. Total hip arthroplasty. An investigation of factors related to postoperative urinary retention. Clin Orthop Relat Res 1985;194:280–2.
32. Irvine R, Johnson BL Jr, Amstutz HC. The relationship of genitourinary tract procedures and deep sepsis after total hip replacements. Surg Gynecol Obstet 1974;139(5):701–6.

33. Wroblewski BM, del Sel HJ. Urethral instrumentation and deep sepsis in total hip replacement. Clin Orthop Relat Res 1980;146:209–12.
34. Bodker B, Lose G. Postoperative urinary retention in gynecologic patients. Int Urogynecol J Pelvic Floor Dysfunct 2003;14(2):94–7.
35. Haylen BT, Krishnan S, Schulz S, et al. Has the true prevalence of voiding difficulty in urogynecology patients been underestimated? Int Urogynecol J Pelvic Floor Dysfunct 2007;18(1):53–6.
36. Kulacoglu H, Dener C, Kama NA. Urinary retention after elective cholecystectomy. Am J Surg 2001;182(3):226–9.
37. Shea JA, Berlin JA, Bachwich DR, et al. Indications for and outcomes of cholecystectomy: a comparison of the pre and postlaparoscopic eras. Ann Surg 1998;227(3):343–50.
38. Manchana T, Sirisabya N, Lertkhachonsuk R, et al. Long term complications after radical hysterectomy with pelvic lymphadenectomy. J Med Assoc Thai 2009;92(4):451–6.
39. Uccella S, Laterza R, Ciravolo G, et al. A comparison of urinary complications following total laparoscopic radical hysterectomy and laparoscopic pelvic lymphadenectomy to open abdominal surgery. Gynecol Oncol 2007;107(Suppl 1): S147–9.
40. Axelsen SM, Petersen LK. Urogynaecological dysfunction after radical hysterectomy. Eur J Surg Oncol 2006;32(4):445–9.
41. Zaheer S, Pemberton JH, Farouk R, et al. Surgical treatment of adenocarcinoma of the rectum. Ann Surg 1998;227(6):800–11.
42. Petrelli NJ, Nagel S, Rodriguez-Bigas M, et al. Morbidity and mortality following abdominoperineal resection for rectal adenocarcinoma. Am Surg 1993;59(7): 400–4.
43. Cunsolo A, Bragaglia RB, Manara G, et al. Urogenital dysfunction after abdominoperineal resection for carcinoma of the rectum. Dis Colon Rectum 1990; 33(11):918–22.
44. Tekkis PP, Cornish JA, Remzi FH, et al. Measuring sexual and urinary outcomes in women after rectal cancer excision. Dis Colon Rectum 2009;52(1):46–54.
45. Doyle PT, Briscoe CE. The effects of drugs and anaesthetic agents on the urinary bladder and sphincters. Br J Urol 1976;48(5):329–35.
46. Combrisson H, Robain G, Cotard JP. Comparative effects of xylazine and propofol on the urethral pressure profile of healthy dogs. Am J Vet Res 1993;54(12): 1986–9.
47. Matsuura S, Downie JW. Effect of anesthetics on reflex micturition in the chronic cannula-implanted rat. Neurourol Urodyn 2000;19(1):87–99.
48. Orko R, Rosenberg PH. Comparison of some postanaesthetic effects of atropine and glycopyrrolate with particular emphasis on urinary problems. Acta Anaesthesiol Scand 1984;28(1):112–5.
49. Kamphuis ET, Ionescu TI, Kuipers PW. Recovery of storage and emptying functions of the urinary bladder after spinal anesthesia with lidocaine and with bupivacaine in men. Anesthesiology 1998;88(2):310–6.
50. Axelsson K, Mollefors K, Olsson JO, et al. Bladder function in spinal anaesthesia. Acta Anaesthesiol Scand 1985;29(3):315–21.
51. Ringdal M, Borg B, Hellstrom AL. A survey on incidence and factors that may influence first postoperative urination. Urol Nurs 2003;23(5):341–6, 354.
52. Petros JG, Bradley TM. Factors influencing postoperative urinary retention in patients undergoing surgery for benign anorectal disease. Am J Surg 1990; 159(4):374–6.

53. Ryan JA Jr, Adye BA, Jolly PC, et al. Outpatient inguinal herniorrhaphy with both regional and local anesthesia. Am J Surg 1984;148(3):313–6.
54. Mulroy MF, Salinas FV, Larkin KL, et al. Ambulatory surgery patients may be discharged before voiding after short-acting spinal and epidural anesthesia. Anesthesiology 2002;97(2):315–9.
55. Faas CL, Acosta FJ, Campbell MD, et al. The effects of spinal anesthesia vs epidural anesthesia on 3 potential postoperative complications: pain, urinary retention, and mobility following inguinal herniorrhaphy. AANA J 2002;70(6):441–7.
56. Kau YC, Lee YH, Li JY, et al. Epidural anesthesia does not increase the incidences of urinary retention and hesitancy in micturition after ambulatory hemorrhoidectomy. Acta Anaesthesiol Sin 2003;41(2):61–4.
57. Jellish WS, Thalji Z, Stevenson K, et al. A prospective randomized study comparing short- and intermediate-term perioperative outcome variables after spinal or general anesthesia for lumbar disk and laminectomy surgery. Anesth Analg 1996;83(3):559–64.
58. McLain RF, Kalfas I, Bell GR, et al. Comparison of spinal and general anesthesia in lumbar laminectomy surgery: a case-controlled analysis of 400 patients. J Neurosurg Spine 2005;2(1):17–22.
59. Jensen P, Mikkelsen T, Kehlet H. Postherniorrhaphy urinary retention—effect of local, regional, and general anesthesia: a review. Reg Anesth Pain Med 2002;27(6):612–7.
60. Klein SM, Greengrass RA, Weltz C, et al. Paravertebral somatic nerve block for outpatient inguinal herniorrhaphy: an expanded case report of 22 patients. Reg Anesth Pain Med 1998;23(3):306–10.
61. Wynd CA, Wallace M, Smith KM. Factors influencing postoperative urinary retention following orthopaedic surgical procedures. Orthop Nurs 1996;15(1):43–50.
62. Boulis NM, Mian FS, Rodriguez D, et al. Urinary retention following routine neurosurgical spine procedures. Surg Neurol 2001;55(1):23–7 [discussion: 27–8].
63. Verhamme KM, Sturkenboom MC, Stricker BH, et al. Drug-induced urinary retention: incidence, management and prevention. Drug Saf 2008;31(5):373–88.
64. Joelsson-Alm E, Nyman CR, Lindholm C, et al. Perioperative bladder distension: a prospective study. Scand J Urol Nephrol 2009;43(1):58–62.
65. Campbell ED. Prevention of urinary retention after anorectal operations. Dis Colon Rectum 1972;15(1):69–70.
66. Bailey HR, Ferguson JA. Prevention of urinary retention by fluid restriction following anorectal operations. Dis Colon Rectum 1976;19(3):250–2.
67. Place R, Hyman N, Simmang C, et al. Practice parameters for ambulatory anorectal surgery. Dis Colon Rectum 2003;46(5):573–6.
68. Kozol RA, Mason K, McGee K. Post-herniorrhaphy urinary retention: a randomized prospective study. J Surg Res 1992;52(2):111–2.
69. Petros JG, Mallen JK, Howe K, et al. Patient-controlled analgesia and postoperative urinary retention after open appendectomy. Surg Gynecol Obstet 1993;177(2):172–5.
70. Hershberger JM, Milad MP. A randomized clinical trial of lorazepam for the reduction of postoperative urinary retention. Obstet Gynecol 2003;102(2):311–6.
71. Feliciano T, Montero J, McCarthy M, et al. A retrospective, descriptive, exploratory study evaluating incidence of postoperative urinary retention after spinal anesthesia and its effect on PACU discharge. J Perianesth Nurs 2008;23(6):394–400.

72. Petersen TK, Husted SE, Rybro L, et al. Urinary retention during i.m. and extradural morphine analgesia. Br J Anaesth 1982;54(11):1175–8.
73. Durant PA, Yaksh TL. Drug effects on urinary bladder tone during spinal morphine-induced inhibition of the micturition reflex in unanesthetized rats. Anesthesiology 1988;68(3):325–34.
74. Wren KR, Wren TL. Postsurgical urinary retention. Urol Nurs 1996;16(2):45–7 [quiz: 48–49].
75. Gallo S, DuRand J, Pshon N. A study of naloxone effect on urinary retention in the patient receiving morphine patient-controlled analgesia. Orthop Nurs 2008;27(2):111–5.
76. O'Riordan JA, Hopkins PM, Ravenscroft A, et al. Patient-controlled analgesia and urinary retention following lower limb joint replacement: prospective audit and logistic regression analysis. Eur J Anaesthesiol 2000;17(7):431–5.
77. Cepeda M. Addition of ultralow dose naloxone to postoperative morphine PCA: unchanged analgesia and opioid requirement but decreased incidence of opioid side effects. Pain 2004;107(1-2):41–6.
78. Dolin SJ, Cashman JN. Tolerability of acute postoperative pain management: nausea, vomiting, sedation, pruritis, and urinary retention. Evidence from published data. Br J Anaesth 2005;95(5):584–91.
79. Marret E, Remy C, Bonnet F, et al. Meta-analysis of epidural analgesia versus parenteral opioid analgesia after colorectal surgery. Br J Surg 2007;94(6): 665–73.
80. Rawal N, Mollefors K, Axelsson K, et al. An experimental study of urodynamic effects of epidural morphine and of naloxone reversal. Anesth Analg 1983; 62(7):641–7.
81. Kuipers PW, Kamphuis ET, van Venrooij GE, et al. Intrathecal opioids and lower urinary tract function: a urodynamic evaluation. Anesthesiology 2004;100(6): 1497–503.
82. Basse L, Werner M, Kehlet H. Is urinary drainage necessary during continuous epidural analgesia after colonic resection? Reg Anesth Pain Med 2000;25(5): 498–501.
83. Dray A. Epidural opiates and urinary retention: new models provide new insights. Anesthesiology 1988;68(3):323–4.
84. Grass JA. Fentanyl: clinical use as postoperative analgesic–epidural/intrathecal route. J Pain Symptom Manage 1992;7(7):419–30.
85. Kim JY, Lee SJ, Koo BN, et al. The effect of epidural sufentanil in ropivacaine on urinary retention in patients undergoing gastrectomy. Br J Anaesth 2006;97(3): 414–8.
86. Singh SK, Agarwal MM, Batra YK, et al. Effect of lumbar-epidural administration of tramadol on lower urinary tract function. Neurourol Urodyn 2008;27(1):65–70.
87. Marret E, Kurdi O, Zufferey P, et al. Effects of nonsteroidal antiinflammatory drugs on patient-controlled analgesia morphine side effects: meta-analysis of randomized controlled trials. Anesthesiology 2005;102(6):1249–60.
88. Etches RC, Warriner CB, Badner N, et al. Continuous intravenous administration of ketorolac reduces pain and morphine consumption after total hip or knee arthroplasty. Anesth Analg 1995;81(6):1175–80.
89. Fletcher D, Negre I, Barbin C, et al. Postoperative analgesia with i.v. propacetamol and ketoprofen combination after disc surgery. Can J Anaesth 1997;44(5 Pt 1): 479–85.
90. Andersson KE, Ek A, Persson CG. Effects of prostaglandins on the isolated human bladder and urethra. Acta Physiol Scand 1977;100(2):165–71.

91. Javery KB, Ussery TW, Steger HG, et al. Comparison of morphine and morphine with ketamine for postoperative analgesia. Can J Anaesth 1996;43(3):212–5.
92. Pfisterer MH, Griffiths DJ, Schaefer W, et al. The effect of age on lower urinary tract function: a study in women. J Am Geriatr Soc 2006;54(3):405–12.
93. Resnick NM, Elbadawi A, Yalla SV. Age and the lower urinary tract: what is normal? Neurourol Urodyn 1995;14:577–9.
94. Taylor JA 3rd, Kuchel GA. Detrusor underactivity: clinical features and pathogenesis of an underdiagnosed geriatric condition. J Am Geriatr Soc 2006; 54(12):1920–32.
95. Diokno AC, Brock BM, Brown MB, et al. Prevalence of urinary incontinence and other urological symptoms in the noninstitutionalized elderly. J Urol 1986;136(5): 1022–5.
96. Rotkin ID. Epidemiology of Benign Prostatic Hypertrophy: Review and Speculations. In: Grayhack JT, Wilson D, Scherbenski MJ, editors. Benign Prostatic Hyperplasia, Washington, D.C.: U.S. Government Printing Office; 1976. p. 105, 106–117.
97. Kebapci N, Yenilmez A, Efe B, et al. Bladder dysfunction in type 2 diabetic patients. Neurourol Urodyn 2007;26(6):814–9.
98. Liang CC, Lee CL, Chang TC, et al. Postoperative urinary outcomes in catheterized and non-catheterized patients undergoing laparoscopic-assisted vaginal hysterectomy—a randomized controlled trial. Int Urogynecol J Pelvic Floor Dysfunct 2009;20(3):295–300.
99. Michelson JD, Lotke PA, Steinberg ME. Urinary-bladder management after total joint-replacement surgery. N Engl J Med 1988;319(6):321–6.
100. Kotwal R, Hodgson P, Carpenter C. Urinary retention following lower limb arthroplasty: analysis of predictive factors and review of literature. Acta Orthop Belg 2008;74(3):332–6.
101. Pavlin DJ, Rapp SE, Polissar NL, et al. Factors affecting discharge time in adult outpatients. Anesth Analg 1998;87(4):816–26.
102. Gosling JA, Kung LS, Dixon JS, et al. Correlation between the structure and function of the rabbit urinary bladder following partial outlet obstruction. J Urol 2000;163(4):1349–56.
103. Gabella G, Uvelius B. Reversal of muscle hypertrophy in the rat urinary bladder after removal of urethral obstruction. Cell Tissue Res 1994;277(2):333–9.
104. Skelly JM, Guyatt GH, Kalbfleisch R, et al. Management of urinary retention after surgical repair of hip fracture. CMAJ 1992;146(7):1185–9.
105. Benoist S, Panis Y, Denet C, et al. Optimal duration of urinary drainage after rectal resection: a randomized controlled trial. Surgery 1999;125(2):135–41.
106. Livne PM, Kaplan B, Ovadia Y, et al. Prevention of post-hysterectomy urinary retention by alpha-adrenergic blocker. Acta Obstet Gynecol Scand 1983; 62(4):337–40.
107. Lose G, Lindholm P. Prophylactic phenoxybenzamine in the prevention of postoperative retention of urine after vaginal repair: a prospective randomized double-blind trial. Int J Gynaecol Obstet 1985;23(4):315–20.
108. Evron S, Magora F, Sadovsky E. Prevention of urinary retention with phenoxybenzamine during epidural morphine. Br Med J (Clin Res Ed) 1984;288(6412): 190.
109. Gonullu NN, Dulger M, Utkan NZ, et al. Prevention of postherniorrhaphy urinary retention with prazosin. Am Surg 1999;65(1):55–8.
110. Gottesman L, Milsom JW, Mazier WP. The use of anxiolytic and parasympathomimetic agents in the treatment of postoperative urinary retention following

anorectal surgery. A prospective, randomized, double-blind study. Dis Colon Rectum 1989;32(10):867–70.

111. Hindley RG, Brierly RD, Thomas PJ. Prostaglandin E2 and bethanechol in combination for treating detrusor underactivity. BJU Int 2004;93(1):89–92.
112. Madeiro AP, Rufino AC, Sartori MG, et al. The effects of bethanechol and cisapride on urodynamic parameters in patients undergoing radical hysterectomy for cervical cancer. A randomized, double-blind, placebo-controlled study. Int Urogynecol J Pelvic Floor Dysfunct 2006;17(3):248–52.

# Postoperative Cognitive Dysfunction in the Elderly

Ramesh Ramaiah, MD, FCARCSI, FRCA[a,*], Arthur M. Lam, MD, FRCPC[a,b]

**KEYWORDS**

• Elderly • Cognitive • Post operative • Dysfunction
• General anesthesia • Non cardiac

J.R. was a 72-year-old man who presented for elective replacement of his right hip. He was still working as an accountant and had been physically active, including playing tennis, until osteoarthritis in the right hip became painful. His medical history included hypertension controlled with diltiazem, and hypercholesterolemia that was well controlled with simvastatin. On physical examination he was alert and calm, and was originally encountered telling jokes to the nurses in the preoperative area. After discussion with his anesthesiologist, he underwent his procedure under general anesthesia. The postoperative course was uncomplicated and he was discharged to a rehabilitation facility on postoperative day 3, returning home 10 days later. About 1 month later, the orthopedic surgeon mentions that the patient has had serious problems adding numbers and has had to give up working as an accountant. The surgeon questions whether the procedure should have been done under regional anesthesia.

The United States population is aging rapidly as the life expectancy advances, and by 2020 the number of people older than 65 years is expected to increase by 53% compared with 2001. Half of all the surgical procedures currently performed are in elderly patients 65 years or older, and this number is expected to increase.[1] Despite improvement in surgical techniques, anesthetic management, and intensive care, a significant number of elderly patients develop postoperative cognitive decline. Postoperative cognitive dysfunction (POCD) is a postoperative memory or thinking impairment that has been corroborated by neuropsychological testing.[2] The International Classification of Disease has not yet recognized a diagnostic code for this condition, but clinicians are beginning to use the term POCD as a general description of patients who complain of memory and thought process impairment in the postoperative period. According to the *Diagnostic and Statistical Manual of Mental Disorder, Fourth*

[a] Anesthesiology and Pain Medicine, University of Washington, Harborview Medical Center, Box 359724, 325 Ninth Avenue, Seattle, WA 98104-8009, USA
[b] Cerebrovascular Laboratory, Harborview Medical Center, Box 359724, 325 Ninth Avenue, Seattle, WA 98104-8009, USA
* Corresponding author.
*E-mail address:* ramaiahr@u.washington.edu (R. Ramaiah).

Anesthesiology Clin 27 (2009) 485–496
doi:10.1016/j.anclin.2009.07.011
**anesthesiology.theclinics.com**
1932-2275/09/$ – see front matter 

*Edition* (DSM-IV), POCD is considered a mild neurocognitive disorder. The symptoms typically include difficulty staying focused on a task, difficulty with completing more than one task at the same time, problems recalling information recently heard or read, and difficulty with finding words. Postoperative cognitive dysfunction should not be confused with delirium, which is a transient and fluctuating disturbance of consciousness that tends to occur shortly after surgery, whereas POCD is a more persistent problem of a change in cognitive performance. POCD has been reported after a variety of surgical procedures, but until recently most research in this field had focused on cardiac surgery, in which the incidence seems to be highest (30%–80%). In general, POCD is associated with a decline in performance of activities of daily living in elderly patients, and can cause substantial damage to the family and social support system. In this article POCD and delirium are defined, and the physiology of aging discussed. The incidence and mechanism of POCD are outlined, and methods to reduce the incidence of this complication discussed.

## DELIRIUM

Delirium is a common deleterious complication after surgery in elderly patients. Delirium is defined as an acute change in mental status, with inattention and altered level of consciousness that tend to fluctuate during the course of the day.[3] Delirium often exhibits perceptual disturbances, psychomotor or memory impairment, and disorganized thought processes. The overall incidence of postoperative delirium in all age groups is estimated to be between 5% and 10%. The incidence also varies with the type of surgery, occurs in 10% to 45% of elderly patients, and is associated with increased morbidity and mortality, greater length of hospital stay, and increased costs.[4,5] Preoperative variables associated with the development of delirium include older age, decreased albumin level, lower hematocrit, functional and cognitive impairment, electrolyte disturbances, and history of alcohol abuse. Intraoperative variables include hypotension, hypoxemia, blood transfusion, and use of multiple drugs.[5,6] The surgical procedures most associated with delirium include aortic aneurysm repair, and thoracic, cardiac, and orthopedic procedures. Among anesthetic agents, anticholinergic medications that cross the blood-brain barrier (eg, atropine and scopolamine) are classic pharmacologic causes of postoperative confusion.[7] Delirium is a complicated and costly problem in the elderly population, and Medicare expenditure for its diagnosis and treatment exceeds US$4 billion per year (1994 dollars).[8] Perioperative geriatric programs involving pre- and postoperative assessment with identification and treatment of superimposed illness or infection, postoperative supplemental oxygen therapy, and maintenance of systolic blood pressure above 90 mm Hg have been suggested as methods to reduce this risk.[9]

## PHYSIOLOGY OF AGING

Normal aging is associated with progressive loss of functional reserve in all organ systems. The extent and onset of these changes are highly variable from person to person. During normal aging, the brain undergoes extensive structural and physiologic changes reflected by a decrease in the volume of both gray and white matter.[10] The decrease in volume is thought to be secondary to neuronal shrinkage as opposed to neuronal loss. Brain weight decreases on average 2 to 3 g per year after 60 years, whereas hemispheric volume decreases 2% to 3.5% per decade after age 20.[11] These changes are easily seen on computed tomography and magnetic resonance scans as prominent enlargement of the ventricles, increased space between the surface of the brain and the skull, and sulcal widening. It is controversial whether the aging process alters synaptic density in the cortex. However, data from nonhuman primates suggest significant regional reductions in the neurotransmitters dopamine, acetylcholine, norepinephrine, and serotonin with aging.[12] On the other hand, the level of glutamate, which is the primary neurotransmitter in the cortex, seems not to be affected by age. Older adults experience minor impairment in memory and speed of cognitive processing, but the extent of impairment is variable, and is influenced by years of education and level of physical activity. The sensorimotor system can also deteriorate. Impairment in vision, hearing, and vibratory sense in the lower extremity are common, along with decrease in motor speed. Physical activity has a beneficial effect on motor speed and cognitive performance, thus an elderly person with physically active lifestyle will have better motor speed and cognitive ability than a person with sedentary lifestyle.[13] The cerebrovascular system is also affect by aging. Arteriosclerosis and atherosclerosis are more prevalent in elderly persons, with associated increased risk for stroke. Cerebral blood flow decreases with age and cerebral metabolic rate remains stable in healthy elderly subjects. Cerebral autoregulation and carbon dioxide responsiveness seem to be relatively well preserved with aging.

## INCIDENCE AND RISK FACTORS FOR THE DEVELOPMENT OF POSTOPERATIVE COGNITIVE DYSFUNCTION

Adverse effects of anesthesia in old people were first described over 6 decades ago. A retrospective study published by Bedford[14] in 1955 indicated that anesthesia could have lasting effects. This study prompted Bedford to speculate that anesthetic agents themselves may be partially responsible for the cognitive decline. However, subsequent studies failed to confirm this hypothesis.[15,16] Most research has focused on patients undergoing cardiac surgery, in whom the incidence is estimated be between 30% and 80% 1 week after surgery, and approximately 60% several months after surgery.[17–20] A large prospective, randomized controlled study conducted by ISPOCD1 (the International Study on Postoperative Cognitive Function) reported that the incidence of POCD in the first week after major noncardiac surgery was 23% in patients between 60 and 69 years old, and 29% in patients older than 70 years.[15] Cognitive dysfunction was still present in 14% of patients older than 70 years at 3 months after surgery,[15,21,22] indicating that increasing age is a major risk factor for the development of POCD. This rate was significantly higher than the control group of healthy volunteers, in whom the incidence was 3.4% at 1 week and 2.8% at 3 months. POCD is a known complication after both cardiac and noncardiac surgery. Canet and colleagues investigated patients undergoing minor surgery under general anesthesia and the incidence of POCD. These investigators reported that the incidence of POCD at 1 week is significantly lower (7%) in elderly patients undergoing minor surgery than undergoing major surgery.[23] Canet and colleagues also found a lower incidence in day-case setting than hospitalized patients.[23] One study reports that POCD may persist beyond 1 year in approximately 1% of elderly patients, and also suggest that POCD is a reversible condition in the majority of elderly patients.[24]

The causes for postoperative cognitive decline are likely to be multifactorial, and include age, educational level, duration of anesthesia, postoperative infection, second operation,[15] preoperative symptoms of depression, and mild cognitive decline. Age, however, is the least controversial risk factor for the development of POCD, with a proven relationship with increasing age.[15,25] The mechanism by which increasing age is related to POCD remains unknown. Elderly patients may have preexisting conditions or limited cognitive reserve to cope with the physiologic challenges of anesthesia and surgery. Progressive atherosclerosis linked to silent cardiovascular disease associated with the risk of embolization may be an acceptable explanation in cardiac surgery.[17] POCD is also reported in adult patient populations following noncardiac surgery. Patients in all age groups have improvements in cognitive function by 3 months after surgery, but the prevalence of late POCD is significantly higher in the elderly than in the young or middle-aged patients.[25] Another important risk factor for POCD is years of formal education. A low level of education has been shown to predispose cognitive decline, whereas high education levels seem to protect against cognitive decline following surgical procedures involving open heart surgery. One proposed theory for this relationship involves the concept of cerebral cognitive reserve; however, it is not clear how a greater number of years of education translates to a cognitive reserve. Education presumably increases the synaptic density in the neocortex by recruiting neurons, increasing neuronal communication, and minimizing the signs of cognitive and functional impairment.[26] Alternatively, patients with high levels of cognitive reserve are more likely to pursue and complete higher education, thus the educational level serves as a marker of cognitive reserve. Elderly patients with preoperative mental comorbidities including depression and presurgical cognitive impairment may also be at increased risk for the development of POCD.[27]

There is no longer any doubt that cognitive impairment occurs in some elderly patients after uncomplicated anesthesia and surgery. What remains unclear is the cause of this complication. Anesthesia itself may be the obvious factor; however, there is no convincing evidence to support this. The noble gas xenon has been demonstrated to exert substantial neuroprotective properties in animal studies, but when it was studied in humans there was no significant difference in the incidence of POCD in comparison to propofol.[28] On the other hand, use of nitrous oxide in clinically relevant concentrations in elderly patients is not associated with an increased incidence of delirium or POCD.[29] The fact that the incidence of prolonged POCD is apparently similar regardless of the anesthetic technique used (regional anesthesia decreases the incidence of POCD early after surgery)[30] suggests that nonanesthetic factors are likely to be important.[31] Earlier hypotheses attribute the development of POCD to perioperative hypotension and hypoxia, but more recent evidence does not support this. For example, even though pulse oximetry identifies arterial desaturation in most of the patients during anesthesia, cognitive outcome is not improved by pulse oximetry-guided supplemental oxygen administration.[32]

### *Normotensive Versus Hypotensive Anesthesia*

Several earlier studies have shown that controlled hypotension during surgery is not associated with increased risk for the development of POCD in elderly patients.[33] Williams-Russo and colleagues, in their prospective randomized study of elderly patients (mean age, 72 years) undergoing elective primary total hip replacement under epidural anesthesia, found no difference in early or long-term cognitive decline between two groups of patients randomized to a mean arterial pressure of 45 to 55 mm Hg or 55 to 75 mm Hg.[34] The first international study of postoperative cognitive dysfunction (ISPOCD1) by Moller revealed that neither perioperative hypotension (mean arterial pressure < 60% of reference for >30 minutes) nor hypoxia (pulse oximetry < 80% for >2 minutes) were significant risk factors for the development of POCD 3 months after surgery.[15] However, a recent post hoc analysis demonstrates that in elderly hypertensive patients undergoing lumbar laminectomy or microdiscetomy, a lower intraoperative mean arterial pressure (as a fraction of baseline mean arterial pressure [MAP]) is associated with poor cognitive performance at 1 day and 3 months after surgery. Cerebral ischemia may occur secondary to decreased cerebral perfusion over an extended period of time, but in this study the investigators did not incorporate the time component in the minimum MAP measurement.[35]

### *Normocapnia Versus Hypocapnia*

The effect of hypocapnia and cognitive performance was investigated in one study.[36] Elderly patients undergoing cataract surgery were assigned to either ventilation targeting mean arterial carbon dioxide tension ($PaCO_2$) of 4.9 kPa (37 mm Hg), hyperventilation to a mean $PaCO_2$ of 2.9 kPa (22 mm Hg), or local anesthesia. There was no decline in the cognitive performance in any group after surgery, and no difference was found between groups. Studies in orthopedic surgery suggest that the mechanism for cognitive decline may be in the form of microemboli that have been identified using transcranial Doppler studies of the middle cerebral artery during surgery. Other studies in which transcranial Doppler was used in orthopedic surgery did not find any relation between the number of microemboli and changes in neuropsychological performance.[37,38] Intraoperative cerebral oxygen desaturation monitored by cerebral oximetry is associated with an increased risk of POCD in cardiac bypass surgery.[39]

## GENERAL ANESTHESIA, SURGERY, AND THE DEVELOPMENT OF POCD

There is a general agreement that POCD is likely to be multifactorial, although it remains unclear whether its occurrence is a result of surgery or general anesthesia. In 1955 Bedford[14] published a retrospective review of 1193 elderly patients, concluding that anesthesia could have lasting effects on cognitive function, and speculating that anesthetic agents may be partially responsible for the cognitive decline. This study was controversial, as many of the anesthetic records were incomplete. In a later study, Simpson and colleagues[40] prospectively investigated physical and mental changes after elective surgery in elderly patients, and concluded that anesthesia had no effects on either physical or mental performance. Moreover, most recent studies using objective cognitive measures report no significant difference in the incidence of long-term POCD after either general anesthesia or regional anesthesia in elderly patients.[16,30]

### *Anesthetic Agents*

Volatile anesthetics are widely used in clinical anesthesia, and researchers have made considerable progress in understanding how anesthetics affect central nervous system function, although the molecular and neuronal substrates remain a matter of debate.[41] Unfortunately, there are no studies on the anesthetic effects without surgery in elderly volunteers. However, there are some studies with small numbers of young and healthy subjects from which one can make inferences. In one study, seven young men (mean age, 25 years) were anesthetized with halothane for 14 minimal alveolar concentration hours.[42] The investigators reported generalized electroencephalogram slowing, reduction in a frequency, and increase in posterior d activity, which persisted for 6 to 8 days following halothane anesthesia. A rare sharp wave activity developed in 3 subjects along with psychological impairment in the first week following anesthesia. The investigators attribute this impairment to the persistence in the circulation of unchanged halothane. In another study, neither enflurane nor halothane had any negative effects on intelligence or perceptual motor function in healthy young adult men.[43] However, volunteers who received halothane did experience difficulty in remembering things and had difficulty concentrating, as well as faintness or dizziness and having to do things slowly to complete them correctly. These symptoms did not persist beyond 2 weeks. Although both studies show that even after protracted exposure to halothane central nervous system effects were absent after 2 weeks, they also show that lipid soluble anesthetics can reside in the nervous tissue for many days. Anesthetic agents paradoxically have also been shown to improve cognitive performance. A recent experiment was performed on male mice (age 4–5 months) to evaluate the effects of isoflurane anesthesia without surgery on cognitive function, cellular processes of learning and memory, and protein expression.[44] Compared with control animals, it was observed that: (1) isoflurane anesthesia improves cognitive performance and long-term potentiation in the CA1 region in hippocampal slices; (2) isoflurane anesthesia induces a selective upregulation of functional NR2B receptors in the hippocampus; and (3) isoflurane anesthesia induces NR2B-dependent long-term potentiation and NR2B-dependent improvement of learning and memory. Moreover, in humans a deeper level of general anesthesia, as defined by a median bispectral index score BIS level of 39 compared with BIS of 51 was associated with better cognitive performance 4 to 6 weeks postoperatively, particularly with respect to the ability to process information.[45] The investigators speculate that deeper levels of isoflurane anesthesia might have had a neuroprotective effect, perhaps by decreasing the cerebral metabolic rate. Important cellular mechanisms of isoflurane neuroprotection also occur through a calcium-mediated decrease in glutamate release, as well as through the preservation of the important neuronal regulatory enzyme CaMKIIB.[46] Benzodiazepines and POCD in elderly patients was investigated by Rasmussan and colleagues,[47] who examined the influence of long-acting benzodiazepines in a selected group of patients undergoing abdominal surgery using diazepam-based anesthesia. The incidence of POCD was 48% and therefore these patients appeared to be at increased risk. However, the researchers could not find any significant relationship between blood concentrations of benzodiazepines and change in the cognitive function 1 week after surgery. Propofol and fentanyl were compared for cerebral oxygenation during normothermic cardiopulmonary bypass and POCD.[48] Both propofol and fentanyl preserved cerebral oxygenation as estimated by jugular venous oxygenation during cardiopulmonary bypass, and propofol did not affect the cognitive performance following surgery.

### *Surgical Factors*

Surgical stress causes release of neuroendocrine hormones, and triggers an inflammatory response with release of cytokines that may be responsible for changes in brain function and recovery. There is corroborating evidence that minor surgical procedures are associated with decreased surgical stress, and results in less cognitive decline than after major surgery.[23] A relationship between the inflammatory mediator interleukin-6 and late functional recovery has also been reported.[49] The pattern of diurnal variation in cortisol level after major surgery is another important factor, as it is significantly associated with the occurrence of POCD.[50]

## PREVENTION OF POSTOPERATIVE COGNITIVE DYSFUNCTION

At present, there is no single therapy that can be recommended for treating postoperative cognitive decline, thus primary prevention is the most effective strategy.[8] Several preventive strategies have been investigated to reduce the occurrence of postoperative cognitive decline. Hypothermia (32°C) may be effective in reducing the cognitive dysfunction following cardiac surgery.[51] One may assume that avoiding cardiopulmonary bypass may cause less cognitive decline in cardiac surgery. However, a recent prospective randomized study reports that off-pump coronary artery bypass graft surgery did not result in decreased cognitive decline.[52] Regarding noncardiac surgical procedures, Gustafson and colleagues investigated several interventions on the occurrence of acute confusional state. These procedures included pre- and postoperative geriatric assessments, oxygen therapy, and early surgery, prevention of perioperative hypotension, and treatment of postoperative complications. The investigators compared this study to their earlier study as a historical control group, and found a decreased incidence of acute confusional state in the intervention study group compared with the historical control group. Furthermore, they reported that the acute confusional state that occurred in the intervention group was less severe and of shorter duration compared with that in the control group.[9,53] The concept of multimodal postoperative rehabilitation using well-defined perioperative management with adequate postoperative analgesia including epidurals, early oral nutrition, and early mobilization was investigated in elderly patients undergoing hip fracture surgery.[54] The investigators reported that, despite multimodal interventions, acute POCD was prevalent among hip fracture patients following surgery. Preoperative administration of vitamins and their effects on POCD was studied by Day and colleagues.[55] These investigators randomized 2 groups undergoing surgery for a fractured femur; one group received intravenous vitamins (B complex and C) whereas the control group received no supplement. Day and colleagues assessed participants on three occasions, 7, 14, and 84 days postoperatively, and found no decline and no difference between groups on any assessment.[55] Thus, at the present time, beyond the sound principles of maintaining good oxygenation and cerebral perfusion, and providing adequate analgesia and emotional support perioperatively, there is no proven effective strategy to prevent the development of POCD.

## ASSESSMENT OF POSTOPERATIVE COGNITIVE DYSFUNCTION

Several neuropsychological test batteries have been administered to evaluate cognitive changes over time or assess the effects of clinical interventions. Cognitive function is an evaluation of memory, sensorimotor speed, cognitive flexibility, and various aspects of motor performance. Preoperative and postoperative cognition is tested using basic tests described here.

### *Mini Mental State Examination*

Described in detail by Folstein and colleagues,[56] this test is a frequently used measure of general cognitive status that examines orientation (time and space) and memory, the ability to follow instructions, name objects, and write a sentence, as well as attention. The Mini Mental State Examination can be administered within 10 minutes, and a score of between 28 and 30 indicates intact cognitive functions (guidelines are in the reference[56]). A postoperative low score in comparison with the preoperative score is a concern, and may require enhanced postoperative follow-up and neurologic or neuropsychological consultations.

### *Clock Drawing Test*

The clock drawing test is administered to measure attention, planning, and organization. In this test, patients are asked to draw the face of a clock, put in all the numbers, and set the hands to 10 after 11 using paper and a pencil. This test assesses several tasks: the patient has to remember how the clock looks like, plan the clock face, appropriately align the numbers, and simultaneously remember the instructions while drawing the hands to the appropriate time. The task of setting the hands at 10 after 11 itself requires the patient to ignore the competing visual "10" while setting the hand to the appropriate number "2." The scoring involves the number of errors measured during the test.[57] This is a simple test and evaluates the patient's cognitive decline by comparing his or her performance before and after surgery.

### *List-Learning Test*

This test is an assessment of learning and retention of information using a sample of words. There are several list-learning tests available in clinical practice, and they differ regarding the number of words available and age appropriateness. For example, the Hopkins Verbal Learning test assesses an individual's ability to learn a list of 12 words over 3 different learning trials, whereas in the ISPOCD1 study, a 15-word list was used for the cognitive assessment. This test has multiple forms, which are valuable for repeat testing.

### *Paragraph or Story Memory Test*

Another way of assessing learning and memory is by paragraph or story memory tests. This test involves reading a paragraph or a story to an individual, and asking him or her to repeat the story both immediately and after a set time delay. A well-known story memory measure is the logical memory subtest from the Wechsler memory scale.

### *Other Tests*

There are additional tests used for the assessment of cognitive function. With the concept-shifting test the participant is required to alternate between letters and digits to assess processing speed. In the Stroop Color Word Interference Test, words spelling out a color are printed in contrasting ink color (eg, blue printed with red ink) and the participant is asked to tell the printed color of the word rather than the actual meaning of the word. This test assesses the patient's ability to concentrate and ignore distracting stimuli. In the Letter Digit Coding Test, the participants are asked to match letters with digits. This test estimates mental processing speed and concentration. Finally, the service of a neuropsychologist is valuable, as he or she is able not only to administer tests but also provide the comprehensive assessment and written documentation of the findings.

## BRAIN IMAGING

Brain magnetic resonance imaging (MRI) conducted preoperatively can provide baseline images to compare with postoperative MRI, and may also identify neuroanatomic risk factors for stroke. Brain functional MRI can identify eloquent areas involved in motor and language function in surgical patients, and can evaluate the risk of postoperative neurologic deficit. For example, patients with preexisting white matter lesions may have a greater risk of acute cognitive decline after surgery. Moreover, patients with preexisting white matter lesions and lacunae are associated with an increased risk of postoperative stroke.[58] In elderly patients white matter changes observed with increasing age are considered to be benign, but they are also seen in abundance in vascular dementia and may increase the risk for the development of postoperative cognitive decline.[59] Therefore, preoperative brain MRI theoretically may be helpful in assessing the risk versus benefit for a given elective surgical procedure in an elderly patient. However, the cost-effectiveness of preoperative MRI has not been studied, and it is highly unlikely that such a preoperative screening test would be covered by insurance.

## CONSEQUENCES OF POSTOPERATIVE COGNITIVE DYSFUNCTION

Postoperative cognitive dysfunction has been an underestimated complication after surgery, yet it is not only devastating to the patients but also the caregivers. Patients who have developed cognitive decline following surgery require more nursing care and longer hospital stay, resulting in additional hospital costs. Long-term postoperative cognitive decline correlates significantly with reduced activity of daily living, which indicates that patients with postoperative cognitive dysfunction need more assistance and attention with all activities compared with before surgery.[15] A recent prospective multicenter cohort study was conducted by Steinmetz and colleagues,[60] examining the long-term consequences of postoperative cognitive dysfunction. A total of 701 patients were followed up for a median of 8.5 years. It was reported that patients who had cognitive decline 3 months after noncardiac surgery were associated with an increased mortality. Furthermore, Steinmetz and colleagues also observed that patients showing cognitive decline at 1 week had an increased risk of leaving the labor market prematurely and a higher prevalence of time spent receiving social transfer payments. The investigators believe that the increased all-cause mortality among patients who had cognitive decline 3 months after surgery could be mediated through the inability to seek and follow up on medical treatment and care, leading to reduced preservation of their physical health.[60] Persistence of postoperative cognitive dysfunction 5 years after cardiac surgery has been noted to have a major effect on quality of life, as well as important social and financial implications.[26]

## FUTURE RESEARCH

The challenge of future research in POCD will likely focus on the following. (1) Elucidation of the mechanism responsible for age-related increased incidence. Fruitful approaches might include proteomics and genomics in search of the relevant single-nucleotide polymorphism. (2) Identification of the phenotypic expression that predisposes elderly patients to the development of POCD. This method may include preoperative screening with sophisticated brain imaging techniques. (3) Institution of perioperative intervention techniques. These techniques may include preoperative "mental exercise training," as well as postoperative therapy. POCD is a problem that will acquire increasing importance as the population ages, and a multidisciplinary approach involving neuroscientists, geriatricians, molecular biologists, neuropsychologists, in addition to anesthesiologists, will be needed.

## SUMMARY

Improvement in surgical technique, anesthesia, and intensive care has made it possible for elderly patients to undergo major surgical procedures that successfully prolong life. However, the occurrence of postoperative cognitive decline may affect their quality of life. POCD is multifactorial in origin, with increasing age as the leading risk factor, yet the mechanism is not fully understood. There is no convincing evidence to suggest general anesthesia causes occurrence of POCD, as the incidence of POCD is equivalent between patients receiving general and regional anesthesia. At the present time it is impossible to recommend an ideal anesthetic technique that will change cognitive outcome until further evidence accumulates. All available data support the concept that maintenance of adequate tissue oxygenation and hemodynamic stability, as well as a well planned anesthetic, might improve cognitive outcome in elderly patients. Anesthesiologists should inform the concerned patients and their families about the nature and risk of postoperative cognitive problems.

## REFERENCES

1. Etzioni DA, Liu JH, Maggard MA, et al. The aging population and its impact on surgery work force. Ann Surg 2003;238:170–7.

2. Fong HK, Sands LP, Leung JM. The role of postoperative analgesia in delirium and cognitive decline in elderly patients: a systematic review. Anesth Analg 2006;102:1255–66.
3. Inouye SK, Van Dyck CH, Alessi CA, et al. Clarifying confusion: the confusion assessment method. A new method for detection of delirium. Ann Intern Med 1990;113(12):941–8.
4. Parikh SS, Chung F. Postoperative delirium in the elderly. Anesth Analg 1995;80: 1223–32.
5. Robinson TN, Raeburn CD, Tran ZV, et al. Postoperative delirium in the elderly: risk factors and outcomes. Ann Surg 2009;249:173–8.
6. Marcantonio ER, Goldman L, Orav EJ, et al. The association of intraoperative factors with the development of postoperative delirium. Am J Med 1998;105:380–4.
7. Simpson KH, Smith RJ, Davies LF, et al. Comparison of the effects of atropine and glycopyrrolate on cognitive function following general anesthesia. Br J Anaesth 1987;59:966–9.
8. Bekker AY, Weeks EJ. Cognitive function after anaesthesia in the elderly. Best Pract Res Clin Anaesthesiol 2003;17:259–72.
9. Gustafson Y, Brännström B, Berggren D, et al. A geriatric-anesthesiologic program to reduce acute confusional states in elderly patients treated for femoral neck fractures. J Am Geriatr Soc 1991;39(7):655–62.
10. Ge Y, Grossman RI, Babb JS, et al. Age-related total gray matter and white matter changes in normal adult brain. Part II: quantitative magnetization transfer ratio histogram analysis. AJNR Am J Neuroradiol 2002;23:1334–41.
11. Mrak RE, Grifin ST, Graham DI, et al. Aging-associated changes in human brain. J Neuropathol Exp Neurol 1997;56:1269–75.
12. Peters A. Structural changes that occur during normal aging of primate cerebral hemispheres. Neurosci Biobehav Rev 2002;26:733–41.
13. Diehl M. Everyday competence in later life: current status and future directions. Gerontology 1998;38:422–33.
14. Bedford PD. Adverse cerebral effects of anesthesia on old people. Lancet 1955; 269:259–63.
15. Moller JT, Cluitmans P, Rasmussen LS, et al. Long-term postoperative cognitive dysfunction in the elderly ISPOCD1 study. ISPOCD investigators. International Study of Post-Operative Cognitive Dysfunction. Lancet 1998;351:857–61.
16. Williams-Russo P, Sharrock NE, Mattis S, et al. Cognitive effects after epidural vs general anesthesia in older adults. A randomized trial. JAMA 1995;274:44–50.
17. Arrowsmith JE, Grocott HP, Reves JG, et al. Central nervous system complications of cardiac surgery. Br J Anaesth 2000;84(3):378.
18. Newman M, Kirchner JL, Phillips-Bute B, et al. Longitudinal assessment of neurocognitive function after coronary-artery bypass surgery. N Engl J Med 2001;344: 395–402.
19. Savageau JA, Stanton BA, Jenkins CD, et al. Neuropsychological dysfunction following elective cardiac operation. II. A six-month reassessment. J Thorac Cardiovasc Surg 1982;84:595–600.
20. Savageau JA, Stanton BA, Jenkins CD, et al. Neuropsychological dysfunction following elective cardiac operation. I. Early assessment. J Thorac Cardiovasc Surg 1982;84:585–94.
21. Laalou FZ, Carre AC, Forestier C, et al. Pathophysiology of post-operative cognitive dysfunction: current hypotheses. J Chir (Paris) 2008;145:323–300 [in French].
22. Rasmussen LS, Moller JT. Central nervous system dysfunction after anesthesia in the geriatric patient. Anesthesiol Clin North America 2000;18:59–70.

23. Canet J, Raeder J, Rasmussen LS, et al. Cognitive dysfunction after minor surgery in the elderly. Acta Anaesthesiol Scand 2003;47(10):1204–10.
24. Abildstrom H, Rasmussen LS, Rentowl P, et al. Cognitive dysfunction 1-2 years after non-cardiac surgery in the elderly. Acta Anaesthesiol Scand 2000;44: 1246–51.
25. Monk TG, Weldon BC, Garvan CW, et al. Predictors of cognitive dysfunction after major noncardiac surgery. Anesthesiology 2008;108:18–30.
26. Newman MF, Grocott HP, Mathew JP, et al. Report of the substudy assessing the impact of neurocognitive function on quality of life 5 years after cardiac surgery. Stroke 2001;32:2874–81.
27. Veliz-Reissmuller G, Aguero Torres H, van der Linden J, et al. Pre-operative mild cognitive dysfunction predicts risk for post-operative delirium after elective cardiac surgery. Aging Clin Exp Res 2007;19:172–7.
28. Hocker J, Stapelfeldt C, Leiendecker J, et al. Postoperative neurocognitive dysfunction in elderly patients after xenon versus propofol anesthesia for major noncardiac surgery: a double-blinded randomized controlled pilot study. Anesthesiology 2009;110:1068–76.
29. Leung JM, Sands LP, Vaurio LE, et al. Nitrous oxide does not change the incidence of postoperative delirium or cognitive decline in elderly surgical patients. Br J Anaesth 2006;96:754–60.
30. Rasmussen LS, Johnson T, Kuipers HM, et al. Does anaesthesia cause postoperative cognitive dysfunction? A randomised study of regional versus general anaesthesia in 438 elderly patients. Acta Anaesthesiol Scand 2003;47:260–6.
31. Rasmussen LS. Postoperative cognitive dysfunction: incidence and prevention. Best Pract Res Clin Anaesthesiol 2006;20:315–30.
32. Moller JT, Svennild I, Johannessen NW, et al. Perioperative monitoring with pulse oximetry and late postoperative cognitive dysfunction. Br J Anaesth 1993;71: 340–7.
33. Rollason WN, Robertson GS, Cordiner CM, et al. A comparison of mental function in relation to hypotensive and normotensive anesthesia in the elderly. Br J Anaesth 1971;43:561–6.
34. Williams-Russo P, Sharrock NE, Mattis S, et al. Randomized trial of hypotensive epidural anesthesia in older adults. Anesthesiology 1999;91:926–35.
35. Yocum GT, Gaudet JG, Teverbaugh LA, et al. Neurocognitive performance in hypertensive patients after spine surgery. Anesthesiology 2009;110:254–61.
36. Jhaveri RM. The effects of hypocapnic ventilation on mental function in elderly patients undergoing cataract surgery. Anaesthesia 1989;44:635–40.
37. Koch S, Forteza A, Lavernia C, et al. Cerebral fat microembolism and cognitive decline after hip and knee replacement. Stroke 2007;38:1079–81.
38. Rodriguez RA, Tellier A, Grabowski J, et al. Cognitive dysfunction after total knee arthroplasty: effects of intraoperative cerebral embolization and postoperative complications. J Arthroplasty 2005;20:763–71.
39. Slater JP, Guarino T, Stack J, et al. Cerebral oxygen desaturation predicts cognitive decline and longer hospital stay after cardiac surgery. Ann Thorac Surg 2009; 87:36–44.
40. Simpson BR, Williams M, Scott JF, et al. The effects of anaesthesia and elective surgery on old people. Lancet 1961;2:887–93.
41. Urban BW. Current assessment of targets and theories of anesthesia. Br J Anaesth 2002;89:167–83.
42. Bruchiel KJ, Stockard JJ, Calverley RK, et al. Electroencephalographic abnormalities following halothane anesthesia. Anesth Analg 1978;57:244–51.

43. Storms LH, Stark AH, Calverley RK, et al. Psychological functioning after halothane or enfluran anesthesia. Anesth Analg 1980;59:245–9.
44. Rammes G, Starker LK, Haseneder R, et al. Isoflurane anaesthesia reversibly improves cognitive function and long-term potentiation (LTP) via an up-regulation in NMDA receptor 2B subunit expression. Neuropharmacology 2009;56:626–36.
45. Farag E, Chelune GJ, Schubert A, et al. Is depth of anesthesia, as assessed by the Bispectral Index, related to postoperative cognitive dysfunction and recovery? Anesth Analg 2006;103:633–40.
46. Blanck TJ, Haile M, Xu F, et al. Isoflurane pretreatment ameliorates postischemic neurologic dysfunction and preserves hippocampal $Ca^{2+}$/calmodulin-dependent protein kinase in a canine cardiac arrest model. Anesthesiology 2000;93:1285–93.
47. Rasmussen LS, Steentoft A, Rasmussen H, et al. Benzodiazepines and postoperative cognitive dysfunction in the elderly. ISPOCD Group. International Study of Postoperative Cognitive Dysfunction. Br J Anaesth 1999;83:585–9.
48. Kadoi Y, Saito S, Kunimoto F, et al. Comparative effects of propofol versus fentanyl on cerebral oxygenation state during normothermic cardiopulmonary bypass and postoperative cognitive dysfunction. Ann Thorac Surg 2003;75:840–6.
49. Hall G, Peerbhoy D, Shenkin A, et al. Relationship of the functional recovery after hip arthroplasty to the neuroendocrine and inflammatory response. Br J Anaesth 2001;87:537–42.
50. Rasmussen LS, O'Brien JT, Silverstein JH, et al. Is peri-operative cortisol secretion related to post-operative cognitive dysfunction? Acta Anaesthesiol Scand 2005;49:1225–31.
51. Regragui I. The effects of cardiopulmonary bypass temperature on neuropsychologic outcome after coronary artery operations: A prospective randomized trial. J Thorac Cardiovasc Surg 1996;112(4):1036–45.
52. Jensen BO, Rasmussen LS, Steinbruchel DA. Cognitive outcomes in elderly high-risk patients 1 year after off-pump versus on-pump coronary artery bypass grafting. A randomized trial. Eur J Cardiothorac Surg 2008;34:1016–21.
53. Gustafson Y, Berggren D, Brännström B, et al. Acute confusional state in elderly patients treated for femoral neck fracture. J Am Geriatr Soc 1988;36(6):525–30.
54. Bitsch MS, Foss NB, Kristensen BB, et al. Acute cognitive dysfunction after hip fracture: frequency and risk factors in an optimized, multimodal, rehabilitation program. Acta Anaesthesiol Scand 2006;50:428–36.
55. Day J, Bayer AJ, McMahon M, et al. Thiamine status, vitamin supplements and postoperative confusion. Age Ageing 1988;17(1):29–34.
56. Folstein M, Fostein SE, McHugh PR, et al. "Mini Mental State". A practical method for grading the cognitive state of patients for the clinician. J Psychiatr Res 1975;12:189–98.
57. Libon D. Further analysis of clock drawings among demented and non demented subjects. Arch Clin Neuropsychol 1996;11:193–205.
58. Floyd TF, Shah PN, Price CC, et al. Clinically silent cerebral ischemic events after cardiac surgery: their incidence, regional vascular occurrence, and procedural dependence. Ann Thorac Surg 2006;81:2160–6.
59. Roman GC. Vascular dementia may be the most common form of dementia in the elderly. J Neurol Sci 2002;203–204:7–10.
60. Steinmetz J, Christensen KB, Lund T, et al. Long-term consequences of postoperative cognitive dysfunction. Anesthesiology 2009;110:548–55.

# Diastolic Dysfunction, Cardiovascular Aging, and the Anesthesiologist

David Sanders, MD, Michael Dudley, MD, Leanne Groban, MD*

**KEYWORDS**

• Diastolic dysfunction • Cardiovascular aging
• Echocardiography • Tissue doppler imaging • Perioperative

A 74-year-old woman presented to the preoperative assessment clinic (PAC) before elective, right shoulder arthroplasty. Her past medical history was significant for hypertension, osteoarthritis, and mild chronic obstructive pulmonary disease. She denied any cardiovascular symptoms with the exception of increasing exertional shortness of breath while walking her dog up the hill to her house. She attributed this change in exercise tolerance to getting older and out of shape. The patient quit smoking 25 years ago and regularly takes her antihypertensive regimen of hydrochlorothiazide and lisinopril. In the PAC her vital signs were as follows: blood pressure 158/64 mmHg, pulse 78 beats/min, and room air oxygen saturation 100%. Auscultation of her chest revealed clear lung sounds and a regular cardiac rate and rhythm with a midgrade (3–4/6) systolic ejection murmur radiating to her carotid arteries. A 12-lead electrocardiogram showed normal sinus rhythm and nonspecific S-T wave changes. A transthoracic echocardiogram was obtained which revealed a normal ejection fraction of 65%, impaired left ventricular relaxation, moderate concentric left ventricular hypertrophy, moderate left atrial enlargement, and severe aortic valve stenosis (aortic valve atresia [AVA] = 0.9 $cm^2$; peak gradient 60 mmHg) with mild aortic regurgitation. The patient was referred to cardiology and subsequently underwent a coronary and right heart catheterization, which showed nonobstructive coronary disease, a peak left ventricular pressure gradient of 75 mmHg, and an end-diastolic pressure of 22 mmHg.

The patient was scheduled for aortic valve replacement surgery with cardiopulmonary bypass (CPB). Intraoperative anesthetic and surgical care of the patient were

Supported in part by grants to L. Groban from the Hartford Foundation Project, American Geriatrics Society, Anesthesia Initiative on Aging Education: Geriatrics for Specialists Initiative and Paul Beeson Award, National Institutes of Aging K08 AG-026764-04.
Department of Anesthesiology, Wake Forest University School of Medicine, Medical Center Boulevard, Winston-Salem, NC 27157-1009, USA
* Corresponding author.
*E-mail address:* lgroban@wfubmc.edu (L. Groban).

Anesthesiology Clin 27 (2009) 497–517
doi:10.1016/j.anclin.2009.07.008 **anesthesiology.theclinics.com**

uneventful; she was managed with an isoflurane- and fentanyl-based anesthetic, and muscle relaxation was achieved with cisatracurium. A 23-mm stentless, bioprosthetic aortic valve was inserted and the patient was weaned from CPB without inotropes. Following closure of her sternum, transient episodes of hypotension (80/60 mmHg) occurred with concomitant echocardiographic evidence of left ventricular (LV) underfilling that responded to volume loading with colloid. The patient was hemodynamically stable on transfer to the intensive care unit (ICU), sedated with dexmedetomidine, and on a low dose infusion of phenylephrine. During the first 6 hours in the ICU, the patient's cardiac index dipped below 2.0 which corresponded to her low cardiac filling pressure (left ventricular end diastolic pressure [LVEDP] < 18 mmHg) and labile blood pressure. Because of the minimal chest tube drainage and hemodynamic lability, a bedside transesophageal echocardiogram (TEE) was performed which was negative for evidence of cardiac tamponade, but it did confirm a relative hypovolemia. The patient responded well to volume resuscitation and her hemodynamics stabilized at an LVEDP 24 mmHg. She was subsequently weaned from the ventilator on the morning of postoperative day (POD) 1 and remained hemodynamically stable and cognitively intact before transfer to a floor bed on POD 2.

On POD 3 her family remarked that she was not herself and somewhat disoriented. Her oxygen requirements had increased over the preceding 24 hours, and her physical examination and chest radiograph were consistent with pulmonary edema. An electrocardiogram revealed atrial fibrillation. Her blood pressure was 95/60 mmHg. The patient was transferred to the ICU for closer observation, and for reintubation after low oxygen saturation did not respond to face shield oxygen or Bi-level Positive Airway Pressure (BiPAP). Her cardiac rhythm was medically converted with amiodarone, and she was carefully diuresed with furosemide before extubation a day later. She progressed slowly and was discharged to a rehabilitation facility on POD 8 before returning to her home.

The above case represents a common scenario. Changes in the epidemiology of patients undergoing cardiac and major noncardiac surgery,[1–3] coupled with the growing number of older persons with HF,[4,5] may make future perioperative care more difficult.[6] Although our patient reached hospital discharge with no long-term sequelae, her postoperative course was prolonged and complicated. She exemplifies the limited physiologic reserve that characterizes many persons in her cohort. The question of how to recognize and manage this situation arises and is best addressed through an examination of the physiology of the early spectrum of cardiovascular disease, specifically that of aging and diastolic dysfunction. The valvular lesion that was discovered should not distract the reader from the physiologic derangements that were exposed after aortic valve repair; this patient's hemodynamic lability, poor tolerance of volume shifts, cardiac arrhythmia, and eventual reintubation and ICU recidivism occurred despite normal systolic indices and a well-functioning aortic valve prosthesis. In addition, this patient could revisit the same set of perioperative issues when she returns for her shoulder arthroplasty.

This review focuses on the physiology and management of the patient with diastolic dysfunction from the standpoint of the cardiac anesthesiologist, echocardiographer, and general anesthesiologist. Diastolic dysfunction, the precursor of diastolic HF, has been called the great masquerader.[7] Because its clinical presentation may erroneously be ascribed to chronic obstructive pulmonary disease or to normal aging, diastolic heart disease may remain undiagnosed or ignored. Other than exercise intolerance,[8,9] symptoms associated with isolated diastolic HF in the elderly include weakness, anorexia, fatigue, and mental confusion. One clue in identifying this disorder is the diastolic dysfunction phenotype; that is, the 65-year-old, postmenopausal, hypertensive female patient.[10] Indeed, diastolic dysfunction represents a part of the physiologic spectrum that progresses from normal aging to advanced cardiovascular disease. Although the perioperative risk for the healthy, elderly patient with isolated diastolic dysfunction is not yet known,[11,12] extrapolations from cardiac surgery and cardiology data suggest that it is associated with increased morbidity and mortality.[13–17] Therefore, the perioperative physician is obliged to understand age-related changes in the heart and vasculature that affect diastolic function and to become knowledgeable on the diagnostic and prognostic echocardiographic measures of diastolic function so that perioperative management can be modified in a way that may improve outcomes in the elderly.

## PHYSIOLOGIC CHANGES OF AGING AND DIASTOLIC DYSFUNCTION

Several changes in cardiac structure and function occur with aging that contribute to diastolic dysfunction. On the structural level, there is a decrease in myocyte number, an increase in myocyte size, and an increase in the amount of connective tissue matrix.[18,19] Myocyte number decreases because of cell necrosis and apoptosis. As myocytes are lost they are replaced with fibroblasts, and the remaining myocytes hypertrophy. As the fibroblasts produce collagen, interstitial fibrosis occurs and the heart becomes stiffer and less compliant. The stiffer and less compliant ventricle affects diastolic relaxation as well as systolic contraction. Chronically elevated afterload from stiff vasculature leads to left ventricular hypertrophy (LVH) and prolongation in systolic contraction time. Prolonged systolic contraction, in turn, impinges on early diastole.[20–23]

The two main consequences of age-related arterial stiffening are decreased aortic distensibility and increased pulse wave velocity.[24,25] The aorta is responsible for cushioning the pulse energy generated by the heart and converting it into stored energy through the elastic recoil of the vessel. The loss of distensibility during systole results in a higher systolic pressure (**Fig. 1**), and less stored energy to augment forward flow during diastole. This loss is manifested by a lower diastolic pressure (**Fig. 2**). The resultant increased pulse pressure is an established risk factor for cardiovascular events.[26–29]

The pulse wave velocity is the speed at which the pressure wave, generated by the contracting heart, travels to the periphery and is responsible for a palpable pulse. As vessels become stiffer, the pulse wave becomes faster. The pressure wave is reflected from the periphery, mainly at arterial branch sites, similar to sound waves reflected as echoes. In the younger adult with compliant vessels, the reflected wave returns to the heart during diastole, which augments aortic diastolic pressure and coronary perfusion. However, as the pulse wave velocity increases with stiffened vessels, the reflected wave returns during late systole, which augments systolic pressure, increasing afterload and the pulse pressure width. This increase is analogous to a mistimed intra-aortic balloon pump (IABP). Inflation of an IABP before aortic valve closure leads to an increase in left ventricular end-diastolic volume (LVEDV), LVEDP, LV wall stress (afterload), and oxygen demand. Thus, the large vessel stiffening of advanced age can lead to greater myocardial stroke work, wall tension, and oxygen consumption in the older heart compared with the younger heart. In addition, these arterial changes contribute to altered diastolic function; afterload directly affects LV relaxation, and is a stimulus for hypertrophy of the myocardium.[30,31]

Although most elderly patients presenting for surgery will have normal ejection fractions (EFs) by echocardiogram, up to a one-third of these patients will have abnormal diastolic function.[14] An understanding of the phases of diastole and associated

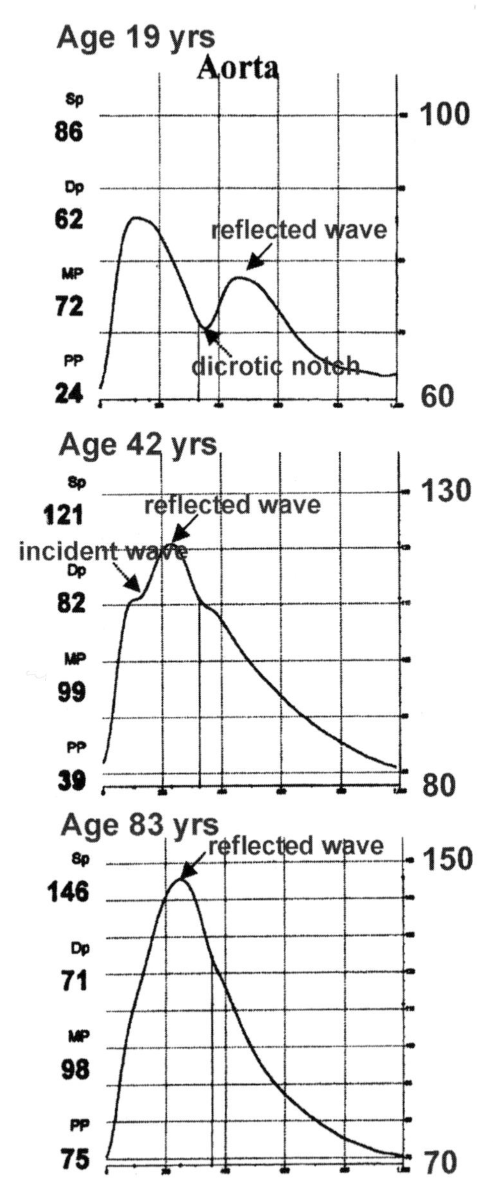


**Fig. 1.** Age-related arterial stiffness and pressure waveform shapes. (*From* Dudley M, Groban L. Cardiovascular changes in the elderly and their anesthetic implications. Curr Rev Clin Anesth 2009;22:266; with permission.)

physiologic determinants is important to understand how age-related changes in cardiac structure and function influence diastology (**Box 1**). At the mechanical level (**Fig. 3**), diastole begins with aortic valve closure when the pressure within the left ventricle begins to decrease, and is called the isovolumic relaxation phase. The LV pressure will continue to decrease even after the opening of the mitral valve. In fact, LV pressure falls below left atrial pressure as a result of elastic recoil, creating a suction effect. Rapid filling of the left ventricle occurs during this phase. Normally, LV

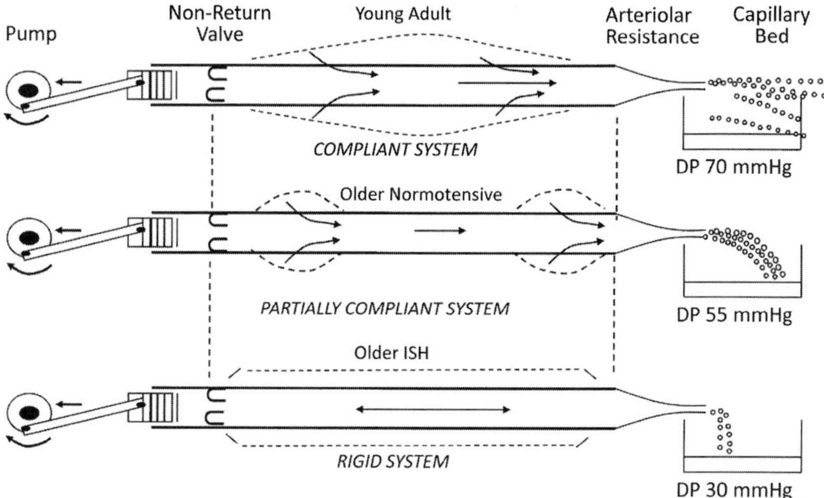


**Fig. 2.** Blood pressure as a result of ejection of blood (eg, stroke volume) into a series of tubes the diameter of which vary with pulsating pressure. In the young adult, the aorta cushions the cardiac pulsation by converting pressure energy into elastic energy through distension. Once the heart ceases ejection and the pressure falls, the walls of the aorta recoil and the elastic energy is reconverted into pressure energy. This conversion reduces the magnitude of pressure change and allows for a steady flow beyond the arterioles, which accounts for the diastolic component of BP. With aging and hypertension, the aorta and other major conduit vessels become rigid, leading to a loss of cushioning of the ejected energy. Accordingly, this loss of stored energy manifests in extremes in pressure; increased pulse pressure and low diastolic pressure. (*Adapted from* Baird RN, Abbott WM. Pulsatile blood-flow in arterial grafts. Lancet 1976;ii:948; with permission.)

relaxation ends in the first third of rapid filling so that most left ventricular filling is dependent on such properties as left ventricular compliance, ventricular interaction (eg, synchronicity), and pericardial restraint. Finally, atrial systole contributes to the rest of LV volume. In the young heart, approximately 80% of LV filling is complete by the end of the passive filling phase, with the remainder occurring during active atrial transport. In contrast, with advanced age, impairments in early diastolic relaxation and ventricular compliance alter filling dynamics such that atrial transport becomes the

**Box 1**
**Principle effects of aging on the cardiovascular system**

- Increased arterial stiffness
- Increased myocardial stiffness
- Impaired β-adrenergic responsiveness
- Impaired endothelial function
- Reduced sinus node function
- Decreased baroreceptor responsiveness
- Net effect: marked reduction in cardiovascular reserve

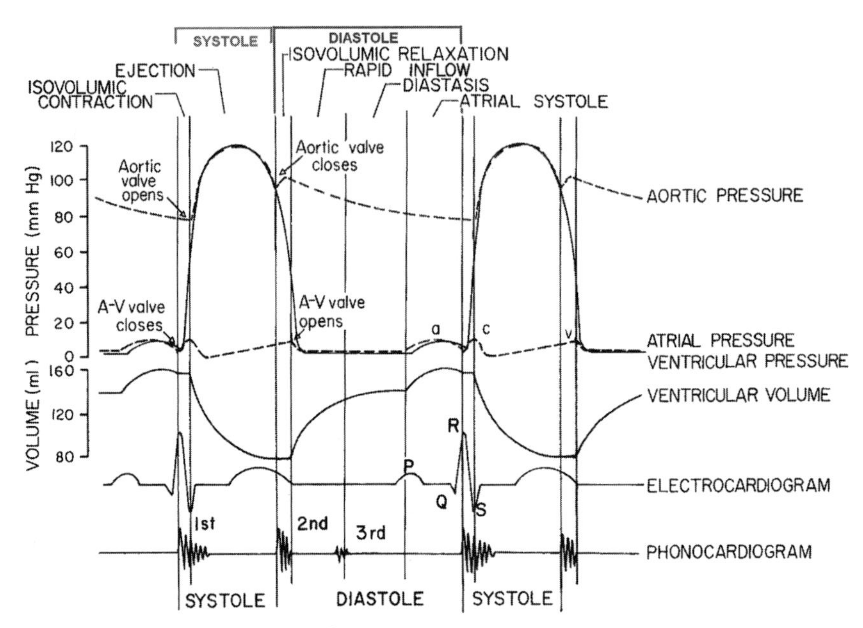


**Fig. 3.** Cardiac cycle with phases of diastole.

more important contributor to diastolic volume. This so-called atrial kick is essential to maintain an adequate preload, particularly if the preceding three phases of diastole are adversely influenced by age-related changes in cardiac structure and function.

The diagnosis of diastolic dysfunction can be made from cardiac catheterization and Doppler LV diastolic filling patterns. Catheterization data show increases in ventricular diastolic pressure (>16 mmHg) with preserved systolic function and normal ventricular volumes. Most Doppler LV diastolic filling patterns can be categorized into 1 of 4 distinct categories (**Fig. 4**). The normal pattern is seen in healthy young and middle-aged persons. In sinus rhythm, there are two peaks in the Doppler diastolic filling profile that occur in response to the pressure gradient between the left atrium (LA) and left ventricle; early in diastole following mitral valve opening when LV pressure falls below LA pressure, and late in diastole when atrial contraction increases LA pressure above LV pressure. The LV filling pattern in healthy young subjects is characterized by predominant rapid filling early in diastole with modest additional filling during atrial contraction. The filling pattern can be quantified by measuring the peak early diastolic flow velocity (E) and the peak flow velocity during atrial contraction (A), and expressing this as E/A ratio (**Fig. 5**). Normally, the E/A ratio in young subjects is greater than one.

The first pattern of altered LV filling is called "delayed relaxation" (see **Fig. 4**). In this pattern there is reduced peak rate and amount of early filling, and the relative importance of atrial filling is enhanced, resulting in a reversed E/A ratio of less than 1 (eg, E<A). This decreased rate of early filling is a result of a decreased early diastolic LA to LV pressure gradient, caused by a slowed rate of LV relaxation. Although a delayed relaxation pattern can be seen in patients with LV hypertrophy, atrial hypertension, and coronary artery disease, it is normally seen in healthy older persons who are free of cardiovascular disease.

The other two patterns (see **Fig. 4**) of altered LV filling are always abnormal, including in the elderly. The first has been called pseudonormalization, as the E/A ratio

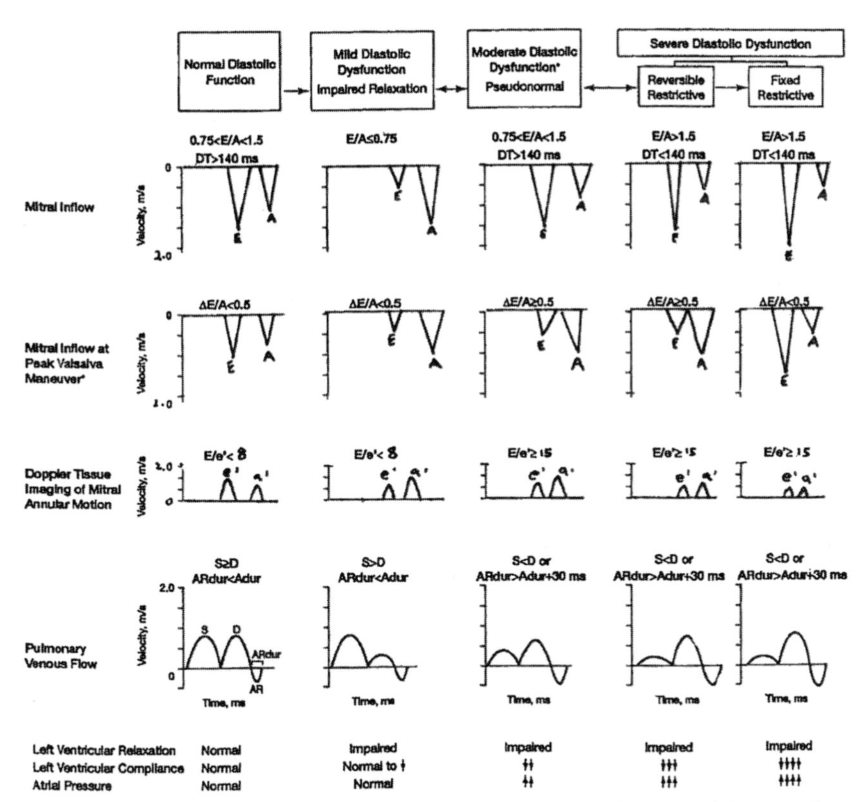


**Fig. 4.** Doppler criteria for classification of diastolic function. (*Reprinted from* Groban L, Dolinski SY. Transesophageal echocardiographic evaluation of diastolic function. Chest 2005;128:3658; with permission.)

is greater than one (as seen in young normals). This pattern results from an increase in LA pressure that compensates for the slowed rate of LV relaxation and restores early diastolic LV pressure gradient to the baseline level seen in younger persons. The left atrium pushes to fill the LV, whereas in the young patient, the left ventricle fills by creating a suction effect. Elevated left atrial pressure results in left atrial enlargement as a result of pressure and volume overload. It has been suggested that left atrial enlargement is associated with age;[32,33] however, there is evidence that increased left atrial size is not a normal result of aging,[34,35] and is more likely a compensatory response to impaired LV relaxation. Left atrial volume increases with progressively worsening diastolic function,[36–38] and is a risk factor for complications including atrial fibrillation and embolic stroke. To differentiate normal from pseudo-normal, the patient's preload can be reduced using nitroglycerin or with the introduction of a Valsalva maneuver, potentially uncovering an E <A pattern and impaired relaxation. Another way to circumvent the preload dependency of transmitral Doppler is the use of myocardial (or annular) velocities by tissue Doppler (TDI) as discussed later.

In the final altered LV filling pattern, called "restrictive," early filling is increased abnormally, even more than that seen in young normals. Moreover, as a result of diminished atrial filling, because of reduced atrial contractility, the E/A ratio is often greater than two. This pattern is seen in patients with severe diastolic dysfunction, pulmonary congestion, and end-stage dilated cardiomyopathy. Similar to

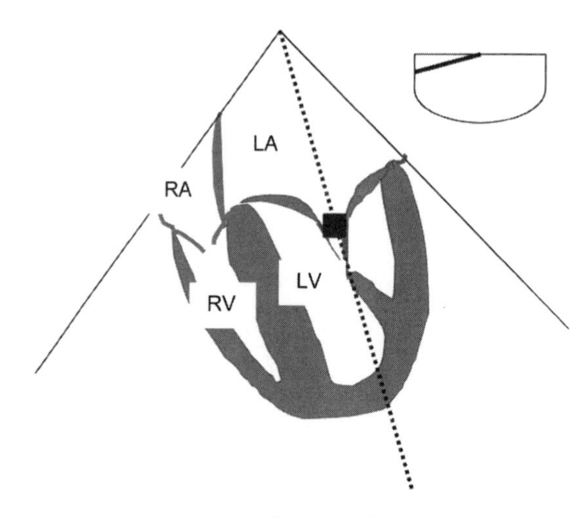


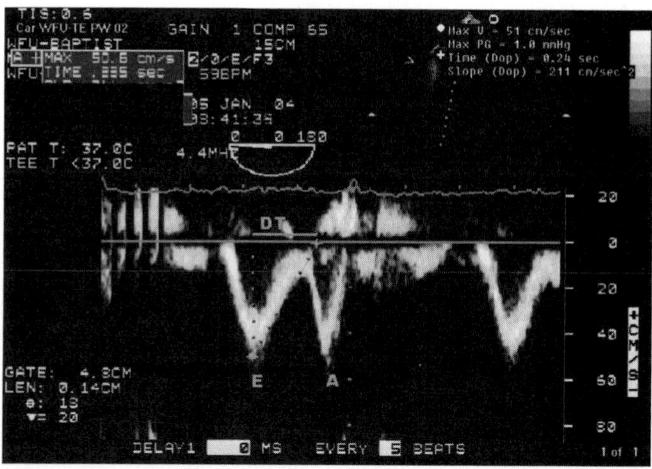


**Fig. 5.** (*Top*) the midesophageal 4-chamber view with pulsed wave Doppler (PWD) imaging sample volume at the level of the tips of the open mitral valve leaflets. (*Bottom*) transmitral blood flow velocity profile obtained with PWD imaging at the midesophageal 4-chamber view. (*Reprinted from* Groban L, Dolinski SY. Transesophageal echocardiographic evaluation of diastolic function. Chest 2005;128:3656; with permission.)

pseudonormalization, reversible and irreversible restrictive disease can be distinguished from each other by Valsalva maneuver. In reversible, restrictive disease the mitral inflow pattern becomes abnormal with the A > E whereas in irreversible, restrictive disease the E wave remains greater than the A wave owing to the stiff ventricle and high filling pressures. Each abnormal filling pattern results from a variable combination of delayed early relaxation, increased LA pressure, and increased LV chamber stiffness. Indeed, these patterns represent a continuum from normal to severe diastolic dysfunction, with progressively increasing LV chamber stiffness.

It is important to distinguish the difference between diastolic dysfunction and diastolic HF (**Box 2**). Diastolic dysfunction is a physiologic or preclinical state in which abnormal relaxation or increased LV stiffness is compensated for by increasing LA pressure so that LV preload remains adequate. These patients may be considered

**Box 2**
**Risk factors for diastolic heart failure**

- Age >70 years, hypertensive woman
- Systolic hypertension, increased pulse pressure (>60 mmHg)
- Diabetes, chronic renal insufficiency
- Echo: normal EF, delayed relaxation, left atrial enlargement (LAE) > 50 mm, LVH
- ECG: previous myocardial ischemia (MI), LVH, atrial fibrillation (AF)
- Recent weight gain (fluid overload)
- Exercise intolerance
- B-type natriuretic peptide (BNP) > 120 (BNP of 200 pg/mL may not be clinically significant in older, postmenopausal women)

American College of Cardiology/American Heart Association (ACC/AHA) stage A or stage B because they are asymptomatic.[39] Progression to diastolic HF, ACC/AHA stage C or D, is characterized by signs and symptoms of HF with normal EF (>50%), the absence of valvular disease, and echocardiographic evidence of diastolic dysfunction. Diastolic HF is a true heart failure syndrome, as neurohormonal activation is triggered in a similar manner to that which occurs in systolic HF.[40,41]

The pathophysiology of diastolic HF is characterized by a low cardiac output state resulting from a stiff, thickened ventricle with a small cavity. Relaxation is slow in early diastole and offers greater resistance to filling in late diastole, so that diastolic pressures are elevated. Elevated left atrial pressure is transmitted backward through the valveless pulmonary veins to the pulmonary capillary bed. Under normal resting conditions, the patient may be asymptomatic. However, periods of activity or stress which increase heart rate, stroke volume, end-diastolic volume or blood pressure (BP) result in pulmonary overload, manifesting as shortness of breath, fatigue, and, most commonly, exertional dyspnea.[8] Accordingly, because patients with diastolic dysfunction are often asymptomatic at rest, it is important to inquire about exercise tolerance.[9] Indeed, the presentation of HF in older patients may be insidious or sudden with the onset of severe shortness of breath usually attributable to pulmonary edema. However, patients may complain only of fatigue or lack of energy, which may be attributable to physical deconditioning. Even though signs/symptoms and clinical examination can provide useful information, such as AF, displaced apex, and jugular venous distension, accurately diagnosing older patients with suspected HF can be difficult. Although it is beyond the scope of this review, investigations for an older patient with suspected HF should include a combination of simple blood tests such as serum electrolytes, 12-lead electrocardiogram, chest radiology, BNP, and echocardiography.

## THE CARDIAC SURGERY PATIENT WITH DIASTOLIC DYSFUNCTION

It is well established that complications following cardiac surgery are encountered in patients of advanced age. Other risk stratification characteristics that are typically encountered include prolonged CPB time, female sex, and diminished systolic function;[42,43] however, there may exist a group of patients who are still at elevated risk for a more complicated hospital course who do not necessarily display these characteristics. Specifically, the echocardiographic identification of diastolic dysfunction and the presence of elevated diastolic filling pressures can yield meaningful information that can help identify these patients and guide perioperative management.

As discussed previously, the LV inflow Doppler is the most commonly used measurement in the echocardiographic examination of diastolic function because transmitral flow patterns and associated deceleration times represent increasing degrees of LV diastolic impairment. Because these measurements, along with the pulmonary venous waveform patterns, change rapidly with preload variations, heart rate (HR) and rhythm disturbances,[44–46] tissue Doppler imaging is considered to be a more sensitive tool in the assessment of diastolic function (**Fig. 6**). Tissue Doppler imaging (TDI) is a modality that measures myocardial velocity, in contrast to traditional Doppler, which measures blood flow velocity and may not represent actual myocardial properties.[47] Mitral annular motion has been shown in experimental animal work and in humans to relate well with invasive indices of relaxation.[48–51] The measurements e′, representing the early diastolic active relaxation phase, and a′, the late diastolic atrial

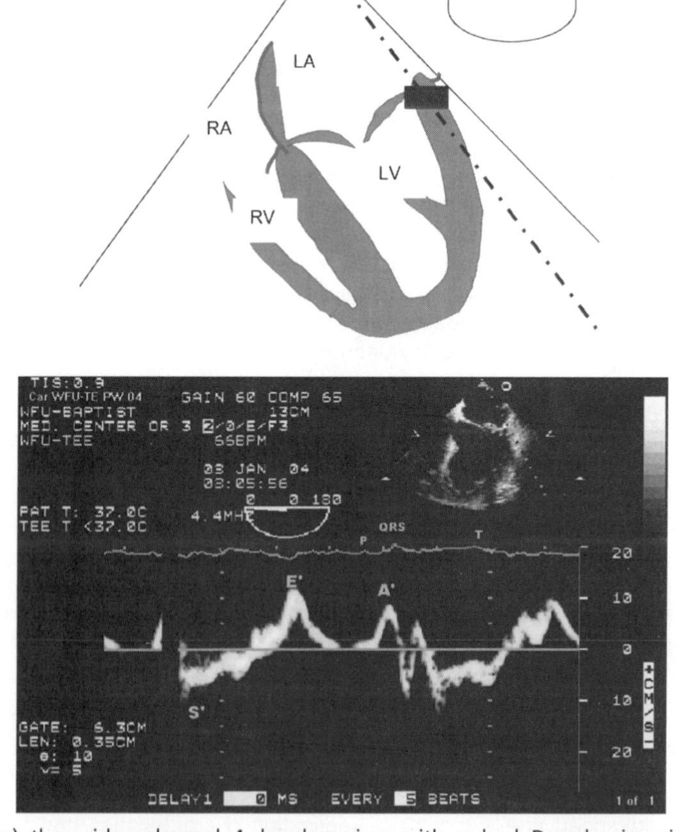


**Fig. 6.** (*Top*) the midesophageal 4-chamber view with pulsed Doppler imaging sample volume located at the lateral mitral annular wall for TDI assessment of diastolic function. (*Bottom*) lateral mitral annular tissue Doppler waveforms for the assessment of left ventricular diastolic function. (*Reprinted from* Groban L, Dolinski SY. Transesophageal echocardiographic evaluation of diastolic function. Chest 2005;128:3660; with permission.)

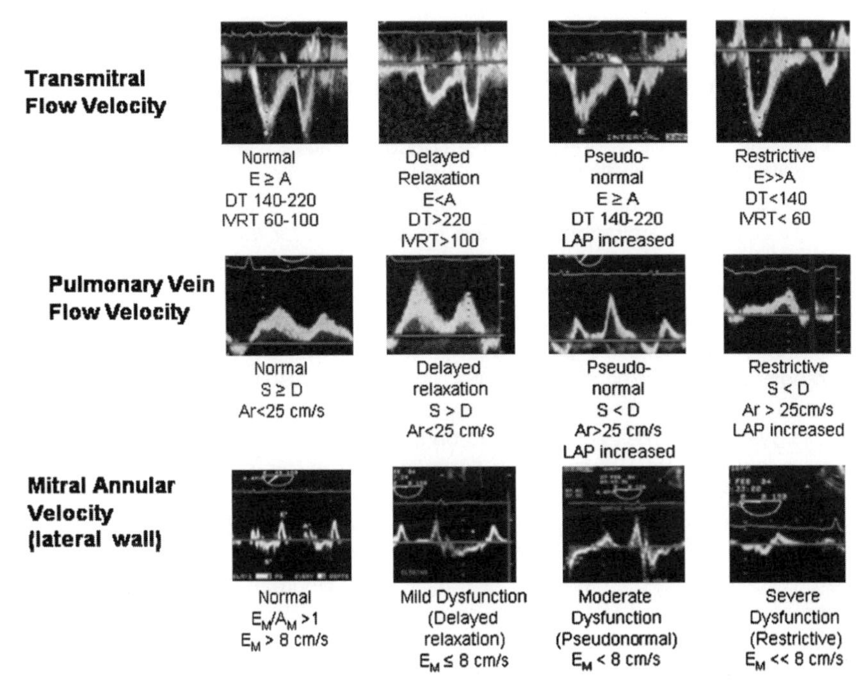


**Fig. 7.** Transmitral Doppler imaging, pulmonary view Doppler imaging, and TDI profiles corresponding to normal, delayed relaxation, pseudonormal, and restrictive filling patterns. (*Reprinted from* Groban L, Dolinski SY. Transesophageal echocardiographic evaluation of diastolic function. Chest 2005;128:3659; with permission.)

contraction phase, can be used to identify and quantify diastolic dysfunction (**Figs. 6** and **7**).

In the normal heart, e′ may be influenced by alterations in preload;[52] however, in the presence of diastolic dysfunction, e′ decreases and becomes preload independent.[53] This allows for the severity of diastolic dysfunction to be quantified by a decreasing e′ value. Age influences the e′ and a′ values; an e′ < 10 cm/s in those less than 50 years of age, and e′ < 8 in those older than 50 years should be considered abnormal.[52] The e′ to a′ ratio verifies abnormal diastolic function (e′/a′ > 1 is considered normal), as an e′/a′ ratio of less than 1 during Valsalva confirms the presence of diastolic dysfunction.[54] Age also influences the e′/a′ ratio, and after the age of 50 e′/a′ < 1 is frequently encountered and should be correlated with other echocardiographic measurements.

A robust quantification of elevated left ventricular filling pressures in diastolic dysfunction is the ratio of transmitral E wave velocity to mitral annular velocity (E/e′).[55–58] This ratio normalizes early transmitral left ventricular filling to mitral annular motion and is used to estimate mean left atrial pressure (with values >15 representing elevated filling pressures, and <8 reflecting normal filling pressures).[17,50,55] Moreover, accuracy of this measurement has been shown to be relatively independent of LV systolic function, rhythm abnormalities (such as tachycardia and AF), LV hypertrophy, and functional mitral regurgitation.[17,50,59–62]

Although e′ relates to global indices of LV relaxation, it must be realized that it is a regional index, as errors can occur in patients with regional wall motion abnormalities at the Doppler sampling site. A limitation to E/e′, a′, and e′ is that myocardial motion at the lateral annulus is higher than the septal annulus, as the septum is tethered to the right ventricle and other structures in the middle of the heart.[55,63] For this reason, and because of its accessibility with transesophageal echocardiography, the lateral mitral annular velocity may be easier to use in the intraoperative transesophageal setting. Although relatively independent of EF, the reliability of E/e′ in predicting pulmonary capillary wedge pressure in decompensated advanced systolic HF has been called into question.[64] The previously mentioned age-related changes and influence of preload in the normal heart when using TDI measures must also be kept in mind. Despite these limitations, TDI is a powerful tool for identifying whether mitral valve inflow velocity patterns represent pseudonormalization and elevated filling pressures.

Doppler echocardiography of diastolic function has proved useful as a diagnostic tool in predicting outcome in patients undergoing cardiac surgery. A recent prospective report of 191 coronary artery bypass graft (CABG) patients found greatly increased mortality (12% vs 0%) following cardiac surgery in patients with significant diastolic dysfunction; risk scores based on systolic function and patient characteristics were less accurate in predicting complications in this patient group than were markers of diastolic dysfunction.[65] Bernard and colleagues[66] identified diastolic dysfunction as an independent predictor of difficult separation from CPB. Liu and colleagues[13] identified that pseudonormal or restrictive transmitral flow patterns were predictive of cardiac events following CABG, whereas left ventricular ejection fraction and the presence of left main coronary artery disease were not independent predictors of poor outcome.

The importance of diastolic dysfunction in cardiac surgery patients is supported by the mechanism of progression of myocardial dysfunction in ischemic heart disease. Diastolic dysfunction has been identified as the earliest potential marker of myocardial ischemia,[67–69] and thereby may represent an early range of the spectrum of myocardial dysfunction that occurs before gross systolic impairment, nonetheless representing a diseased myocardium. An incremental relationship between severity of diastolic dysfunction and outcomes has been demonstrated by Whalley and colleagues,[70] in which nonsurgical congestive HF patients with restrictive diastolic filling patterns had more complications than those with pseudonormal filling patterns or abnormal relaxation. Furthermore, nonsurgical patients with preserved and depressed EF admitted for acute myocardial ischemia (AMI) could be stratified for risk using E/e′ to identify patients with diastolic dysfunction with elevated filling pressures.[17] In that study group, AMI patients were shown to have a higher incidence of HF and poor outcomes with restrictive and pseudonormal LV filling patterns. Elevated filling pressures in that study group were identified by an E/e′ > 15 mmHg, consistent with several previous reports.[17,50,55]

This evidence suggests that elevated LV diastolic filling pressures may be the factor most important in poor outcomes, rather than simply the existence of delayed relaxation.[71] Elevated filling pressures have also been found to be a predictor of mortality in cardiac surgery patients independent of systolic function.[16] In that group, those patients identified as having LV filling pressures more than 22 mmHg were found to have twice the mortality of patients with filling pressures less than 14 mmHg.

There is some indication that elevated LV filling pressures may predict a prolonged and more complicated ICU or hospital stay following cardiac surgery. In a retrospective study of 205 cardiac surgery patients, a 12% increase in hospital length of stay was observed in those patients who had tissue Doppler–based evidence of elevated filling pressures as defined by E/e′ > 17.[72] EF and patient comorbidities were equal between groups. Also, in a study of ICU readmissions following cardiac surgery, ICU recidivism has been shown to be more likely in those with diastolic dysfunction.

This analysis examined 41 ICU readmissions and their likelihood of requiring reintubation. With similar EF, age, baseline BP, HR, and renal function, those who required reintubation were observed to have worse diastolic function, increased E/e′, and increased left atrial size on the preoperative echocardiogram.[17]

Diastolic dysfunction and elevated filling pressures should alert the clinician that the cardiac surgery patient may be more challenging than appreciated, even if systolic function is normal. The increased sensitivity of the cardiovascular system to acute changes in loading conditions, and thus the need for strict management of volume status, is of critical importance. The speed with which intravenous fluids are administered may be more significant, with patients of poor diastolic function less able to tolerate rapid volume shifts. Myocardial protection strategies are, as always, of paramount importance, but may need to be reexamined on a patient-by-patient basis in the presence of diastolic dysfunction to ensure an optimal strategy. Myocardial calcium regulation is abnormal in diastolic dysfunction, and may affect the choice to use an inotrope, or to administer specific agents. Lusitropic agents such as milrinone may be of particular benefit in weaning off cardiopulmonary bypass. Although there is no directed strategy for acutely improving diastolic function, these are a few strategies that have been used in the management of these patients.

The newer, TDI-based diastolic variables e′, a′, and E/e′ are simple to incorporate into the echocardiographic examination, and can give valuable information with respect to postoperative complications following cardiac surgery. These measures are easy to obtain, and can identify patients without traditional predictors of complications following cardiac surgery who still may be at high risk.

## PERIOPERATIVE IMPLICATIONS AND ANESTHETIC MANAGEMENT OF DIASTOLIC DYSFUNCTION FOR THE GENERAL SURGICAL PATIENT

Given the cardiovascular changes that occur with diastolic dysfunction and in the elderly (**Table 1**), the perioperative management of these patients can be challenging. A thorough preoperative assessment is needed to risk-stratify these patients. Particularly in the elderly, it is important to inquire about functional capacity as individuals unable to climb a flight of stairs (four metabolic equivalents [METs]), walk indoors around the house, or do light house work (one MET), are at an increased risk for complications. The functional capacity evaluation may further alert the anesthesiologist to signs of clinically significant diastolic dysfunction. Because an HF history, independent of coronary artery disease is associated with increased morbidity and mortality after noncardiac surgery,[73] risk factors for HF should be sought in the preoperative evaluation. Although not specific to the elderly, the reader should refer to the latest ACC/AHA published guidelines for a complete discussion of perioperative care and evaluation of cardiac patients undergoing noncardiac surgery.[74] In brief, patients with asymptomatic heart disease can safely undergo elective noncardiac surgery without first requiring angioplasty or coronary bypass grafting to lower the risk for surgery. Noninvasive and invasive preoperative cardiac testing should not necessarily be performed unless results will affect patient management. Patients with severe or symptomatic cardiovascular disease or active cardiac conditions should undergo evaluation by a cardiologist and treatment before noncardiac surgery. Statins should not be discontinued before surgery. If a cardiac intervention is required before elective noncardiac surgery, then the patient should have angioplasty with the use of a bare-metal stent followed by 4 to 6 weeks of antiplatelet therapy plus aspirin.

During anesthesia, the cardiovascular changes discussed in the preceding sections predispose the elderly patient to greater hemodynamic instability and

**Table 1**
**Age-related cardiovascular changes and implications**

| Age-Related Change | Mechanism | Consequences | Anesthetic Implications |
|---|---|---|---|
| Myocardial hypertrophy | Apoptotic cells are not replaced and there is compensatory hypertrophy of existing cells; reflected waves during late systole create strain on myocardium leading to hypertrophy | Increased ventricular stiffness, prolonged contraction and delayed relaxation | Failure to maintain preload leads to an exaggerated decrease in CO; excessive volume more easily increases filling pressures to congestive failure levels; dependence on sinus rhythm and low-normal HR |
| Myocardial stiffening | Increased interstitial fibrosis, amyloid deposition | Ventricular filling dependent on atrial pressure | — |
| Reduced LV relaxation | Impaired calcium homeostasis; reduced β receptor responsiveness, early reflected wave | Diastolic dysfunction | — |
| Reduced β receptor responsiveness | Diminished coupling of β receptor to intracellular adenylate cyclase activity, decreased density of β receptors | Increased circulating catecholamines; limited increase in HR and contractility in response to endogenous and exogenous catecholamines; impaired baroreflex control of BP | Hypotension from anesthetic blunting of sympathetic tone, altered reactivity to vasoactive drugs; increased dependence on Frank-Starling mechanism to maintain CO; labile BP, more hypotension |
| Conduction system abnormalities | Apoptosis, fibrosis, fatty infiltration, and calcification of pacemaker and His-bundle cells | Conduction block, sick sinus syndrome, AF, decreased contribution of atrial contraction to diastolic volume | Severe bradycardia with potent opioids, decreased CO from decrease in end-diastolic volume |
| Stiff arteries | Loss of elastin, increased collagen, glycosylation cross linking of collagen | Systolic hypertension<br>Arrival of reflected pressure wave during end-ejection leads to myocardial hypertrophy and impaired diastolic relaxation | Labile BP; diastolic dysfunction, sensitive to volume status |
| Stiff veins | Loss of elastin, increased collagen, glycosylation cross linking of collagen | Decreased buffering of changes in blood volume impairs ability to maintain atrial pressure | Changes in blood volume cause exaggerated changes in cardiac filling |

greater sensitivity to volume status.[6,19,22,75] Several mechanisms can explain the hemodynamic instability. First, the elderly have a higher resting sympathetic tone and have altered β receptor sensitivity. Removal of the baseline sympathetic tone with the induction of general or neuraxial anesthesia often results in hypotension. Second, older patients have a greater sensitivity to volume status. They often arrive on the day of surgery with a depleted intravascular volume because of more frequent use of diuretics, a decreased thirst response to hypovolemia, and age-related changes in renal function. As they are intensely dependent on preload to fill the left ventricle, the reduction in preload induced by anesthesia may result in profound hypotension. Third, the direct effects of intravenous and volatile anesthetics impair cardiac inotropy and lusitropy, and produce arterial and venous vasodilatation.

Anesthetic management of the elderly patient must be planned on a case-by-case basis. Instead of a specific type of anesthetic for the older patient, the authors offer suggestions on a set of principles that address the problems often encountered with the elderly patient. Monitoring volume status is critical to management of the older patient. For patients with known HF, coronary artery disease, or moderate diastolic dysfunction (eg, delayed relaxation with indications of elevated filling pressures), the decision to place an intra-arterial cannula for invasive BP measurement and frequent blood sampling is based on the same considerations applied to the younger patient. Certainly, age-related alterations and coexisting disease may persuade the experienced anesthesiologist to institute such monitoring. However, because no clear evidence exists to specifically recommend this practice before or after induction of anesthesia, the timing of direct arterial pressure monitoring is best based on experience and local practice. For major surgery or vascular surgery, it is imperative that normovolemia be maintained. In such cases, consider use of central venous catheter, pulmonary artery catheter, or transesophageal echocardiography for intraoperative monitoring. Because evidence regarding the efficacy of central venous pressure, pulmonary artery pressure, or transesophageal echocardiographic monitoring as a means to evaluate intravascular volume in the elderly has not been specifically addressed in the perioperative setting, it is not possible to recommend any of these for routine monitoring at this time. Moreover, given the inability of several noninvasive devices, such as the esophageal Doppler or arterial pulse contour, to measure pressures in the central circulation, their usefulness in patients for whom there is concern about the development of pulmonary edema, remains limited.[76] Indeed, future studies are warranted to determine their potential benefit in the elderly surgical patient when combined with an intraoperative goal-directed fluid strategy.

Induction of anesthesia should be accomplished in a smooth and controlled manner. The elderly require a reduced dose of any given induction agent to produce unconsciousness. The induction dose of most agents is decreased by 30% to 50% in the elderly. In addition, induction may be prolonged because of a slow circulation time. Therefore, consider titrating induction agents and waiting for an effect before administering additional doses. It is also important to prevent hypoxemia and hypercarbia, as these patients are prone to pulmonary hypertension. Adequate mask ventilation should be initiated as early as possible. Control of the patient's BP is also essential. It is reasonable to maintain the systolic BP within 10% of the baseline. At the same time, diastolic BP must be maintained, as a low diastolic BP can lead to myocardial ischemia. An attempt should be made to keep the pulse pressure less than the diastolic BP; an increased pulse pressure indicates increased aortic impedance which, as described earlier, will increase wall stress, alter ventricular contraction time, and impair early diastolic filling.

Simultaneous infusions of low dose nitroglycerin and titrated phenylephrine can help to alleviate these physiologic alterations. Administered alone, however, these agents may worsen cardiac function in the elderly. For example, phenylephrine stiffens the vasculature and increases the return of the reflective wave (manifested by an increase in the pulse pressure), potentially impinging on systole and increasing myocardial work. Nitroglycerin alone decreases vascular tone and preload; ultimately reducing cardiac output. However, in contrast to phenylephrine, nitroglycerin decreases the amplitude of the reflected wave and, when used under normovolemic conditions, it reduces the pulse pressure.[77] Thus, the benefits of using combination low dose infusions of phenylephrine and nitroglycerine in the elderly are: (1) the preservation of vascular distensibility; (2) avoidance of reductions in preload and coronary perfusion pressure; and (3) maintenance of stroke volume with minimal cardiac work. In addition, HR should be maintained in the low to normal range (60–70 bpm). At this rate, there is adequate time in diastole to fill the noncompliant ventricle. In general, these principles can be remembered by using the Rule of 70s. For patients age > 70 years, maintain diastolic blood pressure (DBP) > 70, pulse pressure < 70, and HR = 70.

In the early postoperative period, patients with known diastolic heart disease should be watched over closely. As illustrated by this case scenario, elderly patients with diastolic dysfunction can acutely decompensate after initially appearing stable. Hypoxemia or AF are among the most common complications these patients may encounter in the postoperative anesthesia care unit as a consequence of volume overload. Importantly, when vascular sympathetic tone is restored on emergence from general anesthesia or resolution of neuraxial blockade, the noncompliant heart may not be able to tolerate the increased shift in central blood volume thus resulting in pulmonary edema or AF. Indeed, maintaining the low dose infusion of nitroglycerin (eg, 25 μg/min), as discussed previously, may mitigate this from occurring because of its advantageous actions on the pulmonary vasculature. Nonetheless, the assessment of the postoperative patient with suspected HF should include an electrocardiogram for signs of ischemia, LV hypertrophy, AF, and left bundle branch block. If the ECG is abnormal, a further objective assessment of the patient is required. In most cases, this would involve an echocardiogram. Echocardiography is the ideal investigation as information can be obtained about cardiac valves as well as ventricular function. Particularly in older patients, obstructive valvular disease can be detected and other factors influencing the LV preload, including diastolic dysfunction. If echocardiography is not readily available, a chest radiograph may be obtained to provide information about the presence or absence of cardiomegaly and the presence of pulmonary fluid. Also, before treatment commences, additional blood tests such as arterial blood gas, serum electrolytes, and complete blood count (CBC) should be performed in the older patient with confirmed HF. Although treatment options include a carefully chosen dose of intravenous diuretic therapy, a β blocker or calcium channel blocker for HR control, and a venodilator such as nitroglycerin (if tolerated), treatment is best when delivered as part of a multidisciplinary team.

## SUMMARY

As the number of persons aged 65 years and older continues to increase, the anesthesiologist will more frequently encounter this demographic. Cardiovascular changes that occur in this patient population present difficult anesthetic challenges and place these patients at high risk of perioperative morbidity and mortality. The anesthesiologist should be knowledgeable about these age-related cardiovascular changes, the pathophysiology underlying them, and the appropriate perioperative management.

Whether presenting for cardiac or general surgery, the anesthesiologist must identify patients with altered physiology as a result of aging or diastolic dysfunction and be prepared to modify the care plan accordingly. With a directed preoperative assessment that focuses on certain aspects of the cardiovascular system, and the assistance of powerful echocardiographic tools such as tissue Doppler, this can be achieved.

## REFERENCES

1. Engoren M, Arslanian-Engoren C, Steckel D, et al. Cost, outcome, and functional status in octogenarians and septuagenarians after cardiac surgery. Chest 2002; 122:1309–15.
2. Fruitman DS, MacDougall CE, Ross DB. Cardiac surgery in octogenarians: can elderly patients benefit? Quality of life after cardiac surgery. Ann Thorac Surg 1999;68:2129–35.
3. Inpatient Procedures. Fast Stats A-Z, National Center for Health Statistics, US Department for Health and Human Services, Centers for Disease Control. 2009. Available at: http://www.cdc.gov/nchs/fastats/insurg.htm. Accessed March 30, 2009.
4. Bhatia RS, Tu JV, Lee DS, et al. Outcome of heart failure with preserved ejection fraction in a population-based study. N Engl J Med 2006;355:260–9.
5. Kitzman DW, Gardin JM, Gottdiener JS, et al. Importance of heart failure with preserved systolic function in patients > or = 65 years of age. CHS Research Group. Cardiovascular Health Study. Am J Cardiol 2001;87:413–9.
6. Priebe HJ. The aged cardiovascular risk patient. Br J Anaesth 2000;85:763–78.
7. White SE. Anesthesiology: perioperative medicine or "when the anesthetic is a diuretic". J Clin Anesth 2004;16:130–7.
8. Kitzman DW, Groban L. Exercise intolerance. Heart Fail Clin 2008;4:99–115.
9. Little WC, Kitzman DW, Cheng CP. Diastolic dysfunction as a cause of exercise intolerance. Heart Fail Rev 2000;5:301–6.
10. Masoudi FA, Havranek EP, Smith G, et al. Gender, age, and heart failure with preserved left ventricular systolic function. J Am Coll Cardiol 2003;41:217–23.
11. Hernandez AF, Whellan DJ, Stroud S, et al. Outcomes in heart failure patients after major noncardiac surgery. J Am Coll Cardiol 2004;44:1446–53.
12. Hammill BG, Curtis LH, Bennett-Guerrero E, et al. Impact of heart failure on patients undergoing major noncardiac surgery. Anesthesiology 2008;108: 559–67.
13. Liu J, Tanaka N, Murata K, et al. Prognostic value of pseudonormal and restrictive filling patterns on left ventricular remodeling and cardiac events after coronary artery bypass grafting. Am J Cardiol 2003;91:550–4.
14. Phillip B, Pastor D, Bellows W, et al. The prevalence of preoperative diastolic filling abnormalities in geriatric surgical patients. Anesth Analg 2003;97:1214–21.
15. Vaskelyte J, Stoskute N, Kinduris S, et al. Coronary artery bypass grafting in patients with severe left ventricular dysfunction: predictive significance of left ventricular diastolic filling pattern. Eur J Echocardiogr 2001;2:62–7.
16. Salem R, Denault AY, Couture P, et al. Left ventricular end-diastolic pressure is a predictor of mortality in cardiac surgery independently of left ventricular ejection fraction. Br J Anaesth 2006;97:292–7.
17. Møller JE, Pellikka PA, Hillis GS, et al. Prognostic importance of diastolic function and filling pressure in patients with acute myocardial infarction. Circulation 2006; 114:438–44.

18. Lakatta EG. Arterial and cardiac aging: major shareholders in cardiovascular disease enterprises: part III: cellular and molecular clues to heart and arterial aging. Circulation 2003;107:490–7.
19. Groban L. Diastolic dysfunction in the older heart. J Cardiothorac Vasc Anesth 2005;19:228–36.
20. Gillebert TC, Leite-Moreira AF, De Hert SG. Load dependent diastolic dysfunction in heart failure. Heart Fail Rev 2000;5:345–55.
21. Leite-Moreira AF, Correia-Pinto J, Gillebert TC. Afterload induced changes in myocardial relaxation: a mechanism for diastolic dysfunction. Cardiovasc Res 1999;43:344–53.
22. Chen CH, Nakayama M, Nevo E, et al. Coupled systolic-ventricular and vascular stiffening with age: implications for pressure regulation and cardiac reserve in the elderly. J Am Coll Cardiol 1998;32:1221–7.
23. Kawaguchi M, Hay I, Fetics B, et al. Combined ventricular systolic and arterial stiffening in patients with heart failure and preserved ejection fraction: implications for systolic and diastolic reserve limitations. Circulation 2003;107:714–20.
24. Lakatta EG, Levy D. Arterial and cardiac aging: major shareholders in cardiovascular disease enterprises: part I: aging arteries: a "set up" for vascular disease. Circulation 2003;107:139–46.
25. Mitchell GF, Parise H, Benjamin EJ, et al. Changes in arterial stiffness and wave reflection with advancing age in healthy men and women: the Framingham Heart Study. Hypertension 2004;43:1239–45.
26. Meaume S, Benetos A, Henry OF, et al. Aortic pulse wave velocity predicts cardiovascular mortality in subjects >70 years of age. Arterioscler Thromb Vasc Biol 2001;21:2046–50.
27. Chae CU, Pfeffer MA, Glynn RJ, et al. Increased pulse pressure and risk of heart failure in the elderly. JAMA 1999;281:634–9.
28. Franklin SS, Khan SA, Wong ND, et al. Is pulse pressure useful in predicting risk for coronary heart disease? The Framingham Heart Study. Circulation 1999;100:354–60.
29. Domanski M, Norman J, Wolz M, et al. Cardiovascular risk assessment using pulse pressure in the first National Health and Nutrition Examination Survey (NHANES I). Hypertension 2001;38:793–7.
30. Abhayaratna WP, Barnes ME, O'Rourke MF, et al. Relation of arterial stiffness to left ventricular diastolic function and cardiovascular risk prediction in patients > or =65 years of age. Am J Cardiol 2006;98:1387–92.
31. Najjar SS, Scuteri A, Lakatta EG. Arterial aging: is it an immutable cardiovascular risk factor? Hypertension 2005;46:454–62.
32. Nikitin NP, Witte KK, Thackray SD, et al. Effect of age and sex on left atrial morphology and function. Eur J Echocardiogr 2003;4:36–42.
33. Triposkiadis F, Tentolouris K, Androulakis A, et al. Left atrial mechanical function in the healthy elderly: new insights from a combined assessment of changes in atrial volume and transmitral flow velocity. J Am Soc Echocardiogr 1995;8:801–9.
34. Pearlman JD, Triulzi MO, King ME, et al. Left atrial dimensions in growth and development: normal limits for two-dimensional echocardiography. J Am Coll Cardiol 1990;16:1168–74.
35. Thomas L, Levett K, Boyd A, et al. Compensatory changes in atrial volumes with normal aging: is atrial enlargement inevitable? J Am Coll Cardiol 2002;40:1630–5.
36. Leung DY, Boyd A, Ng AA, et al. Echocardiographic evaluation of left atrial size and function: current understanding, pathophysiologic correlates, and prognostic implications. Am Heart J 2008;156:1056–64.

37. Tsang TS, Barnes ME, Gersh BJ, et al. Left atrial volume as a morphophysiologic expression of left ventricular diastolic dysfunction and relation to cardiovascular risk burden. Am J Cardiol 2002;90:1284–9.
38. Osranek M, Seward JB, Buschenreithner B, et al. Diastolic function assessment in clinical practice: the value of 2-dimensional echocardiography. Am Heart J 2007; 154:130–6.
39. Hunt SA, American College of Cardiology, American Heart Association Task Force on Practice Guidelines (Writing Committee to Update the 2001 Guidelines for the Evaluation and Management of Heart Failure). ACC/AHA 2005 guideline update for the diagnosis and management of chronic heart failure in the adult: a report of the American College of Cardiology/American Heart Association Task Force on Practice Guidelines (Writing Committee to Update the 2001 Guidelines for the Evaluation and Management of Heart Failure). J Am Coll Cardiol 2005;46:e1–82.
40. Schunkert H, Jackson B, Tang SS, et al. Distribution and functional significance of cardiac angiotensin converting enzyme in hypertrophied rat hearts. Circulation 1993;87:1328–39.
41. Flesch M, Schiffer F, Zolk O, et al. Angiotensin receptor antagonism and angiotensin converting enzyme inhibition improve diastolic dysfunction and Ca(2+)-ATPase expression in the sarcoplasmic reticulum in hypertensive cardiomyopathy. J Hypertens 1997;15:1001–9.
42. Royster RL, Butterworth JF IV, Prough DS, et al. Preoperative and intraoperative predictors of inotropic support and long-term outcome in patients having coronary artery bypass grafting. Anesth Analg 1991;72:729–36.
43. Rao V, Ivanov J, Weisel RD, et al. Predictors of low cardiac output syndrome after coronary artery bypass. J Thorac Cardiovasc Surg 1996;112:38–51.
44. Garcia MJ, Smedira NG, Greenberg NL, et al. Color M-mode Doppler flow propagation velocity is a preload insensitive index of left ventricular relaxation: animal and human validation. J Am Coll Cardiol 2000;35:201–8.
45. Hurrell DG, Nishimura RA, Ilstrup DM, et al. Utility of preload alteration in assessment of left ventricular filling pressure by Doppler echocardiography: a simultaneous catheterization and Doppler echocardiographic study. J Am Coll Cardiol 1997;30:459–67.
46. Møller JE, Poulsen SH, Søndergaard E, et al. Preload dependence of color M-mode Doppler flow propagation velocity in controls and in patients with left ventricular dysfunction. J Am Soc Echocardiogr 2000;13:902–9.
47. Maurer MS, Spevack D, Burkhoff D, et al. Diastolic dysfunction: can it be diagnosed by Doppler echocardiography? J Am Coll Cardiol 2004;44:1543–9.
48. Oki T, Tabata T, Yamada H, et al. Clinical application of pulsed Doppler tissue imaging for assessing abnormal left ventricular relaxation. Am J Cardiol 1997; 79:921–8.
49. Sohn DW, Chai IH, Lee DJ, et al. Assessment of mitral annulus velocity by Doppler tissue imaging in the evaluation of left ventricular diastolic function. J Am Coll Cardiol 1997;30:474–80.
50. Ommen SR, Nishimura RA, Appleton CP, et al. Clinical utility of Doppler echocardiography and tissue Doppler imaging in the estimation of left ventricular filling pressures: a comparative simultaneous Doppler-catheterization study. Circulation 2000;102:1788–94.
51. Nagueh SF, Sun H, Kopelen HA, et al. Hemodynamic determinants of the mitral annulus diastolic velocities by tissue Doppler. J Am Coll Cardiol 2001; 37:278–85.

52. Skubas N. Intraoperative Doppler tissue imaging is a valuable addition to cardiac anesthesiologists' armamentarium: a core review. Anesth Analg 2009;108:48–66.
53. Firstenberg MS, Greenberg NL, Main ML, et al. Determinants of diastolic myocardial tissue Doppler velocities: influences of relaxation and preload. J Appl Phys 2001;90:299–307.
54. Dumesnil JG, Paulin C, Pibarot P, et al. Mitral annulus velocities by Doppler tissue imaging: practical implications with regard to preload alterations, sample position, and normal values. J Am Soc Echocardiogr 2002;15:1226–31.
55. Nagueh SF, Middleton KJ, Kopelen HA, et al. Doppler tissue imaging: a noninvasive technique for evaluation of left ventricular relaxation and estimation of filling pressures. J Am Coll Cardiol 1997;30:1527–33.
56. Groban L, Dolinski SY. Transesophageal echocardiographic evaluation of diastolic function. Chest 2005;128:3652–63.
57. Dokainish H, Zoghbi WA, Lakkis NM, et al. Optimal noninvasive assessment of left ventricular filling pressures: a comparison of tissue Doppler echocardiography and B-type natriuretic peptide in patients with pulmonary artery catheters. Circulation 2004;109:2432–9.
58. Paulus WJ, Tschöpe C, Sanderson JE, et al. How to diagnose diastolic heart failure: a consensus statement on the diagnosis of heart failure with normal left ventricular ejection fraction by the Heart Failure and Echocardiography Associations of the European Society of Cardiology. Eur Heart J 2007;28:2539–50.
59. Nagueh SF, Kopelen HA, Quiñones MA. Assessment of left ventricular filling pressures by Doppler in the presence of atrial fibrillation. Circulation 1996;94: 2138–45.
60. Nagueh SF, Mikati I, Kopelen HA, et al. Doppler estimation of left ventricular filling pressure in sinus tachycardia. A new application of tissue Doppler imaging. Circulation 1998;98:1644–50.
61. Bruch C, Stypmann J, Gradaus R, et al. Usefulness of tissue Doppler imaging for estimation of filling pressures in patients with primary or secondary pure mitral regurgitation. Am J Cardiol 2004;93:324–8.
62. Nagueh SF, Lakkis NM, Middleton KJ, et al. Doppler estimation of left ventricular filling pressures in patients with hypertrophic cardiomyopathy. Circulation 1999; 99:254–61.
63. Hadano Y, Murata K, Tanaka N, et al. Ratio of early transmitral velocity to lateral mitral annular early diastolic velocity has the best correlation with wedge pressure following cardiac surgery. Circ J 2007;71:1274–8.
64. Mullens W, Borowski AG, Curtin RJ, et al. Tissue Doppler imaging in the estimation of intracardiac filling pressure in decompensated patients with advanced systolic heart failure. Circulation 2009;119:62–70.
65. Merello L, Riesle E, Alburquerque J, et al. Risk scores do not predict high mortality after coronary artery bypass surgery in the presence of diastolic dysfunction. Ann Thorac Surg 2008;85:1247–55.
66. Bernard F, Denault A, Babin D, et al. Diastolic dysfunction is predictive of difficult weaning from cardiopulmonary bypass. Anesth Analg 2001;92:291–8.
67. Higashita R, Sugawara M, Kondoh Y, et al. Changes in diastolic regional stiffness of the left ventricle before and after coronary artery bypass grafting. Heart Vessels 1996;11:145–51.
68. Castello R, Pearson AC, Kern MJ, et al. Diastolic function in patients undergoing coronary angioplasty: influence of degree of revascularization. J Am Coll Cardiol 1990;15:1564–9.

69. Kunichika H, Katayama K, Sakai H, et al. The effect of left ventricular chamber compliance on early diastolic filling during coronary reperfusion. Jpn Circ J 1995;59:762–71.
70. Whalley GA, Doughty RN, Gamble GD, et al. Pseudonormal mitral filling pattern predicts hospital re-admission in patients with congestive heart failure. J Am Coll Cardiol 2002;39:1787–95.
71. Møller JE, Søndergaard E, Poulsen SH, et al. Pseudonormal and restrictive filling patterns predict left ventricular dilation and cardiac death after a first myocardial infarction: a serial color M-mode Doppler echocardiographic study. J Am Coll Cardiol 2000;36:1841–6.
72. Sanders D, Houle T, Kon N, et al. Diastolic dysfunction predicts adverse outcome after cardiac surgery [abstract]. Anesthesiology 2008;109(Suppl):A1592.
73. Lee TH, Marcantonio ER, Mangione CM, et al. Derivation and prospective validation of a simple index for prediction of cardiac risk of major noncardiac surgery. Circulation 1999;100:1043–9.
74. American College of Cardiology/American Heart Association Task Force on Practice Guidelines (Writing Committee to Revise the 2002 Guidelines on Perioperative Cardiovascular Evaluation for Noncardiac Surgery), American Society of Echocardiography, American Society of Nuclear Cardiology, Heart Rhythm Society, Society of Cardiovascular Anesthesiologists, Society for Cardiovascular Angiography and Interventions, Society for Vascular Medicine and Biology, Society for Vascular Surgery, Fleisher LA, Beckman JA, Brown KA, et al. ACC/AHA 2007 guidelines on perioperative cardiovascular evaluation and care for noncardiac surgery: executive summary: a report of the American College of Cardiology/American Heart Association Task Force on Practice Guidelines (Writing Committee to Revise the 2002 Guidelines on Perioperative Cardiovascular Evaluation for Noncardiac Surgery). Anesth Analg 2008;106:685–712.
75. Rooke GA. Cardiovascular aging and anesthetic implications. J Cardiothorac Vasc Anesth 2003;17:512–23.
76. Funk DJ, Moretti EW, Gan TJ. Minimally invasive cardiac output monitoring in the perioperative setting. Anesth Analg 2009;108:887–97.
77. Pauca AL, Kon ND, O'Rourke MF. Benefit of glyceryl trinitrate on arterial stiffness is directly due to effects on peripheral arteries. Heart 2005;91:1428–32.

# Aortic Valve Stenosis

Charles Z. Zigelman, MD[a,*], Patti M. Edelstein, MD, FAAP, FAAMA[b]

**KEYWORDS**

- Aortic valve stenosis • Anesthesia • Elderly
- Geriatric • Management

A.C. is a 98-year-old woman who suffered an acute retinal detachment and presented for vitrectomy. Her medical history was significant for asthma, severe aortic stenosis (AS), hypothyroidism, and paroxysmal atrial fibrillation. Her aortic valve area was calculated to be 0.8 $cm^2$. Yearly surveillance by transthoracic echocardiography showed progression of her disease, yet she was not referred for surgical replacement. The patient and her treating physicians believed that her advanced age and coexisting medical conditions made her a poor surgical candidate. Preoperative pulmonary function studies were deferred as the risk of increasing the retinal detachment was felt to outweigh the benefits of the study. A baseline arterial blood gas determination was drawn on room air (pH 7.38; $pCO_2$ 46 mm Hg; $pO_2$ 68 mm Hg). Preoperative chest roentgenogram showed no active acute disease, and was consistent with her chronic cardiac and pulmonary diseases. Electrolyte determination and electrocardiogram were unchanged from her previous examinations 6 months before surgery. As it was determined that her medical and physiologic condition was unlikely to be improved, and given the patient's desire for restoration of full vision if possible, informed consent was obtained and surgery was scheduled. Propofol and rocuronium were used for induction of anesthesia. After uneventful intubation, anesthesia was maintained using continuously infused remifentanil and inhalational isoflurane in air and oxygen. The procedure lasted 70 minutes and the patient was extubated before transfer to the postanesthesia care unit (PACU). The immediate postoperative course was stormy. In the PACU the patient developed pulmonary edema and T-wave inversions in chest leads $V_{4-6}$. The patient improved and was discharged home on the fifth postoperative day. She returned to full activity and leads an active life 16 months after her ophthalmologic surgery.

Acquired AS is primarily a disease of the elderly. For patients with tricuspid aortic valves, symptoms typically manifest in the eighth decade of life. Classically, patients develop the 3 "S" rule of AS: Shortness of breath, Syncope, and Sudden death. To this triad, chest pain as angina pectoris is an additional clinical symptom in most patients with severe AS.[1] AS is the most common of the valvular diseases. Anywhere from

[a] Post Anesthesia Care Unit, Department of Anesthesia, Shaare Zedek Medical Center, POB 3235, Jerusalem 91031, Israel
[b] Department of Anesthesia, Shaare Zedek Medical Center, POB 3235, Jerusalem 91031, Israel
* Corresponding author.
*E-mail address:* ziggy@szmc.org.il (C.Z. Zigelman).

Anesthesiology Clin 27 (2009) 519–532
doi:10.1016/j.anclin.2009.07.012 **anesthesiology.theclinics.com**

1% to 2% of the population are born with a bicuspid aortic valve, an anatomic variant that frequently evolves into stenosis.[2] In a study of aortic valves excised from patients with isolated AS, Stephan and colleagues noted that 50% of all excised valves studied were bicuspid or unicuspid. Seventy-five percent of excised valves were congenitally bicuspid or unicuspid in those younger than 65 years old.[3] Tricuspid aortic valves tend to stenose with age, increasing the prevalence of AS in the geriatric population. In persons older than 65 years, 25% have calcific aortic valve disease. It is this population pool that leads to more than 50,000 aortic valve replacements per year in the United States alone.[4] Calcific aortic valve disease ranges from aortic valve sclerosis, with no obstruction to flow, to severe, symptomatic AS. Aranow and colleagues prospectively studied 1881 women and 924 men with a mean age of 81. Using Doppler echocardiography, AS was demonstrated in 17% of the women and 15% of the men, with no statistical difference between the genders.[5]

## PATHOPHYSIOLOGY OF AORTIC STENOSIS

AS, as a discrete pathologic entity, is characterized by obstruction to left ventricular (LV) outflow. Other conditions may cause LV outflow obstruction (LVOO), thereby sharing some of the same signs, symptoms, and physiologic derangements. As a slowly progressive disease, AS allows for compensatory mechanisms to develop as the LVOO worsens. The normal valve area of 3 to 4 $cm^2$ incorporates significant physiologic reserve so that there is little hemodynamic consequence as the valve narrows to half that area.[1,2,6] As LVOO increases, energy is expended as the fluid column of blood makes its way distal to the stenotic lesion. Flow is kinetic energy whereas pressure is potential energy. This decrease in energy level is translated into the pressure drop and gradient across the stenotic valve. The generated pressure in the ventricle is higher than the blood pressure in the aorta. The myocardium responds to this increased pressure load by hypertrophying concentrically. Left ventricular (LV) pressure overload causes increased LV wall thickness to maintain normal, transmural wall stress.[7] With LV stiffness increasing secondary to hypertrophy, LV compliance decreases and LV end-diastolic pressure rises to maintain LV end diastolic volume. As the process progresses, oxygen delivery to the LV myocardium decreases and diastolic dysfunction sets in.[1,2,7,8] Left untreated, congestive heart failure ensues. As oxygen demand outstrips supply, angina pectoris may develop. The ability to increase cardiac output as a response to a drop in systemic vascular resistance (SVR) is impaired as physiologic cardiac reserves and compensatory mechanisms are taxed to the limit. A decrease in SVR in this situation may result in syncope or arrhythmia. The physiologic changes described here easily account for the classic clinical symptoms of AS.

Rheumatic AS, although now less common in developing countries, remains a problem worldwide. The pathologic small orifice results from calcific nodules on both sides of vascularized leaflets, and adherent or fused commissures and cusps. The cusps' nonpliable free edges frequently cause concurrent aortic insufficiency. Rheumatic aortic valve disease is often associated with rheumatic mitral valves.[1]

Patients with congenital bicuspid AS are 4 times more likely to be male and present with severe calcific AS after age 50 years. Bicuspid AS is thought to manifest clinically approximately 2 decades earlier than tricuspid AS because of increased leaflet stress and turbulent flow attributed to the abnormal architecture of the aortic valve. In addition, a higher percentage of congenital bicuspid aortic valves develop LVOO with time compared with the normal tricuspid aortic valve. The mechanical forces are believed to be responsible for the morphologic changes in the valve apparatus.[9] Tissue abnormalities in patients with bicuspid aortic valves extend beyond the valve leaflets. These patients have an increased risk of aortic aneurysm, with a risk of aortic dissection up to nine times that of the general population. The enhanced likelihood of aortic dissection remains high even after the bicuspid valve is replaced. This association has led some investigators to postulate that the presence of a bicuspid aortic valve may reflect an underlying systemic connective tissue disorder.[10] Nonetheless, histopathological changes as well as hemodynamic derangements are essentially the same for tricuspid AS and the congenital bicuspid variant. Therefore, this entity, along with the AS associated with the tricuspid aortic valve, can currently be understood as calcific aortic valve disease.[1,6,9]

Calcific AS, although progressive and age associated, should no longer be regarded as senile or degenerative. In addition to the mechanism of mechanical stress there appears to be a significant inflammatory component. As a prolonged latent period in the evolution of AS exists, it is possible to isolate a precursor entity, aortic sclerosis. Aortic sclerosis progresses to varying degrees of AS in many patients. Faggiano and colleagues[11] demonstrated that approximately 1 in 3 patients with echocardiographically defined aortic sclerosis developed AS. The study had a mean duration of follow-up of 4 years. Of the patients who developed AS during the study period, 10% were diagnosed as severe. Aortic sclerosis may be identified echocardiographically as focal areas of valve thickening with no hemodynamic alterations across the aortic valve. Thus, leaflet motion, valve opening, and flow velocities across the valve are normal.[9] These areas of thickening seem to be composed of plaquelike lesions on the aortic side of the valve leaflet. Accumulated within these lesions are proinflammatory and inflammatory components similar to those seen in atherosclerotic lesions. This observation, coupled with the similarity of risk factors for both AS and atherosclerotic coronary artery disease, has spurred immense interest in investigating potential modulating therapies of AS.[12–19] Among the components of early aortic sclerotic plaques are extracellular lipids, apolipoproteins, and angiotensin-converting enzyme (ACE). Proinflammatory agents may encourage monocyte migration into the leaflet itself. These monocytes differentiate into macrophages and later foam cells and, together with T lymphocytes, are responsible for the expression of a variety of proinflammatory cytokines. Osteopontin derived from these macrophages is responsible for bone matrix formation, fibroblast, and myofibroblast proliferation in the valve leaflet. This calcification, bone deposition, and cellular changes affect the mechanical functioning of the valve and cause hemodynamic deterioration.[9] Evidence of an inflammatory process involved in the pathogenesis of AS opens the theoretical consideration that genetic factors may have a role in AS development.

In 2006, the American College of Cardiology/American Heart Association Task Force on Practice Guidelines (ACC/AHA Practice Guidelines) published,[20] in collaboration with the Society of Cardiovascular Anesthesiologists, guidelines for the management of patients with valvular heart disease. A classification of severity that incorporates 3 measurable factors in AS was proposed. Estimation of aortic valvular area, maximum aortic velocity of the blood column during systole, as well as peak and mean pressure gradients across the stenotic valve can be achieved using Doppler echocardiography. Initial evaluation includes transthoracic echocardiography (TTE).[6] If inadequate, quantitative evaluation of the degree of AS may be achieved using transesophageal echocardiography (TEE).[21] Determination of the aortic valve may be estimated using planimetry. The valve area is manually traced at the level of the orifice, and the computer calculates the circumference of the trace. Accuracy of the information obtained requires aiming the echo beam at an angle that minimizes the error of measurement. The error of measurement using this method is potentially significant for calcific AS, as the computer assumes a circle for area calculation as well as the difficulties in delineating the orifice. The annulus has been described as "crown shaped," the "tips of the crown representing the outermost points of coaptation between the leaflets."[21] Planimetric measurements of the aortic valve area are no longer popular. Using Doppler wave echocardiography, velocity of the blood column may be calculated as the echo beam is reflected off the erythrocytes in motion. The beam should be aimed parallel to the flow measured for maximal accuracy. Knowledge of the velocities in different areas allows for calculation of the aortic valve area because of the Law of Conservation of Mass. Simply stated, multiplying the velocity ($V_1$) by the area ($A_1$) must equal the product of velocity ($V_n$) and area ($A_n$) throughout the fluid column. Therefore, the unknown area of the aortic valve is derived by knowing the velocities of the blood column across the valve as well as in the aorta and the aortic area. Pressure gradients may be measured using the echocardiographic velocity or by direct pressure measurements during cardiac catheterization. A modification of the Bernoulli equation is applied to determine the pressure gradient echocardiographically: Pressure Gradient = 4 × (maximal blood velocity).[2] There is a tendency for pressure gradients derived by echo data to be larger than those directly measured using invasive cardiac catheters. This phenomenon may be explained by "pressure recovery," a process whereby some of the kinetic energy as expressed by velocity reverts to potential energy as expressed by pressure at a distance from the stenotic valve.[21] The pressure measured directly by a catheter at some distance from the aortic valve will be greater than the pressure immediately distal to the stenotic aortic valve. This overestimation is eliminated when calculating the mean transvalvular gradient.[21]

Small differences in valvular area calculation have been observed when comparing TTE and TEE.[22,23] In severe AS the acoustic window for both TEE and TTE may be technically difficult. For those patients in whom echocardiographic interrogation of the aortic valve is critical, measurements and determinations may be of less than optimal quality. When LV outflow tract measurements are questionable or difficult, there are recently developed and reported calculations that may be employed.[23]

## CLASSIFICATION CRITERIA FOR AORTIC STENOSIS

AS is graded as mild by the ACC/AHA Practice Guidelines for a valve area greater than 1.5 $cm^2$, moderate for areas between 1.0 and 1.5 $cm^2$, and severe for a valve area less than 1.0 $cm^2$. When analyzing measured jet velocity in meters per second, the criteria for mild, moderate, and severe AS are less than 3.0, 3.0 to 4.0, and greater than 4.0, respectively. A mean gradient across the valve of less than 25 mm Hg is classified as mild AS, with severe AS defined by a mean pressure drop greater than 40 mm Hg. Moderate AS occupies the niche between mild and severe valvular disease.[20]

Defining the severity of AS by mean gradient measurements requires an evaluation of forward flow and cardiac index. Many patients with significant AS have elements of heart failure, which when improved may lead to changes in the mean gradient. In a subset of 6 patients treated with a nitroprusside infusion, a significant increase in stroke volume led to a corresponding increase in the mean pressure gradient across the valve. Aortic valve area in these patients remained unchanged.[24] Classification by dynamic criteria in patients with systolic dysfunction underestimated the severity of the AS when compared with the anatomic criteria of valve areas. It is important, therefore, to remember that the classification system is for convenience and does not eliminate the current understanding of the dynamic nature with which patients may respond, or the smooth continuum of the disease entity.[20]

## PHYSICAL EXAMINATION AND CLINICAL PRESENTATION

The diagnosis of AS is often made after physical examination reveals a systolic murmur that subsequently triggers an echocardiographic examination. Classically, the murmur of AS is described as a crescendo-decrescendo murmur heard over the aortic area (right sternal border, second intercostal space) radiating to the neck. The murmur is the result of turbulent flow across the partially obstructed aortic valve. In addition, assessment of the carotids for a slow and delayed carotid upstroke belies a delay in the pressure wave, as it is impeded during systole by the affected aortic valve. This physical finding is referred to as the "parvus and tardus" carotid impulse, and is specific for AS.[1,6,25] The finding is not sensitive, however, and its absence does not preclude severe stenosis. The loss of the second systolic heart sound or its softening correlates with an aortic valve that no longer opens and closes well.[2]

Physical examination by an experienced cardiologist performed on 123 patients[25] (70% male, mean age 63 $\pm$ 16 years, range 22–84 years) with initially asymptomatic AS found that only carotid upstroke amplitude predicted outcome. All patients had systolic murmurs, grade 1 through 4. Several physical findings present in the majority of patients correlated with severity of AS as diagnosed by Doppler echocardiography. Murmur intensity and time to peak murmur intensity, single second heart sound (present in 65%), delayed carotid upstroke (present in 89%), and decreased carotid amplitude (present in 85%) were all noted. A fourth heart sound was audible in only a few patients. It is significant that carotid amplitude and upstroke delay, a single S2, systolic murmur grade, time of peak intensity, and radiation of the murmur were all univariate predictors of clinical outcome. Munt and colleagues concluded that echocardiography is necessary for the exclusion of a diagnosis of severe AS.

Once the diagnosis of AS has been established, the physical examination should center on detection of symptomatic AS. Symptoms are clinically relevant in that they imply a progression of the disease and a need to consider therapy. Clinical signs and symptoms include dyspnea on exertion, shortness of breath, angina pectoris, syncope, and arrhythmia. Bleeding associated with AS is due to impaired platelet function and acquired von Willebrand syndrome, and is reversible after aortic valve replacement (AVR).

## NATURAL PROGRESSION AND COURSE OF AORTIC STENOSIS

Having established that AS is a spectrum of disease ranging from sclerosis with no detectable LVOO to symptomatic, severe AS requiring AVR, it is important to shed light on the natural course of AS. Rosenhek and colleagues[26] identified 128 consecutive patients with severe AS with an aortic jet velocity of 5.0 $\pm$ 0.6 m/s and followed them prospectively for 22 $\pm$ 18 months. An event was defined as either death (8 patients) or AVR. The AVR was performed on symptomatic patients. At 1 year two-thirds of the patients remained event free, and by 4 years only a third remained event free. The severity of aortic valve calcification was an independent predictor of event-free survival. Absence or minimal valvular calcification predicted a 75% event-free survival at 4 years. Only 20% of those with moderate to severe calcification remained event free at 4 years. The presence of hypertension, coronary artery disease, diabetes mellitus, age, sex, and hypercholesterolemia did not independently predict an event as defined here. Of those patients whose aortic jet velocity increased by more than 0.3 meters per second per year, 80% died or underwent AVR within 2 years. Surveillance of the aortic valve area for calcification and deterioration of the AS as monitored by jet velocity seemed clinically helpful in identifying a population of AS patients at risk. Aortic valve calcification (AVC) as a predictor of worsened clinical outcome was verified in a prospective study of 50 patients.[15] For patients with moderate to severe AVC undergoing dialysis, aortic jet velocity increased by 0.37 ± 0.36 m/s over a 12-month follow-up.[27] Although conducted on only 55 patients, this study, in light of the significant morbidity and mortality noted earlier for AVC, pointed to a poor prognosis for those suffering the comorbidity of chronic renal failure on dialysis. A larger study of 622 patients[28] with severe, asymptomatic AS as defined by a peak jet velocity of greater than 4 m/s confirmed and largely agreed with the previous findings of Rosenhek and colleagues. At 5-year follow-up only 25% of the patients remained free of surgery or cardiac death. Of the patients studied, one-third developed cardiac symptoms of angina, syncope, or dyspnea before surgery within 2 years. By 5 years only one-third remained symptom free. This study was large enough to identify a statistical risk of sudden death of approximately 1% per year in unoperated patients. Patients with higher peak jet velocities, which imply more significant AS, had an increased risk of developing symptoms, cardiac death, or surgery. This study identified a group of 90 patients who during the course of the study period, became symptomatic, were identified as such, and did not undergo surgery. This significant group represents a large body of patients with untreated severe, symptomatic AS who require care in the face of their severe AS.

For patients older than 80 years, the rate of progression of mild to moderate AS as determined by decreasing aortic valve area is twice that of matched controls 20 years their junior.[29] Although a small study, it is possible that elderly patients older than 80 years experience a natural progression of AS that differs from that of younger patients.

The rate of progression of AS in the individual patient remains variable. The presence of aortic valve sclerosis and varying degrees of stenosis are associated with an increased incidence of mortality from both cardiovascular and all causes. For elderly patients, there exists an approximately 50% increased risk of cardiovascular death and myocardial infarction in those with aortic valvular pathology.[30] While the mechanism of this association is unclear, increased vigilance is recommended for all patients in whom calcific aortic valve disease is identified.[20]

## MODULATING THERAPIES AND STRATEGIES IN AORTIC STENOSIS

Observations of shared common risk factors such as hypertension, hyperlipidemia, diabetes mellitus, smoking, male gender, and age, in addition to similar histopathological changes in calcific AS and in atherosclerotic heart disease, lead to the supposition that a common pathway exists for these disease entities.[9,12] That the aortic valve is in direct contact with, and a continuation of aortic endothelium contributes to this line of reasoning. To date, there is no conclusive evidence to support medical management in the therapy for AS. As there is a strong theoretical basis for the use of 3-hydroxy-3-methylglutaryl-coenzyme A reductase inhibitors (statins) in the attempt to prevent or slow the progression of AS to the severe, symptomatic presentation, the subject continues to be the source of study and possibly conflicting results. Early, retrospective studies appeared to point to a therapeutic advantage. For those patients receiving statin therapy, the rate of deterioration of the aortic valve seemed slowed.[13,31,32]

Prospectively studying the effects of atorvastatin in a double-blind, placebo-controlled trial, Cowell and colleagues discovered a significant lipid-lowering effect of the study limb when compared with placebo controls. The investigators were unable to demonstrate any significant differences between the groups for progression of AVC or aortic jet velocity.[12] Inclusion of patients with severe AS in the study, as well as relatively short treatment and follow-up periods, may have prevented the demonstration of a potential benefit in therapy. A second, prospective, randomized, placebo-controlled study[15] assessed the use of atorvastatin in a lower dosing regimen. Here, too, AVC progression and the rate of hemodynamic deterioration were not significantly different between placebo and drug limbs. The "magic bullet" clearly was not found.

In a retrospective study[14] distinguishing patients with aortic valve sclerosis and mild AS from those with moderate AS, investigators attempted to identify patients with early, asymptomatic disease in an effort to assess the possible benefits of statin administration. For those with aortic valve sclerosis and mild AS receiving statin therapy, progression of the disease was significantly slower, as assessed by peak aortic jet velocities, compared with those not receiving statin therapy. This effect was not demonstrable in the moderate AS patients. The mean follow-up of this study was 5.6 $\pm$ 3.2 years.

In 2007, Moura and colleagues[33] prospectively studied 121 patients with AS. There were 61 patients who, in addition to moderate to severe, asymptomatic AS had hyperlipidemia (low-density lipoprotein [LDL] 159.7 $\pm$ 33.4 mg/dL). These patients received 20 mg of rosuvastatin every day. The control group of 60 patients had normal blood levels of LDL (118.6 $\pm$ 37.4 mg/dL) and received no statin therapy. There was no significant difference in degree of AS between the groups as measured by peak aortic valve velocity and valve area. The patients were followed for 18 months. For those receiving lipid-lowering therapy, a significantly slower progression of AS was observed in both degression of valve area and increasing peak aortic valve jet velocity. This study was prospective but not blinded. Further studies are required, and are in progress, to attempt to answer the following questions. Is there a therapeutic benefit in statin therapy for the treatment of AS? What is the optimal timing for initiation of such treatment assuming a benefit can be demonstrated? Is the dosing regimen dependent on the drugs' lipid lowering effects? Are investigators observing an additional anti-inflammatory aspect to the drug which requires monitoring other factors, ie, C-reactive protein (CRP)? The current ACC/AHA guidelines do not advocate the use of statins for altering the course and natural progression of AS.[20]

The presence of angiotensin II and ACE have been demonstrated in the sclerotic aortic valve.[9] As with the statins, the common presence of angiotensin-ACE in atherosclerotic lesions and sclerotic aortic valves allows for the postulation that interference with the angiotensin mechanism may favorably alter the progression of AS. Retrospectively studied and published in 2004, ACE inhibition was not demonstrated to alter the course of AS.[13] As with the statins, there exists theoretical involvement of the angiotensin-ACE pathway in the process of calcific aortic valve disease. Proof that modification of this mechanism modulates the disease and its progression is lacking.

The inflammatory marker, CRP, is elevated in patients with AS.[34] Two studies[17,18] reported CRP levels that were double for patients who exhibited rapid progression of disease compared with those with documented slow progression. In these studies, aortic valve area and peak aortic jet velocity were used to assess AS severity and its course. The role of the inflammatory cascade in calcium deposition and bone formation in the aortic valve can theoretically be used in monitoring patients with AS as well as being prognostically useful. A direct correlation exists between AVC and outcome.[15] However, when studying inflammatory markers and calcification, Fox and colleagues[16] found that coexisting conditions of hypertension and diabetes could account for the observed correlation of AVC and inflammation, and that these were not independent factors.

Much promise remains for the development of modulating therapies in AS. To date, however, because of lack of clarity and definitive data, some of which are summarized in this article, the ACC/AHA Practice Guidelines clearly state that "there are no medical treatments proven to prevent or delay the disease process in the aortic valve leaflets."[20]

Bacterial endocarditis is associated with serious morbidity and significant mortality. Therefore, a Class I recommendation for antibiotic prophylaxis exists for all patients with AS.[20] The antibacterial agents of choice depend on the potential pathogens reasonably expected to be encountered, and patient history for allergy and possible untoward reactions to the agent in question.

## AORTIC VALVE REPLACEMENT

AVR is indicated for patients with symptomatic, severe AS, those with severe AS undergoing coronary artery bypass graft, and for those undergoing other heart valve surgery. Similarly, patients with LV systolic dysfunction, indicated by a low ejection fraction, are currently candidates for AVR. For those with asymptomatic AS, AVR may be considered beneficial if symptoms are elicited during exercise testing or if rapid progression of disease is likely.[20] As a rule, asymptomatic patients are best monitored carefully by echo and diligent follow-up, as the risk of surgery outweighs the benefit.[35] The immediate in-hospital mortality for AVR, as reported by a large observational study,[36] is 4%. For octogenarians undergoing AVR the immediate mortality is 10%.[37] Despite the mortality, the number of patients older than 80 years undergoing AVR is significant. In a retrospective study of 9 patients 90 years or older undergoing AVR at a single tertiary care center, one patient died in the immediate postoperative period.[38] No AVR was performed during the 1990s at this medical center for nonagenarians. As the population ages, and without an alternative therapeutic option, surgery in these high-risk patients continues. For patients with severe AS who refuse surgery, the average survival is 2 years or less.[9] Of the octogenarians surviving the initial postoperative period of 60 days, two-thirds survived 3 years or longer, and 40% were alive 5 or more years after surgery.[37] Because symptomatic AS is an indication for surgery, alleviation of symptoms postoperatively is a factor in assessing surgical risk and benefit. In the elderly, relief of symptoms may be of even greater importance than long-term survival data. Patients and physicians alike are therefore willing to undertake AVR even in light of significant immediate mortality.

Myocardial repair and remodeling are apparent shortly after surgery for AVR.[39] The initial improvement in LVOO allows for myocyte hypertrophy to reverse as the pressure generated by the left ventricle decreases. As the systolic dysfunction reverts to a more normal situation, LV hypertrophy and diastolic dysfunction improve. The severity of AS correlates inversely with the degree of myocardial blood flow in the subendocardium, even in the presence of normal coronary arteries.[40] After AVR, the microcirculation tends to allow for increased LV blood flow, the mechanism of which is not related to decreasing LV mass, but to other mechanisms not identified.[41] Although ejection fraction increases as LV remodeling progresses, there is microscopic fibrosis, scarring, and damage, the clinical relevance of which is unclear.[42] Remodeling and improved function of the left ventricle may affect mitral valve function and reduce the regurgitant volume, if present, by reducing end-diastolic volume.[43] Changes in ascending aortic distensibility due to AS revert to normal within a year of AVR.[44] Possible explanations include reduced endothelial and microvascular trauma to the aorta after AVR, allowing for remodeling of the aorta.

Surgical AVR is the standard technique for treating AS when intervention is indicated. The anesthetic considerations for open heart surgery can be summarized by accounting for and understanding the mechanisms, progression, physiology, and pathology of AS as outlined earlier. As a general rule, hypotension, bradycardia, and tachycardia should be avoided so as to preserve cardiac output without unduly deranging the compensatory mechanisms of LV hypertrophy, increased preload, and increased afterload.

Percutaneous aortic valve replacement (PAVR) is a new and evolving technology. The techniques, available bioprostheses, anesthetic management, and considerations have recently been reviewed.[45–47] At present, two approaches are feasible. The antegrade approach, originally performed via the femoral vein, avoids manipulating a large-bore delivery device through an often tortuous, atheromatous, and relatively inelastic arterial tree. From the inferior vena cava to the right atrium, the left atrium is accessed. The delivery device crosses the mitral valve, and can be delivered through the left ventricle into the LV outflow tract. This early approach has been largely abandoned as the technique risks damage to the anterior leaflet of the mitral valve. Acute mitral regurgitation in patients with long-standing LVOO can be disastrous.[45] At present, for patients in whom the retrograde approach is not advisable, antegrade access is possible via a transapical approach. The LV apex is accessed via a small left anterior thoracotomy. Cardiopulmonary bypass is not required. Complications include postoperative bleeding, cardiac tamponade, and recurrent pleural effusions. The retrograde approach requires advancing a large-bore delivery device via the femoral and iliac arteries into the aorta. For all techniques, anesthesia is helpful in allowing TEE assistance and rapid ventricular pacing for the correct positioning and deployment of the valve. Here, as elsewhere, the anesthesiologist is challenged to allow effective therapy while continuing to provide patient comfort and minimizing the physiologic derangements caused by the therapy during the perioperative period.

A small, prospective study[48] advocates a combined approach. Twenty-nine patients were consecutively enrolled for PAVR. Patients were referred for transapical AVR in the presence of peripheral vascular disease, porcelain aorta, small bore, or calcification of the ileofemoral arteries and horizontal ascending aorta. All others were treated with transfemoral PAVR. The mean age of the patients was 84 $\pm$ 7 years and the immediate, 30-day mortality was 8.7%. These preliminary results are encouraging, as these patients were considered poor surgical candidates.

## ANESTHETIC MANAGEMENT FOR NONCARDIAC SURGERY

A large number of patients suffering from symptomatic severe AS do not undergo valve replacement. Reasons vary from patient refusal and severe coexisting comorbidities that reduce the benefit to risk ratio, to advanced, calcified AS that increases the risk of the procedure and threaten its very success. As the incidence of AS in the aging population is high, there are many patients with AS who present for noncardiac surgery. The severity of AS, after discounting confounding cardiac risk factors, remains strongly predictive of perioperative mortality and nonfatal myocardial infarction.[49] The ACC/AHA Guidelines[50] recommend postponing necessary, elective surgery until AVR is performed. Emergency surgery and surgery for those who are not AVR candidates may proceed with the knowledge that perioperative mortality is 10%. The managing physicians may consider balloon valvuloplasty as a way to bridge the patient past the emergency procedure. Balloon valvuloplasty therapies often restenose and therefore cannot be considered as definitive therapeutic options for severe AS.

For patients with severe asymptomatic AS who are closely monitored and have been evaluated within the year, elective surgery may proceed. If evaluation has not been done within the preceding 12-month period, a cardiac consultation and evaluation are required. The recommendations include routine echocardiographic surveillance every 3 to 5 years for mild AS, and every 1 to 2 years for moderate AS. Patients who are monitored may proceed to elective surgery; others should be evaluated to assess the degree of stenosis. Monitoring of asymptomatic patients requires an attempt by history, physical examination and, if necessary, testing to evoke symptoms. It cannot be overstressed that all symptomatic AS requires evaluation for, and consideration of, AVR. All AS patients who undergo relevant noncardiac surgical procedures require antibiotic prophylaxis against bacterial endocarditis.[50,51]

The anesthetic plan should incorporate considerations for the alleviation of postoperative pain and suffering. An acceptable goal for all patients should be the maximum reduction of physiologic trespass and insult that surgery and anesthesia entail. During surgery, the maintenance of cardiac output in the face of AS is facilitated by normal sinus rhythm. Atrial contraction and avoidance of tachycardia allows for sufficient LV end-diastolic volume to maintain forward flow. Tachycardia increases oxygen demand while decreasing diastolic coronary blood flow, and may trigger ischemia. Bradycardia, on the other hand, may excessively tax the hypertrophied left ventricle and cause congestive failure. Sudden changes in SVR and intravascular volume can potentially hinder a patient's ability to maintain cardiac output and vital organ perfusion, and thus are best avoided. To this end, intraoperative TEE is often a useful monitor. The etiology of hypotension and hemodynamic instability in the operative and perioperative settings for the patient with severe AS is a diagnostic challenge requiring accurate and immediate intervention. Hypovolemia, myocardial ischemia with or without infarction, heart failure, and hypertrophic obstructive cardiomyopathy are among the causes of hypotension during surgery for patients with AS. TEE can often be used to differentiate between these differing etiologies.[52] As a useful monitoring modality for surgery in which fluid shifts and blood loss may be anticipated, TEE should be considered. A contraindication for intraoperative TEE is esophageal disease where a risk of perforation exists. Esophageal tumors, tears, bleeding varices, penetrating injuries, and recent gastric and esophageal surgery are examples in which TEE monitoring should be reconsidered. Risk of gastric aspiration is of concern for those patients in whom a "full stomach" is likely. Upper airway compromise and injury, operator expertise, and cervical manipulations are additional factors to be considered before TEE is applied.

A case report[53] advocating the use of total intravenous anesthesia (TIVA) using the short-acting agents, remifentanil and propofol, has recently been published. These agents have the advantage of tight control and allow for backtracking if inadvertently undesired drug effects appear. There is no evidence advocating TIVA as the preferred method of anesthesia for patients with AS undergoing general anesthesia. The use of monitored anesthesia care for patients undergoing procedures with local anesthetic allows for availability of a skilled practitioner dedicated to hemodynamic monitoring. For the elderly, the risk of postoperative delirium is increased by the use of benzodiazepines and meperidine, and avoidance of these agents as adjuvants or sedatives might be prudent.[54] A retrospective study[55] identified 22 patients for hip arthroplasty with epidural anesthesia and AS. No complications attributable to the anesthetic technique were identified. No one in the study group suffered from severe AS. Regional anesthesia techniques have not been studied specifically in the population of patients with severe AS.

## SUMMARY

AS is a disease in evolution. Primarily a disease of the elderly, calcific AS has characteristic features that are biomechanical as well as systemic and inflammatory in nature, with risk factors and histopathology similar to atherosclerosis. Congenital bicuspid valves account for a significant number of patients with AS. To date, no medical therapy has been shown to conclusively alter the progression of the disease, although there are potential interventions under investigation. Fortunately, no invasive interventional therapy is required until symptoms develop. Factors that may alert the physician to an accelerated progression of calcific aortic valvular disease toward severe symptomatic AS include moderate or greater AVC, chronically dialyzed patients, and patients 80 years and older. AVR is indicated for symptomatic patients, and various new techniques and approaches are being developed. There remains significant morbidity and mortality associated with AVR. For those who undergo successful AVR the long-term prognosis is good. Symptoms are relieved, and cardiac function improves due to ventricular and aortic remodeling. A substantial number of patients with symptomatic AS present for anesthesia care. A thorough, modern understanding of AS and its course are necessary for the anesthesiologist to steer the patient through the perioperative period, with the least physiologic and pharmacologic trespass and best possible outcome.

## REFERENCES

1. Otto CM, Bonow RO. Valvular heart disease. In: Libby P, Bonow RO, Mann DL, editors. Braunwald's heart disease: a textbook of cardiovascular medicine. 8th edition. Philadelphia: WB Saunders; 2007. p. 1625–33.
2. Carabello BA. Aortic stenosis. N Engl J Med 2002;346(9):677–82.
3. Stephan PJ, Henry CH III, Hebeler RF Jr, et al. Comparison of age, gender, number of aortic valve cusps, concomitant coronary artery bypass grafting, and magnitude of left ventricular-systemic arterial peak systolic gradient in adults having aortic valve replacement for isolated aortic valve stenosis. Am J Cardiol 1997;79:166–72.
4. Rajamannan NM, Otto CM. Targeted therapy to prevent progression of calcific aortic stenosis. Circulation 2004;110:1180–2.
5. Aronow WS, Ahn C, Kronzon I. Comparison of echocardiographic abnormalities in African-American, Hispanic and white men and women aged >60 years. Am J Cardiol 2001;87:1131–3.
6. Grimard BH, Larson JM. Aortic stenosis: diagnosis and treatment. Am Fam Physician 2008;78(6):717–24.
7. Grossman W, Jones D, McLaurin LP. Wall stress and patterns of hypertrophy in the human left ventricle. J Clin Invest 1975;56:56–64.
8. Aranow WS. Heart disease and aging. Med Clin North Am 2006;90:849–62.
9. Freeman RV, Otto CM. Spectrum of calcific aortic valve disease: pathogenesis, disease progression and treatment strategies. Circulation 2005;111:3316–26.
10. Lewin MB, Otto CM. The bicuspid aortic valve: adverse outcomes from infancy to old age. Circulation 2005;111(7):832–4.
11. Faggiano P, Antonini-Canterin F, Erlicher A, et al. Progression of aortic valve sclerosis to aortic stenosis. Am J Cardiol 2003;91:99–101.
12. Cowell SJ, Newby DE, Prescott RJ, et al. A randomized trial of intensive lipid-lowering therapy in calcific aortic stenosis. N Engl J Med 2005;352:2389–97.
13. Rosenhek R, Rader F, Loho N, et al. Statins but not angiotensin converting enzyme inhibitors delay progression of aortic stenosis. Circulation 2004;110:1291–5.
14. Antonini-Canterin F, Hirsu M, Popescu BA, et al. Stage related effect of statin treatment on the progression of aortic valve sclerosis and stenosis. Am J Cardiol 2008;102:738–42.

15. Dichtl W, Alber HF, Feuchtner GM, et al. Prognosis and risk factors in patients with asymptomatic aortic stenosis and their modulation by atorvastatin (20 mg). Am J Cardiol 2008;102:743–8.
16. Fox CS, Guo CY, Larson MG, et al. Relations of inflammation and novel risk factors to valvular calcification. Am J Cardiol 2006;97:1502–5.
17. Imai K, Okura H, Kume T, et al. C-reactive protein predicts severity, progression, and prognosis of asymptomatic aortic valve stenosis. Am Heart J 2008;156:713–8.
18. Sanchez PL, Santos JL, Kaski JC, et al. Relation of circulating C-reactive protein to progression of aortic valve stenosis. Am J Cardiol 2006;97:90–3.
19. Pedersen TR. Intensive lipid-lowering therapy for patients with aortic stenosis. Am J Cardiol 2008;102:1571–6.
20. Bonow RO, Carabello BA, Chatterjee K, et al. ACC/AHA 2006 guidelines for the management of patients with valvular heart disease: a report of the American College of Cardiology/American Heart Association Task Force on Practice Guidelines (writing committee to develop guidelines for the management of patients with valvular heart disease). Circulation 2006;114:e84–231.
21. Friedrich AD, Shekar PS. Interrogation of the aortic valve. Crit Care Med 2007; 35(8 Suppl):S365–71.
22. Silvestry FE, Kerber RE, Brook MM, et al. Echocardiography-guided interventions. J Am Soc Echocardiogr 2009;22:213–31.
23. Johnson MA, Moss RR, Munt B. Determining aortic stenosis severity: what to do when measuring left ventricular outflow tract diameter is difficult. J Am Soc Echocardiogr 2009;22:452–3.
24. Khot UN, Novaro GM, Popovic ZB, et al. Nitroprusside in critically ill patients with left ventricular dysfunction and aortic stenosis. N Engl J Med 2003;348:1756–63.
25. Munt B, Legget ME, Kraft CD, et al. Physical examination in valvular aortic stenosis: correlation with stenosis severity and prediction of clinical outcome. Am Heart J 1999;137:298–306.
26. Rosenhek R, Binder T, Porenta G, et al. Predictors of outcome in severe, asymptomatic aortic stenosis. N Engl J Med 2000;343:611–7.
27. Kume T, Kawamoto T, Akasaka T, et al. Rate of progression of valvular aortic stenosis in patients undergoing dialysis. J Am Soc Echocardiogr 2006;19:914–8.
28. Pellikka PA, Sarano ME, Nishimura RA, et al. Outcome of 622 adults with asymptomatic hemodynamically significant aortic stenosis during prolonged follow-up. Circulation 2005;111:3290–5.
29. Kume T, Kawamoto T, Okura H, et al. Rapid progression of mild to moderate aortic stenosis in patients older than 80 years. J Am Soc Echocardiogr 2007; 20:1243–6.
30. Barasch E, Gottdiener JS, Marino-Larsen EK, et al. Cardiovascular morbidity and mortality in community-dwelling elderly individuals with calcification of the fibrous skeleton of the base of the heart and aortosclerosis (The Cardiovascular Health Study). Am J Cardiol 2006;97:1281–6.
31. Aronow WS, Ahn C, Kronzon I, et al. Association of coronary risk factors and use of with progression of mild valvular aortic stenosis in older persons. Am J Cardiol 2001;88:693–5.
32. Bellamy MF, Pellikka PA, Klarich KW, et al. Association of cholesterol levels, hydroxymethylglutaryl coenzyme-A reductase inhibitor treatment, and progression of aortic stenosis in the community. J Am Coll Cardiol 2002;40:1723–30.
33. Moura LM, Ramos SF, Zamorano JL, et al. Rosuvastatin affecting aortic valve endothelium to slow the progression of aortic stenosis. J Am Coll Cardiol 2007; 49(5):554–61.

34. Galante A, Pietroiusti A, Vellini M, et al. C-reactive protein is increased in patients with degenerative aortic valve stenosis. J Am Coll Cardiol 2001;38:1078–82.
35. Otto CM. Valvular aortic stenosis: disease severity and timing of intervention. J Am Coll Cardiol 2006;47(11):2141–51.
36. Ambler G, Omar RZ, Royston P, et al. Generic, simple risk stratification model for heart valve surgery. Circulation 2005;112:224–31.
37. Roberts WC, Ko JM, Garner WL, et al. Valve structure and survival in octogenarians having aortic valve replacement for aortic stenosis (± aortic regurgitation) with versus without coronary artery bypass grafting at a single US medical center (1993-2005). Am J Cardiol 2007;100:489–95.
38. Roberts WC, Ko JM, Matter GJ. Aortic valve replacement for aortic stenosis in nonagenarians. Am J Cardiol 2006;98:1251–3.
39. Iwahashi N, Nakatani S, Kanzaki H, et al. Acute improvement in myocardial function assessed by myocardial strain and strain rate after aortic valve replacement for aortic stenosis. J Am Soc Echocardiogr 2006;19:1238–44.
40. Rajappan K, Rimoldi OE, Dutka DP, et al. Mechanisms of coronary microcirculatory dysfunction in patients with aortic stenosis and angiographically normal coronary arteries. Circulation 2002;105:470–6.
41. Rajappan K, Rimoldi OE, Camici PG, et al. Functional changes in coronary microcirculation after valve replacement in patients with aortic stenosis. Circulation 2003;107(25):3170–5.
42. Strotmann JM, Lengenfelder B, Blondelot J, et al. Functional differences of left ventricular hypertrophy induced by either arterial hypertension or aortic valve stenosis. Am J Cardiol 2008;101:1493–7.
43. Unger P, Plein D, Van Camp G, et al. Effects of valve replacement for aortic stenosis on mitral regurgitation. Am J Cardiol 2008;102:1378–82.
44. Nemes A, Galema TW, Geleijnse ML, et al. Aortic valve replacement is associated with improved aortic distensibility at long term follow-up. Am Heart J 2007;153:147–51.
45. Cheung A, Ree R. Transcatheter aortic valve replacement. Anesthesiol Clin 2008;26:465–79.
46. Shook DC, Savage RM. Anesthesia in the cardiac catheterization laboratory and electrophysiology laboratory. Anesthesiol Clin 2009;27:47–56.
47. Chiam PT, Ruiz CE. Percutaneous transcatheter aortic valve implantation: evolution of the technology. Am Heart J 2009;157:229–42.
48. Rodes-Cabau J, Dumont E, LaRochelliere R, et al. Feasibility and initial results of percutaneous aortic valve implantation including selection of the transfemoral or transapical approach in patients with severe aortic stenosis. Am J Cardiol 2008;102:1240–6.
49. Kertai MD, Bountioukos M, Boersma E, et al. Aortic stenosis: an underestimated risk factor for perioperative complications in patients undergoing noncardiac surgery. Am J Med 2004;116:8–13.
50. Fleisher LA, Beckman JA, Brown KA, et al. ACC/AHA 2007 guidelines on perioperative cardiovascular evaluation and care for noncardiac surgery: executive summary a report of the American College of Cardiology/American Heart Association Task Force on Practice Guidelines (writing committee to revise the 2002 guidelines on perioperative cardiovascular evaluation for non cardiac surgery). Circulation 2007;116:1971–96.
51. Mauck KF, Manjarrez EC, Cohn SL. Perioperative cardiac evaluation: assessment, risk reduction, and complication management. Clin Geriatr Med 2008;24:585–605.

52. Porembka DT. Importance of transesophageal echocardiography in the critically ill and injured patient. Crit Care Med 2007;35(8 Suppl):S414–30.
53. Nakamura K. Successful anesthetic management of two high-risk elderly patients using propofol-remifentanil. Masui 2008;57(4):479–82.
54. Bagri AS, Rico A, Ruiz JG. Evaluation and management of the elderly patient at risk for postoperative delirium. Clin Geriatr Med 2008;24:667–86.
55. Ho MC, Beathe JC, Sharrock NE. Hypotensive epidural anesthesia in patients with aortic stenosis undergoing total hip replacement. Reg Anesth Pain Med 2008;33:129–33.

# Fat Embolism

Shamsuddin Akhtar, MD

**KEYWORDS**

- Fat embolism • Geriatric • Fat embolism syndrome
- Acute respiratory distress syndrome • Trauma

S.M. is a 65-year-old ski instructor with a history of hypertension, well controlled with an angiotensin-converting enzyme inhibitor, who was involved in a mid-mountain collision, which resulted in compound fractures of her right and left femurs and her right tibia. She was originally transferred to small local hospital near the slope from which she was transferred to your hospital. On examination she complains of pain at a 7 on a 10-point scale. Preoperative vital signs are pulse 83 bpm, blood pressure 159/98 mmHg, and an $SpO_2$ on room air of 91%. The orthopedic surgeon is planning to use multiple intramedullary rods.

*Is this the appropriate procedure at the right time?*
*Does the choice of anesthetic have any impact on outcome?*

After some discussion, you proceed under general anesthesia. During the initial work on the right femur, you note a decreasing saturation that responds to increases in $FiO_2$ and low levels of positive end-expiratory pressure. By the end of the first femur fixation, you note petechial rash and increasing respiratory pressures. The surgeon asks you what you think. Should you:

*Stop at this time and take the patient to an intensive care unit (ICU) for proper ventilatory care?*
*Ask the surgeon to put external fixators on the other fractures before going to the ICU?*
*Finish the procedure as originally planned?*

The number of orthopedic procedures, especially joint replacement procedures, has risen sharply. By some estimates more than 650,000 hip and knee replacement procedures are being performed annually.[1] As the population's age increases this number is likely to grow. Furthermore, the incidence of hip and pathologic fractures is also likely to increase. The complication rate related to these operations is not trivial, and is associated with significant morbidity. The rate of major adverse events after hip and knee arthroplasty is estimated to be between1.7% and 4.6%.[2] Advanced age is a key factor for these adverse events. Although the rate of complication is lower for elective procedures, it can be greater than 5% for emergency procedures. Most of

Department of Anesthesiology, Yale University School of Medicine, 333 Cedar Street, TMP # 3, New Haven, CT 06520-8051, USA
*E-mail address:* shamsuddin.akhtar@yale.edu

Anesthesiology Clin 27 (2009) 533–550
doi:10.1016/j.anclin.2009.07.018
anesthesiology.theclinics.com

the complications are related to myocardial infarction, deep vein thrombosis, surgical site infection, pneumonia, and pulmonary embolism.[2,3] However, one of the most catastrophic complications is that related to fat embolism and fat embolism syndrome (FES). The exact incidence of fat embolism and FES in this population is unknown, and may be much higher than reported in retrospective studies. The presentation of FES can be nonspecific, with patients progressing to respiratory failure and acute respiratory distress syndrome (ARDS). However, it is clear that as the number of orthopedic interventions provoking fat embolization is increasing, the risk of perioperative cardiorespiratory emergencies is also increasing.[4] Thus, it is important that clinicians be knowledgeable about FES and associated sequelae. Of note, they should consider this in the differential diagnosis of cardiorespiratory and neurologic deterioration after trauma and orthopedic surgery.

## HISTORY

The pathologic significance of fat embolism was first described by Zenker in 1862.[5,6] In 1865, Wagner described the correlation of fat embolism with fractures, and attributed the origin of fat in the lungs to the bone marrow.[5] Von Bergmann is considered the first individual to clinically diagnose fat embolism and report his findings in 1873.[6,7] Seminal work by Sevitt[8] and Peltier and colleagues[9–11] has contributed significantly to the understanding of fat embolism and FES.

## DEFINITION

Fat embolism refers to the presence of fat droplets within the peripheral and lung microcirculation with or without clinical sequelae.[12] However, not all fat emboli progress to FES. FES is a clinically relevant syndrome that occurs in the presence of intravasation of fat in the pulmonary tree, and is characterized by clear signs and symptoms.[6,13,14] FES is a serious manifestation of fat embolism that involves petechial rash, deteriorating mental status, and progressive respiratory insufficiency, usually occurring within 24 hours of injury.[15] At autopsy, presence of fat can be identified in the lung vessels in more than 90% of patients with skeletal trauma,[16] and in pulmonary arterial blood samples in up to 70% of patients with pelvic or long bone fractures.[17] However, the clinical picture of the more clinically relevant FES does not develop in all patients who demonstrate the presence of intravascular or pulmonary fat.

Although various criteria have been used to characterize and define FES (**Table 1**), the criteria suggested by Gurd and Wilson[18] with some modification by Lindeque and colleagues are those that have been most widely adopted.[14,19] The criteria of Gurd and Wilson[18] require the presence of at least two of the following major clinical features: respiratory insufficiency, petechial rash or cerebral involvement, or one major and four of the five minor clinical features, defined as pyrexia, tachycardia, retinal changes, jaundice, renal changes (anuria or oliguria), fat in the urine or sputum, unexplained drop in hematocrit or platelet values, and fat macroglobulinemia. The Gurd and Wilson definition has been criticized for excluding an objective assessment of hypoxemia documented by arterial blood gas, which precedes other clinical symptoms and signs. Lindeque and colleagues[19] included the results of arterial blood gases in the formulation of their criteria. As such, they demonstrated a much higher incidence of FES by using arterial blood gases as part of the criteria (13% vs 29%). Schonfeld proposed a fat embolism index. However, this has limited value in patents with concomitant cerebral, thoracic, or abdominal injuries.[20] The clinical signs and symptoms of FES are nonspecific. Thus the differential diagnosis for each of these signs can be broad, and typically the diagnosis of FES is a diagnosis of exclusion.

**Table 1**
**Three criteria used to define fat embolism syndrome**

| Criterion | Features |
|---|---|
| Gurd and Wilson (FES = 1 major + 4 minor + fat microglobulinemia) | Major criteria<br>Respiratory insufficiency<br>Cerebral involvement<br>Petechial rash<br>Minor criteria<br>Pyrexia<br>Tachycardia<br>Retinal changes<br>Jaundice<br>Renal changes (anuria or oliguria)<br>Thrombocytopenia (a drop of >50% of the admission thrombocyte value<br>High erythrocyte sedimentation rate<br>Fat macroglobulinemia |
| Fat embolism index (FES = 5 or more points) | Diffuse petechiae (5 points)<br>Alveolar infiltrates (4 points)<br>Hypoxemia (<70 mm Hg) (3 points)<br>Confusion (1 point)<br>Fever 38°C<br>Heart rate >120/min<br>Respiratory rate >30/min |
| Lindeque criteria (FES = femur fracture ± tibia fracture + 1 feature) | A sustained $PaO_2$ <60 mm Hg<br>A sustained $PaCO_2$ >55 mm Hg) or pH <7.3<br>A sustained respiratory rate >35/min even after adequate sedation<br>Increased work of breathing judged by dyspnea, use of accessory muscles, tachycardia, and anxiety |

## EPIDEMIOLOGY

As there exist no standard uniform diagnostic and clinical criteria for diagnosing FES, the reported incidence varies widely in the literature. The incidence of posttraumatic FES has been reported to be as low as 0.25%[16] or as high as 35%.[18,19,21] In the perioperative period, some investigators report an incidence of fat embolism with the strategy of early fixation of fractures between 3.5% and 5%.[22,23] Larger series involving 3000 to 17,000 patients have reported an incidence of 0.3% to 1.3% in patients with fractures.[24] The reported incidence of FES has remained constant over the past 2 decades. A retrospective study examining a large database (National Hospital Discharge Survey) reports an incidence of FES of 0.12% in patients presenting with femur, tibia, fibula, pelvis, ribs, humerus, radius, or ulna fractures.[24] FES is also reported during instrumented spine surgery[25–27] and during vertebroplasty.[27–29] The incidence of intraoperative FES is unknown. One study reports an incidence of 0.2%.[5]

Other factors are associated with a higher risk of FES (**Table 2**). The incidence is four-fold higher in men.[24] Younger patients (10–40 years old) are more likely to develop FES than those older than 40 years (0.37% vs 0.05%).[24,30] Children younger than 10 years are less likely to develop FES. This discrepancy may be related to lower fat and olein content in the younger patients. Low incidence of FES in older patients may be because the fractures are due to low impact and involving only the neck of the femur.[24]

**Table 2**
**Risk factors for fat embolism syndrome**

| | |
|---|---|
| General factors | Males<br>Age 10–39 y<br>Posttraumatic hypovolumic state<br>Reduced cardiopulmonary reserve |
| Injury-related factors | Multiple fractures<br>Bilateral femur fractures<br>Femur shaft fractures<br>Lower extremity fractures<br>Traumatic fractures<br>Concomitant pulmonary injury |
| Surgery-related factors | Intramedullary reamed and unreamed nailing after femoral fracture<br>Joint replacement after femoral fracture<br>Bilateral procedures<br>Joint replacement with high-volume prosthesis |

The location of fracture also contributes to the frequency of fat embolization. Patients with long bone fractures are more likely to develop FES. The fracture site most frequently responsible for fat embolism is the femur. The incidence of FES is 7.6% higher in patients with isolated fractures of the femur (excluding neck) than in patients with isolated fractures of the neck.[24] Those with multiple fractures have a higher incidence than those with isolated fractures of the femur (0.06%), and tibia or fibula (0.3%).[24] Patients with bilateral femur fractures have a higher incidence of FES (4.8%–7.5%) than those with single femur fracture.[31] Open fractures are less likely to develop FES compared with closed fractures, as higher pressure is more likely to develop in closed fractures.[22,32] Patients with single fractures similarly are less likely to develop FES compared with those with multiple fractures, as more marrow is available for embolization.[33]

Carcinomas of the breast, lung, and prostate metastasize to the bone. The femur and humerus are one of the most common long bone sites for osseus metastases, and impending or pathologic fractures are uncommon, causing significant pain and disability.[34] Intramedullary rod fixation is a popular fixation technique for these fractures. Pulmonary embolic events are probably more common during intramedullary rod fixation of pathologic fractures than those without metastases.[35]

Delayed stabilization and closed reduction of a fracture is also associated with higher incidence of fat embolization.[36–38] Reamed nailing causes a higher degree of fat embolization than unreamed nailing.[39] However, unreamed nailing is not protective against fat embolization.[40] Reaming also seems to impair immune reactivity.[41] Surgical techniques, such as the use of alignment guides and long-stemmed prosthesis, can also affect the amount of fat embolization. The incidence of FES was higher in older individuals who underwent single-stage bilateral total knee replacement.[42] The incidence of FES is also reported to be higher in patients who underwent single-stage bilateral total knee replacement versus unilateral total knee arthroplasty.[42,43] Although fat can be found in pulmonary vessels after burns or injury to the adipose tissue, only a fraction of those patients develop FES.[30]

## ETIOLOGY

The most common cause of fat embolism is trauma, and it is principally related to two factors: (1) movement of unstable bone fragments and (2) reaming of the medullary cavity with internal fixation devices, which leads to distortion and increased medullary cavity pressure. Movement of the bone fragments leads to disruption of the bone marrow and intravasation of the bone marrow into the circulation. Increased medullary cavity pressure during fixation can force the fat, marrow, and bone fragments into the open venous channels. During hip and knee arthroplasty intramedullary pressure can increase from a normal value of 65 mm Hg to more than 500 mm Hg,[39] and in some studies pressures up to 1400 mm Hg have been reported. The pressures generated can be higher during arthroplasty than after fractures, as intact bone and the concomitant use of cement during arthroplasty can increase pressure within the medullary cavity.[44]

Nontraumatic causes of FE or FES are rare, and the overall incidence of these causes is extremely low.[24] One can divide them into three categories, namely disease-related, drug-related, or procedure-related. Disease-related causes are due to the process of fat or marrow necrosis (osteomyelitis, pancreatitis, panniculitis, sickle cell C variant, bone transplantation, crush injury, alcoholic fatty liver, blast injuries),[45] or by the increased concentration of lipids in the blood. Drug-related causes of FES include infusion of lipids at rates greater than the normal clearance capacity of lipids (ie, 3.8 g/kg per day)[43,46,47] or carbon tetrachloride poisoning.[6] Agglutination of lipid emulsion particles with fibrin and can also cause fat embolism. Procedure-related causes of fat embolism include intraosseous fluid and drug administration,[48] and many cases have been reported. FES has also been associated with extracorporeal circulation such as during extracorporeal membrane oxygenation and cardiopulmonary bypass.

## PATHOPHYSIOLOGY

The exact pathophysiologic mechanism that causes FES is unknown. Two theories have traditionally been proposed to explain the pathologic and clinical manifestations of FES: the mechanical hypothesis[49] and the biochemical hypothesis.[50]

### *Mechanical Hypothesis*

The mechanical hypothesis postulates that an increase in intramedullary pressure (after injury or iatrogenic) forces marrow particles, fat, or bone fragments into the circulation via the open venous sinusoids. This process leads to the embolization of fat particles that cause obstruction of the small pulmonary (20 μm in diameter)[51] and systemic vessels. This obstruction leads to organ dysfunction, and the clinical picture is dictated by the extent of the particular organ affected. Macro- and microemboli in the lungs lead to pulmonary dysfunction, ventilation-perfusion mismatch, low partial pressure of oxygen ($PaO_2$) in the arterial blood, and low oxygen saturation ($SaO_2$). Embolization to cerebral vessels or renal vessels also leads to central nervous system and renal dysfunction, respectively.[52] Central nervous system dysfunction can present as cognitive dysfunction, delirium, or confusion, whereas increases in creatinine and potentially other biochemical markers signify renal injury and dysfunction.

Translocation of the fat particles into the pulmonary circulation through venous channels can be explained physiologically. However, it is unclear how these fat emboli gain access to systemic circulation. In the setting of elevated right heart pressures and acute cor pulmonale, translocation of fat particles into the systemic circulation can be explained as passage through a patent foramen ovale (PFO). However, FES has been demonstrated in patients without echocardiographically proven right to left shunt or a PFO.[53] It is more plausible that acute elevation of right heart pressure forces the deformed fat globules through the pulmonary capillaries into the systemic circulation.[52] Other investigators have proposed the passage of fat through the intrapulmonic pulmonary-bronchial shunt.[5,54,55] Although there has been ample experimental and clinical evidence supporting the mechanical hypothesis, it is also recognized that all patients with large emboli documented by transesophageal echo (TEE) may not develop FES.[56] Therefore, factors other than mechanical obstruction by fat globules are probably involved in the development of FES.

### *Biochemical Hypothesis*

The biochemical theory postulates that physiochemical alteration occurs when fat globules are acted on by lipoprotein lipase, resulting in the release of free fatty acids (FFAs). The toxic intermediates that are produced as a result of this process cause direct injury to the pneumocytes and lung endothelial cells.[11] In turn, the damage to the endothelium leads to increased pulmonary permeability and lung surfactant inactivation, and exacerbates alveolar edema, all contributing to the development of respiratory failure. The clinical picture that develops in the lungs is indistinguishable from that seen in ARDS.[57] Some studies have demonstrated the correlation of hypoxemia with FFAs,[58,59] and inflammatory effects of FFAs in the lungs have been confirmed.[60] However, the exact source of FFAs is unclear. There is some indirect evidence that factors likely to increase the levels of FFAs (ie, decreased hepatic clearance as in shock, sepsis, or decreased plasma concentration of albumin) may also increase the risk of FES.[61,62] In addition to the presence of fatty droplets in the lungs, chemical mediators including platelet-activating factor, phospholipase A2, cyclic guanosine monophosphate, serotonin, and nitric oxide have been implicated in the pathogenesis of FES,[63–66] and these factors may play a role in the pathogenesis of ARDS.[66] The biochemical theory also includes an obstructive component, which postulates that release of mediators from the fracture site triggers coalescence of fat globules and alteration of blood lipid solubility.[50] Larger particles then cause obstruction of the vessels, leading to organ dysfunction. This process may help to explain why nontraumatic injuries can also result in FES.

The pathophysiology of FES cannot be explained solely on the basis of either the mechanical or biochemical hypotheses (**Fig. 1**). It is likely that aspects of both mechanisms contribute to the genesis of the syndrome. Mechanical factors initially may contribute to the embolization of fat (in traumatic FES) into the pulmonary and systemic circulation. FFAs and other mediators subsequently exert their biochemical and toxic effects, which are then associated with vasculitis, pneumonitis, and local inflammatory reaction in the lungs. Other inflammatory factors including activation of the coagulation cascade, disseminated intravascular coagulation, and antifibrinolytic pathways may further contribute to lung injury.[67,68] The resulting systemic inflammatory response and lung injury can quickly progress to ARDS and acute lung injury (ALI), thus making it difficult for the clinician to diagnose and differentiate FES from other causes of ARDS and ALI.

## CLINICAL PRESENTATION

FES usually manifests as a multisystem disorder. A latent period of 12 to 48 hours may precede any clinical manifestations. Tachycardia, tachypnea, and fever are nonspecific clinical signs, and commonly develop 12 to 72 hours following trauma. Some investigators have described FES to have potentially 3 clinical presentations, namely subclinical, nonfulminant subacute, and fulminant acute.[5] This presentation can be distinguished by the time of onset of symptoms after injury and the severity of the presenting clinical picture. Although these clinical presentations can be distinct, the

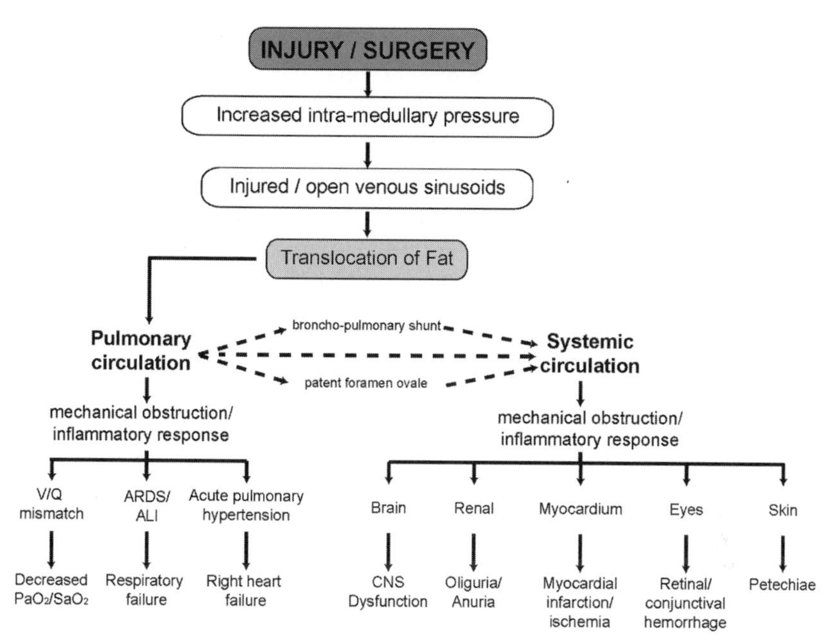


**Fig. 1.** Pathophysiology of fat embolism syndrome. ALI, acute lung injury; ARDS, acute respiratory distress syndrome; CNS, central nervous system; V/Q, ventilation/perfusion.

classification is somewhat artificial, as clinical signs and symptoms often merge or a milder presentation can progress quickly to a more severe form, especially during the manipulation of long bone fractures, insertion of prostheses, and closed reduction of fractures. FES most severely affects the lungs and brain, although there may be cardiovascular and skin involvement as well.

## *Respiratory*

Up to 75% of patients presenting with FES have some degree of respiratory dysfunction, ranging from tachypnea and mild hypoxemia to respiratory failure requiring ventilatory support.[6] Hypoxemia (room air $SaO_2$ <90%) is also common (50%–90%) after major long bone injuries, and is attributed to subclinical FES.[69–71] McCarthy documented the presence of hypoxemia ($PaO_2$ <80mm Hg) in 74% of the patients, and an elevated A-a $O_2$ gradient (>20 mm Hg) in all 50 patients he studied, who presented with uncomplicated extremity fracture.[72] A patient may initially present with tachypnea that may be related to an irritant reflex and increased alveolar dead space. This state may imperceptibly merge into a second stage of marked hypoxemia, impaired gas exchange, and low ventilation/perfusion mismatch.[73] Patients may clinically present with respiratory failure and ARDS (tachypnea, dyspnea, rales, cyanosis). It is uncommon to develop FES in the absence of pulmonary manifestations. Respiratory failure can develop rapidly and may be temporally associated with acute manipulation of fracture, reaming of the medullary cavity, or sudden release of limb tourniquet.[74] In an anesthetized patient, FES can present as respiratory deterioration with hypoxemia, pulmonary edema and decrease in lung compliance,[74] acute cor pulmonale, or acute cardiopulmonary collapse. Although these signs do not solely indicate FES, in the setting of an appropriate clinical scenario the diagnosis of FES must be considered.

### *Central Nervous System*

Perioperative central nervous system dysfunction is yet another nonspecific sign of FES. In an awake patient, cerebral signs are usually nonspecific, nonlateralizing, and mimic diffuse encephalopathy.[75] The initial presentation of drowsiness, acute anxiety, restlessness, and rigidity may progress to include seizures, confusion, stupor, and coma. The lack of cortical involvement and the symmetric appearance of lesions make it improbable that emboli are the sole cause of neurologic manifestations. The neurologic manifestations of FES are attributed to cerebral edema, which is due to injury secondary to hypoxemia, ischemia, or cerebral vascular injury due to toxic effects of FFAs and other inflammatory molecules.[76] Fortunately, these neurologic changes are usually reversible.

### *Cardiovascular*

Cardiovascular changes after pulmonary fat embolization are characterized by an increase in pulmonary artery pressure, systemic arterial hypotension, a decrease in cardiac output, and arrhythmias. The cardiovascular deterioration is often transient but may be fulminant, resulting in full-blown cardiac failure, cardiac arrest, and even death.[4] The increase in pulmonary artery pressure that occurs due to fat embolism is due not only to a mechanical blockage of the pulmonary artery, but may be the result of pulmonary vasoconstriction.[77–79]

### *Skin*

Petechial rash is also associated with FES in 25% to 95% of cases.[5,80] However, the rash is typically located on the upper anterior torso, and is also evident on oral mucous membranes, conjunctiva, skin folds of the neck, and axillae. The rash tends to be transient and disappears within 24 hours. This condition is due to engorgement of dermal vessels and increased endothelial fragility, as well as platelet damage resulting from FFAs.[81]

### *Eyes*

Retinopathy has been reported in 50% of patients with FES[82] and in 4% of patients with long bone fractures presenting with a subclinical syndrome.[32] Typical lesions consist of cotton-wool spots and flamelike hemorrhages, and are attributed to microvascular injury and microinfarction of the retina. Retinal lesions disappear after a few weeks, although scotomas may persist.[83]

### *Platelets*

Thrombocytopenia (platelet count <150,000/ml) and unexplained anemia are not uncommon. A correlation has been demonstrated between increases in A-a gradient and thrombocytopenia, even in asymptomatic fracture patients.[72] This finding has prompted some clinicians to include thrombocytopenia in the differential criteria for the diagnosis of FES.

## DIAGNOSIS

As FES has an extremely heterogeneous pattern of presentation, the precise diagnosis continues to be elusive. In addition, the signs and symptoms of FES are nonspecific. There are no pathognomic signs (except for petechial rash) or specific confirmatory tests. Thus the diagnosis of FES is based on a constellation of clinical and laboratory findings, and exclusion of other potential diagnoses.[6]

### *Laboratory Tests*

A blood gas analysis performed at room air will often reveal a $PaO_2$ of less than 60 mm Hg. Hypoxemia is almost always present in patients with FES, and is considered one of the major criteria for the diagnosis of FES.[19] Hypoxemia can lead to compensatory tachypnea, and on the initial blood gas analysis respiratory alkalosis may be noted. Specific biochemical tests that measure serum lipase or phospholipase A2 were initially thought to aid in the diagnosis of FES. Although these enzymes are increased in patients with FES and lung injury, however, they are not specific and are not considered reliable tests for the diagnosis of FES.[84] Fat globules may be seen in patients with FES on cytologic examination of urine, blood, or sputum. However, none of these tests are reliable and they cannot be used solely for the diagnosis of FES.[84,85] Quantification of cells containing fat droplets in bronchial alveolar lavage (BAL) fluid within the first 24 hours after trauma have also been shown to correlate with clinical fat embolism in some studies.[86–89] In the absence of a high load of exogenously delivered fat, BAL fluid that contains more than 30% macrophages laden with lipid inclusions is very suggestive of FES. However, it may not be possible to obtain an adequate number of macrophages for analysis;[90] obtaining BAL is resource intensive (requires bronchoscopy) and is not specific for FES.[89]

### *Imaging Studies*

Abnormalities on chest radiograph are evident in patients with FES 30% to 50% of the time.[91] However, the abnormalities are nonspecific and demonstrate a lag time about 12 to 24 hours as related to the clinical symptoms. Diffuse, evenly distributed interstitial and alveolar densities are typical findings. Patchy infiltrates in the perihilar and basilar areas resemble pulmonary edema, without vascular congestion and cardiomegaly. Comparable changes on the computed tomography (CT) scan can also be seen with multiple subsegmented (mottled) perfusion defects. Ventilation-perfusion scans also demonstrate subsegmental perfusion defects, and are highly suggestive of FES.[92] These defects may be present even in the absence of any radiographic abnormalities on the chest radiograph. CT scan of the brain may show nonspecific signs of cerebral edema and multiple areas of hemorrhagic infarct.[93] Of clinical note, magnetic resonance imaging (MRI) of the brain seems to be more sensitive in detecting abnormalities in patients with FES.[94–98] Abnormalities in an MRI in patients with FES include hypointense lesions on cerebral T1W images. Conventional T2W sequences typically reveal multiple diffuse foci of hyperintensity in the deep white matter, basal ganglia, corpus callosum, periventricular region, and cerebellar hemisphere. The changes associated with T2W images are associated with vasogenic edema but they may require a few days to develop.[96] The MRI changes seen in acute state can resolve in 3 weeks and are associated with resolution of neurologic symptoms. Although the MRI changes are somewhat nonspecific and can be seen with other conditions like diffuse axonal injury, gliosis, and demyelinating process in conjunction with the clinical picture, FES should be considered in the presence of these findings. Cerebral microemboli after long bone fractures can be detected in vivo and monitored over time by transcranial Doppler (TCD) as well. In a study of 12 patients undergoing elective hip or knee replacement, all patients showed intraoperative cerebral microemboli by TCD.[99] In another study, 41% of the 22 patients studied intraoperatively with TCD showed signals consistent with microemboli.[100] However, the perioperative potential of TCD monitoring needs to be explored further.[101]

Suspected intraoperative pulmonary embolism can be identified most rapidly with use of TEE. In patients with pulmonary embolism large enough to produce hemodynamic instability, TEE has a sensitivity of 80% and a specificity of 100%.[102] Unfortunately, as the echocardiographic appearance of fat and tumor are similar, it is not possible to reliably diagnose fat embolism intraoperatively. Fat embolism can be demonstrated intraoperatively by echocardiography in 60% of the patients undergoing total hip arthroplasty[103] and 80% to 90% of the time during intraoperative medullary manipulation.[25,35] Evidence of echogenic emboli in the right heart by echo and a simultaneous drop in $PaO_2$ can be a specific sign of subclinical FES.

## MANAGEMENT

There is no definitive therapy for FES. Once the full-blown syndrome develops, treatment is most often supportive. Thus the clinical management strategies are generally geared toward prophylactic measures. Three traditional scenarios can be encountered. The first scenario is a patient who is at risk of developing FES and has nonspecific signs of the disease. The second represents a patient who has clinical manifestations of FES and is presenting for surgery. The third involves a patient who develops signs of worsening FES or fulminant FES intraoperatively. The intraoperative scenario can develop during manipulation of the fracture or insertion of a prosthesis.

### *Preventative Measures*

Before any clinical syndrome develops, it is possible to initiate certain measures that may prevent or decrease the severity of FES. Early stabilization of the fracture involving the pelvis or long bones is probably the single most important prophylactic measure that has been shown to result in a decrease in the incidence of FES.[21,104,105] Early rigid fixation of fractures decreases the recurrent bouts of fat embolism. One report shows a 70% reduction in pulmonary complications (relative risk = 0.3, confidence interval 0.22–0.4).[106]

It has been shown that in those patients who are likely to develop FES preoperatively, are also likely to experience exacerbations intraoperatively. Some institutions delay any definitive operative fixation until clinical improvement has been observed.[5] One alternative is to stabilize fractures by external fixation (if possible) initially and then perform the definitive fixation once the clinical situation allows.[106–108] Although early stabilization of fractures is the preferred option in uncomplicated cases, it is unclear whether this is an optimal option in patients who are already showing signs of FES[109] or have sustained significant trauma and lung contusion.[107,110] There is experimental evidence suggesting that femoral nailing can result in significant polymorphonuclear leukocyte activation, pulmonary permeability, and interstitial lung edema compared with external fixation.[110] Pulmonary permeability also appears more enhanced in the setting of lung contusion.[110] However, this has not been confirmed by other studies.[111] Although there is clinical utility in prophylactically placing a Greenfield filter in patients with deep vein thrombosis before surgery, its role in preventing FES in high-risk patients has not been studied and therefore cannot be advocated as a matter of routine practice.

Several surgical strategies have been advanced to reduce the likelihood.[112] Although the signs of intraoperative FES can be nonspecific, sudden development of cardiopulmonary instability, pulmonary edema that is temporarily related to fracture manipulation, and intramedullary nailing of long bone fractures should alert the clinician to the possibility of FES. Depending on the severity of operative procedure planned, the surgery may have to be curtailed. Intraoperative surgical techniques such as venting to prevent high medullary pressure may have a role in decreasing the incidence of FES. However, this technique is not universally adopted, and practice patterns vary widely.[113] Careful surgical technique that focuses on limiting the medullary canal pressurization associated with reaming is helpful. Drilling holes in the cortex to prevent development of high pressures may prevent FES, in some but not all cases.[103] Lavaging the marrow before inserting the prosthesis similarly may decrease the amount of marrow available for embolization.[114] In some situations use of a tourniquet may prevent embolization of the material into the systemic circulation; however, FES can still occur on tourniquet release.[115] Venting before the insertion of prosthesis has also been suggested as one strategy to decrease intramedullary pressure and the incidence of FES.

The use of preventative pharmacologic therapies has been disappointing.[116,117] Although various agents (aspirin, hypertonic saline, low molecular weight dextran, and steroids) have all been suggested, none have been definitively proven to help. Sildenafil has been shown to prevent an increase in pulmonary pressures after bone marrow embolization in one experimental model.[4] In another model, *N*-acetylcysteine attenuated ALI induced by fat embolism.[118] High-dose methylprednisone (90 mg/kg over 4 days) or a lower dose prophylactically (6 mg/kg over 2 days) has shown some clinical efficacy in improving outcomes.[119] Steroids are thought to limit the increase of FFAs, stabilize the membranes, and inhibit complement-mediated leukocyte aggregation. However, high-dose methylprednisolone can also have significant side effects. Therefore, the use or methylprednisolone has not been proved by any large-scale prospective trials and its routine use cannot be advocated.

### *Perioperative Considerations*

The possibility of FES should be entertained in patients with long bone fractures presenting for definitive operative procedures. In most situations the clinical status of patients will be recognized before anesthetizing them for surgery. Intraoperative use of some monitors may help detect and diagnose intraoperative fat embolism. End-tidal $CO_2$ is not sensitive in detecting fat embolism as it is a venous air embolism.[120] For patients who present with significant preoperative cardiopulmonary issues, it may be prudent to monitor their hemodynamics invasively with an arterial line and central line, or a pulmonary artery catheter. Pulmonary artery pressure can increase significantly, though not consistently, with FES.[120] Any sudden increases in pulmonary artery pressure from the baseline should alert the physician to the possibility of an impending FES. Because pulmonary pressures may not change significantly even in the setting of FES, the utility of a pulmonary artery catheter in this setting has been questioned.[121] TEE is a sensitive monitor to detect FES. The embolic particles typically appear as several white flakes flowing through the right atrium. However, rapid infusion of fluids may cause similar visual effects. In addition, TEE can be extremely helpful in excluding significant pulmonary thromboembolism and regional wall motion abnormalities suggestive of myocardial ischemia, and ruling out other causes of intraoperative hemodynamic instability. TCD can be used as a method for detecting and monitoring cerebral microemboli intraoperatively.[100,101] However, the potential diagnostic and therapeutic implications of TCD as a perioperative monitor need to be further explored.[101]

If FES develops perioperatively, there is no definitive treatment. Early recognition and supportive therapy are paramount in optimizing clinical outcomes in patients who develop FES. Once the syndrome develops, the clinical dysfunction is treated symptomatically. Initial respiratory dysfunction is managed using supplemental oxygen to prevent hypoxemia. Respiratory failure (ARDS/ALI) is managed by ventilatory support modes. The use of steroids in the treatment of FES is controversial and is not supported by large, randomized control trials. Inotropes (epinephrine, norepinephrine, vasopressin, phenylephrine) and fluids are typically used to manage intraoperative hypotension and cardiovascular collapse. Management of right heart failure secondary to increased pulmonary hypertension is challenging. In addition to inotropic support, it may require specific pulmonary vasodilators.

No significant differences have been noted in FES outcomes in patients receiving general or regional anesthesia. Although the incidence of deep vein thrombosis is decreased with regional anesthesia, the choice of anesthetic should be decided by the clinical condition of the patient. Anesthesiologists occasionally may encounter mental status changes, significant emergence delirium, irritability, and confused state in the postoperative care unit or postoperatively.[122] In the appropriate clinical setting, the diagnosis FES must be entertained, and patients should be evaluated with an MRI scan to rule out FES.[96] Management of cerebral dysfunction is primarily supportive, with the aim of optimizing the intracranial pressure, cerebral perfusion pressure, and oxygen delivery.

## PROGNOSIS

Most of the morbidity associated with FES is related to pulmonary dysfunction. However, pulmonary presentations of fulminant FES in a multitrauma patient can be identical to the presentation of ARDS in many of the clinical settings. In many cases it may be impossible to differentiate and establish the etiology of ARDS/ALI. Thus it is difficult to determine the exact morbidity and mortality from FES. Bulger and colleagues[36] reported an incidence of 0.9% mortality among patients with long bone fractures, whereas Chan and colleagues[84] reported an incidence of 8.7% in a prospective series of 80 patients. However, most investigators agree that with the improvement in supportive therapy, and early stabilization and definitive fixation of fractures, the overall outcomes of patients with FES has improved. The overall mortality may now be less than 10%[6,12] compared with as high as 30% quoted in older studies. Patients who develop central nervous system dysfunction secondary to FES have a poor prognosis.

## SUMMARY

The pathologic consequences of fat embolism are well recognized. Fat embolism is most often associated with trauma and orthopedic injuries. FES is a serious manifestation of fat embolism that involves a cascade of clinical signs such as petechial rash, deteriorating mental status, and progressive respiratory insufficiency, usually occurring within 24 hours of injury.[15] The diagnosis of FES is based on a constellation of clinical and laboratory findings, and exclusion of other diagnoses.[6] Whereas there is no specific treatment for FES, management strategies are mainly supportive measures. Prophylactic measures such as early stabilization of fractures, and prudent intraoperative techniques, may help decrease the incidence and severity of FES. It is evident that the number of orthopedic interventions provoking fat embolization is increasing, and therefore, the risk of perioperative cardiorespiratory emergencies is also increasing.[4] Thus it is important that clinicians be knowledgeable regarding FES and its associated clinical presentation, and should be considered in the differential diagnosis of cardiorespiratory and neurologic deterioration during and following trauma and orthopedic surgery.

## REFERENCES

1. Kurtz S, Mowat F, Ong K, et al. Prevalence of primary and revision total hip and knee arthroplasty in the United States from 1990 through 2002. J Bone Joint Surg Am 2005;87(7):1487–97.

2. Mantilla CB, Horlocker TT, Schroeder DR, et al. Frequency of myocardial infarction, pulmonary embolism, deep venous thrombosis, and death following primary hip or knee arthroplasty. Anesthesiology 2002;96(5):1140–6.
3. Mahomed NN, Barrett JA, Katz JN, et al. Rates and outcomes of primary and revision total hip replacement in the United States medicare population. J Bone Joint Surg Am 2003;85(1):27–32.
4. Krebs J, Ferguson SJ, Nuss K, et al. Sildenafil prevents cardiovascular changes after bone marrow fat embolization in sheep. Anesthesiology 2007;107(1): 75–81.
5. Capan LM, Miller SM, Patel KP. Fat embolism. Anesthesiol Clin North America 1993;11(1):25–54.
6. Taviloglu K, Yanar H. Fat embolism syndrome. Surg Today 2007;37(1):5–8.
7. Warthin AS. Traumatic lipemia and fatty embolism. Int Clin 1913;4:171–227.
8. Sevitt S. The significance and pathology of fat embolism. Ann Clin Res 1977; 9(3):173–80.
9. Peltier LF. Fat embolism. I. The amount of fat in human long bones. Surgery 1956;40(4):657–60.
10. Boyd HM, Peltier LF, Scott JR, et al. Fat embolism. II. The chemical composition of fat obtained from human long bones and subcutaneous tissue. Surgery 1956; 40(4):661–4.
11. Peltier LF. Fat embolism. III. The toxic properties of neutral fat and free fatty acids. Surgery 1956;40(4):665–70.
12. Turillazzi E, Riezzo I, Neri M, et al. The diagnosis of fatal pulmonary fat embolism using quantitative morphometry and confocal laser scanning microscopy. Pathol Res Pract 2008;204(4):259–66.
13. Schmid A, Tzur A, Leshko L, et al. Silicone embolism syndrome: a case report, review of the literature, and comparison with fat embolism syndrome. Chest 2005;127(6):2276–81.
14. Talbot M, Schemitsch EH. Fat embolism syndrome: history, definition, epidemiology. Injury 2006;37(suppl 4):S3–7.
15. Levy D. The fat embolism syndrome. A review. Clin Orthop Relat Res 1990;(261): 281–6.
16. Peltier LF. Fat embolism. A current concept. Clin Orthop Relat Res 1969;66: 241–53.
17. Lozman J, Deno DC, Feustel PJ, et al. Pulmonary and cardiovascular consequences of immediate fixation or conservative management of long-bone fractures. Arch Surg 1986;121(9):992–9.
18. Gurd AR, Wilson RI. The fat embolism syndrome. J Bone Joint Surg Br 1974; 56(3):408–16.
19. Lindeque BG, Schoeman HS, Dommisse GF, et al. Fat embolism and the fat embolism syndrome. A double-blind therapeutic study. J Bone Joint Surg Br 1987; 69(1):128–31.
20. Schonfeld SA, Ploysongsang Y, DiLisio R, et al. Fat embolism prophylaxis with corticosteroids. A prospective study in high-risk patients. Ann Intern Med 1983;99(4):438–43.
21. Riska EB, Myllynen P. Fat embolism in patients with multiple injuries. J Trauma 1982;22(11):891–4.
22. ten Duis HJ, Nijsten MW, Klasen HJ, et al. Fat embolism in patients with an isolated fracture of the femoral shaft. J Trauma 1988;28(3):383–90.
23. Moore P, James O, Saltos N. Fat embolism syndrome: incidence, significance and early features. Aust N Z J Surg 1981;51(6):546–51.

24. Stein PD, Yaekoub AY, Matta F, et al. Fat embolism syndrome. Am J Med Sci 2008;336(6):472–7.
25. Takahashi S, Kitagawa H, Ishii T. Intraoperative pulmonary embolism during spinal instrumentation surgery. A prospective study using transoesophageal echocardiography. J Bone Joint Surg Br 2003;85(1):90–4.
26. Takahashi Y, Narusawa K, Shimizu K, et al. Fatal pulmonary fat embolism after posterior spinal fusion surgery. J Orthop Sci 2006;11(2):217–20.
27. Syed MI, Jan S, Patel NA, et al. Fatal fat embolism after vertebroplasty: identification of the high-risk patient. AJNR Am J Neuroradiol 2006;27(2):343–5.
28. Chen HL, Wong CS, Ho ST, et al. A lethal pulmonary embolism during percutaneous vertebroplasty. Anesth Analg 2002;95(4):1060–2, table of contents.
29. Benneker LM, Heini PF, Suhm N, et al. The effect of pulsed jet lavage in vertebroplasty on injection forces of polymethylmethacrylate bone cement, material distribution, and potential fat embolism: a cadaver study. Spine 2008;33(23): E906–10.
30. Mokkhavesa S, Shim SS, Patterson FP. Fat embolism: clinical and experimental studies with emphasis on therapeutic aspects. J Trauma 1969;9(1):39–48.
31. Kontakis GM, Tossounidis T, Weiss K, et al. Fat embolism: special situations bilateral femoral fractures and pathologic femoral fractures. Injury 2006; 37(suppl 4):S19–24.
32. Thomas JE, Ayyar DR. Systemic fat embolism. A diagnostic profile in 24 patients. Arch Neurol 1972;26(6):517–23.
33. Rokkanen P, Lahdensuu M, Kataja J, et al. The syndrome of fat embolism: analysis of thirty consecutive cases compared to trauma patients with similar injuries. J Trauma 1970;10(4):299–306.
34. Choong PF. Cardiopulmonary complications of intramedullary fixation of long bone metastases. Clin Orthop Relat Res 2003;(415 suppl):S245–53.
35. Christie J, Robinson CM, Pell AC, et al. Transcardiac echocardiography during invasive intramedullary procedures. J Bone Joint Surg Br 1995;77(3):450–5.
36. Bulger EM, Smith DG, Maier RV, et al. Fat embolism syndrome. A 10-year review. Arch Surg 1997;132(4):435–9.
37. Robert JH, Hoffmeyer P, Broquet PE, et al. Fat embolism syndrome. Orthop Rev 1993;22(5):567–71.
38. Pinney SJ, Keating JF, Meek RN. Fat embolism syndrome in isolated femoral fractures: does timing of nailing influence incidence? Injury 1998;29(2):131–3.
39. Pape HC, Giannoudis P. The biological and physiological effects of intramedullary reaming. J Bone Joint Surg Br 2007;89(11):1421–6.
40. Kropfl A, Davies J, Berger U, et al. Intramedullary pressure and bone marrow fat extravasation in reamed and unreamed femoral nailing. J Orthop Res 1999; 17(2):261–8.
41. Giannoudis PV, Pape HC, Cohen AP, et al. Review: systemic effects of femoral nailing: from Kuntscher to the immune reactivity era. Clin Orthop Relat Res 2002;(404):378–86.
42. Urban MK, Chisholm M, Wukovits B. Are postoperative complications more common with single-stage bilateral (SBTKR) than with unilateral knee arthroplasty: guidelines for patients scheduled for SBTKR. HSS J 2006;2(1):78–82.
43. Ritter M, Mamlin LA, Melfi CA, et al. Outcome implications for the timing of bilateral total knee arthroplasties. Clin Orthop Relat Res 1997;(345):99–105.
44. Kallos T, Enis JE, Gollan F, et al. Intramedullary pressure and pulmonary embolism of femoral medullary contents in dogs during insertion of bone cement and a prosthesis. J Bone Joint Surg Am 1974;56(7):1363–7.

45. Goldhaber SZ. Pulmonary embolism. Lancet 2004;363(9417):1295–305.
46. Haber LM, Hawkins EP, Seilheimer DK, et al. Fat overload syndrome. An autopsy study with evaluation of the coagulopathy. Am J Clin Pathol 1988;90(2):223–7.
47. Kitchell CC, Balogh K. Pulmonary lipid emboli in association with long-term hyperalimentation. Hum Pathol 1986;17(1):83–5.
48. Hasan MY, Kissoon N, Khan TM, et al. Intraosseous infusion and pulmonary fat embolism. Pediatr Crit Care Med 2001;2(2):133–8.
49. Gauss H. The pathology of fat embolism. Arch Surg 1924;9:593–605.
50. Lehmann EP, Moore RM. Fat embolism including experimental production without trauma. Arch Surg 1927;14:621–62.
51. Batra P. The fat embolism syndrome. J Thorac Imaging 1987;2(3):12–7.
52. Findlay JM, DeMajo W. Cerebral fat embolism. Can Med Assoc J 1984;131(7): 755–7.
53. Nijsten MW, Hamer JP, ten Duis HJ, et al. Fat embolism and patent foramen ovale [letter]. Lancet 1989;1(8649):1271.
54. Byrick RJ, Kay JC, Mazer CD, et al. Dynamic characteristics of cerebral lipid microemboli: videomicroscopy studies in rats. Anesth Analg 2003;97(6): 1789–94.
55. Meyer N, Pennington WT, Dewitt D, et al. Isolated cerebral fat emboli syndrome in multiply injured patients: a review of three cases and the literature. J Trauma 2007;63(6):1395–402.
56. Aoki N, Soma K, Shindo M, et al. Evaluation of potential fat emboli during placement of intramedullary nails after orthopedic fractures. Chest 1998;113(1): 178–81.
57. Peltier LF. Fat embolism. A perspective. Clin Orthop Relat Res 1988;(232): 263–70.
58. Riseborough EJ, Herndon JH. Alterations in pulmonary function, coagulation and fat metabolism in patients with fractures of the lower limbs. Clin Orthop Relat Res 1976;(115):248–67.
59. Nixon JR, Brock-Utne JG. Free fatty acid and arterial oxygen changes following major injury: a correlation between hypoxemia and increased free fatty acid levels. J Trauma 1978;18(1):23–6.
60. Parker FB Jr, Wax SD, Kusajima K, et al. Hemodynamic and pathological findings in experimental fat embolism. Arch Surg 1974;108(1):70–4.
61. Moylan JA, Birnbaum M, Katz A, et al. Fat emboli syndrome. J Trauma 1976; 16(5):341–7.
62. Mays ET. The effect of surgical stress on plasma free fatty acids. J Surg Res 1970;10(7):315–9.
63. Roger N, Xaubet A, Agusti C, et al. Role of bronchoalveolar lavage in the diagnosis of fat embolism syndrome. Eur Respir J 1995;8(8):1275–80.
64. Karagiorga G, Nakos G, Galiatsou E, et al. Biochemical parameters of bronchoalveolar lavage fluid in fat embolism. Intensive Care Med 2006;32(1): 116–23.
65. Kao SJ, Chen HI. Nitric oxide mediates acute lung injury caused by fat embolism in isolated rat's lungs. J Trauma 2008;64(2):462–9.
66. Kao SJ, Yeh DY, Chen HI. Clinical and pathological features of fat embolism with acute respiratory distress syndrome. Clin Sci (Lond) 2007;113(6):279–85.
67. King EG, Weily HS, Genton E, et al. Consumption coagulopathy in the canine oleic acid model of fat embolism. Surgery 1971;69(4):533–41.
68. Saldeen T. Fat embolism and signs of intravascular coagulation in a posttraumatic autopsy material. J Trauma 1970;10(4):273–86.

69. Benoit PR, Hampson LG, Burgess JH. Respiratory gas exchange following fractures: the role of fat embolism as a cause of arterial hypoxemia. Surg Forum 1969;20:214–6.
70. Benoit PR, Hampson LG, Burgess JH. Value of arterial hypoxemia in the diagnosis of pulmonary fat embolism. Ann Surg 1972;175(1):128–37.
71. Tachakra SS, Sevitt S. Hypoxaemia after fractures. J Bone Joint Surg Br 1975; 57(2):197–203.
72. McCarthy B, Mammen E, Leblanc LP, et al. Subclinical fat embolism: a prospective study of 50 patients with extremity fractures. J Trauma 1973; 13(1):9–16.
73. Prys-Roberts C. Fat embolism. Anaesthesia 2001;56(7):692–3.
74. Hagley SR. The fulminant fat embolism syndrome. Anaesth Intensive Care 1983; 11(2):167–70.
75. Jacobson DM, Terrence CF, Reinmuth OM. The neurologic manifestations of fat embolism. Neurology 1986;36(6):847–51.
76. Butteriss DJ, Mahad D, Soh C, et al. Reversible cytotoxic cerebral edema in cerebral fat embolism. AJNR Am J Neuroradiol 2006;27(3):620–3.
77. Aebli N, Schwenke D, Davis G, et al. Polymethylmethacrylate causes prolonged pulmonary hypertension during fat embolism: a study in sheep. Acta Orthop 2005;76(6):904–11.
78. Krebs J, Ferguson SJ, Nuss K, et al. Plasma levels of endothelin-1 after a pulmonary embolism of bone marrow fat. Acta Anaesthesiol Scand 2007;51(8): 1107–14.
79. Murphy P, Edelist G, Byrick RJ, et al. Relationship of fat embolism to haemodynamic and echocardiographic changes during cemented arthroplasty. Can J Anaesth 1997;44(12):1293–300.
80. Gossling HR, Pellegrini VD Jr. Fat embolism syndrome: a review of the pathophysiology and physiological basis of treatment. Clin Orthop Relat Res 1982;(165):68–82.
81. Pazell JA, Peltier LF. Experience with sixty-three patients with fat embolism. Surg Gynecol Obstet 1972;135(1):77–80.
82. Adams CB. The retinal manifestations of fat embolism. Injury 1971;2(3):221–4.
83. Chuang EL, Miller FS 3rd, Kalina RE. Retinal lesions following long bone fractures. Ophthalmology 1985;92(3):370–4.
84. Chan KM, Tham KT, Chiu HS, et al. Post-traumatic fat embolism—its clinical and subclinical presentations. J Trauma 1984;24(1):45–9.
85. Peltier LF. Fat embolism. An appraisal of the problem. Clin Orthop Relat Res 1984;(187):3–17.
86. Mimoz O, Edouard A, Beydon L, et al. Contribution of bronchoalveolar lavage to the diagnosis of posttraumatic pulmonary fat embolism. Intensive Care Med 1995;21(12):973–80.
87. Al-Khuwaitir TS, Al-Moghairi AM, Sherbeeni SM, et al. Traumatic fat embolism syndrome. Saudi Med J 2002;23(12):1532–6.
88. Chastre J, Fagon JY, Soler P, et al. Bronchoalveolar lavage for rapid diagnosis of the fat embolism syndrome in trauma patients. Ann Intern Med 1990;113(8): 583–8.
89. Mellor A, Soni N. Fat embolism. Anaesthesia 2001;56(2):145–54.
90. Vedrinne JM, Guillaume C, Gagnieu MC, et al. Bronchoalveolar lavage in trauma patients for diagnosis of fat embolism syndrome. Chest 1992;102(5):1323–7.
91. Greenberg HB. Roentgenographic signs of posttraumatic fat embolism. JAMA 1968;204(6):540–1.

92. Park HM, Ducret RP, Brindley DC. Pulmonary imaging in fat embolism syndrome. Clin Nucl Med 1986;11(7):521–2.
93. Meeke RI, Fitzpatrick GJ, Phelan DM. Cerebral oedema and the fat embolism syndrome. Intensive Care Med 1987;13(4):291–2.
94. Satoh H, Kurisu K, Ohtani M, et al. Cerebral fat embolism studied by magnetic resonance imaging, transcranial Doppler sonography, and single photon emission computed tomography: case report. J Trauma 1997;43(2):345–8.
95. Stoeger A, Daniaux M, Felber S, et al. MRI findings in cerebral fat embolism. Eur Radiol 1998;8(9):1590–3.
96. Chen JJ, Ha JC, Mirvis SE. MR imaging of the brain in fat embolism syndrome. Emerg Radiol 2008;15(3):187–92.
97. Eguia P, Medina A, Garcia-Monco JC, et al. The value of diffusion-weighted MRI in the diagnosis of cerebral fat embolism. J Neuroimaging 2007;17(1):78–80.
98. Sasano N, Ishida S, Tetsu S, et al. Cerebral fat embolism diagnosed by magnetic resonance imaging at one, eight, and 50 days after hip arthroplasty: a case report. Can J Anaesth 2004;51(9):875–9.
99. Koch S, Forteza A, Lavernia C, et al. Cerebral fat microembolism and cognitive decline after hip and knee replacement. Stroke 2007;38(3):1079–81.
100. Barak M, Kabha M, Norman D, et al. Cerebral microemboli during hip fracture fixation: a prospective study. Anesth Analg 2008;107(1):221–5.
101. Forteza AM, Koch S, Romano JG, et al. Transcranial Doppler detection of fat emboli. Stroke 1999;30(12):2687–91.
102. Pruszczyk P, Torbicki A, Pacho R, et al. Noninvasive diagnosis of suspected severe pulmonary embolism: transesophageal echocardiography vs spiral CT. Chest 1997;112(3):722–8.
103. Heinrich H, Kremer P, Winter H, et al. [Transesophageal 2-dimensional echocardiography in hip endoprostheses]. Anaesthesist 1985;34(3):118–23.
104. Svenningsen S, Nesse O, Finsen V, et al. Prevention of fat embolism syndrome in patients with femoral fractures—immediate or delayed operative fixation? Ann Chir Gynaecol 1987;76(3):163–6.
105. Talucci RC, Manning J, Lampard S, et al. Early intramedullary nailing of femoral shaft fractures: a cause of fat embolism syndrome. Am J Surg 1983;146(1): 107–11.
106. Robinson CM. Current concepts of respiratory insufficiency syndromes after fracture. J Bone Joint Surg Br 2001;83(6):781–91.
107. Pape HC. Effects of changing strategies of fracture fixation on immunologic changes and systemic complications after multiple trauma: damage control orthopedic surgery. J Orthop Res 2008;26(11):1478–84.
108. Pape HC, Rixen D, Morley J, et al. Impact of the method of initial stabilization for femoral shaft fractures in patients with multiple injuries at risk for complications (borderline patients). Ann Surg 2007;246(3):491–9 [discussion: 499–501].
109. Tachakra SC, Potts D, Idowu A. Early operative fracture management of patients with multiple injuries [comment]. Br J Surg 1990;77(10):1194.
110. Hildebrand F, Giannoudis P, van Griensven M, et al. Secondary effects of femoral instrumentation on pulmonary physiology in a standardised sheep model: what is the effect of lung contusion and reaming? Injury 2005;36(4): 544–55.
111. Wolinsky P, Tejwani N, Richmond JH, et al. Controversies in intramedullary nailing of femoral shaft fractures. Instr Course Lect 2002;51:291–303.
112. Giannoudis PV, Tzioupis C, Pape HC. Fat embolism: the reaming controversy. Injury 2006;37(suppl 4):S50–8.

113. Dalgorf D, Borkhoff CM, Stephen DJ, et al. Venting during prophylactic nailing for femoral metastases: current orthopedic practice. Can J Surg 2003;46(6): 427–31.
114. Byrick RJ, Bell RS, Kay JC, et al. High-volume, high-pressure pulsatile lavage during cemented arthroplasty. J Bone Joint Surg Am 1989;71(9):1331–6.
115. Hagley SR. The fulminant fat embolism syndrome. Anaesth Intensive Care 1983; 11(2):162–6.
116. Shier MR, Wilson RF, James RE, et al. Fat embolism prophylaxis: a study of four treatment modalities. J Trauma 1977;17(8):621–9.
117. Stoltenberg JJ, Gustilo RB. The use of methylprednisolone and hypertonic glucose in the prophylaxis of fat embolism syndrome. Clin Orthop Relat Res 1979;(143):211–21.
118. Liu DD, Kao SJ, Chen HI. *N*-Acetylcysteine attenuates acute lung injury induced by fat embolism. Crit Care Med 2008;36(2):565–71.
119. Babalis GA, Yiannakopoulos CK, Karliaftis K, et al. Prevention of posttraumatic hypoxaemia in isolated lower limb long bone fractures with a minimal prophylactic dose of corticosteroids. Injury 2004;35(3):309–17.
120. Byrick RJ, Kay JC, Mullen JB. Capnography is not as sensitive as pulmonary artery pressure monitoring in detecting marrow microembolism. Studies in a canine model. Anesth Analg 1989;68(2):94–100.
121. Jules-Elysee KM, Yadeau JT, Urban MK. Pulmonary artery versus central venous catheter monitoring in the outcome of patients undergoing bilateral total knee replacement. HSS J 2009;5(1):27–30.
122. McIntyre K, French S, Rose TH, et al. Case report: acute postoperative neurological impairment from fat embolism syndrome. Can J Anaesth 2007;54(4): 296–300.

# Anesthetic Management of Acute Mesenteric Ischemia in Elderly Patients

Alexander A. Vitin, MD, PhD*, Julia I. Metzner, MD

**KEYWORDS**

- Acute mesenteric ischemia • Elderly • Splanchnic circulation
- Management • Anesthesia

## CLINICAL PRESENTATION

A 76-year-old man is admitted to the hospital because of acute excruciating abdominal pain, nausea, vomiting, shortness of breath, and dizziness. He reports multiple bowel movements, including bloody diarrhea. On admission, his vital signs are: blood pressure (BP) 100/65 mm Hg, heart rate (HR) 110/min irregular, respiratory rate (RR) 18/min, arterial oxygen saturation ($Sa_{O_2}$) 91% on room air. Chest auscultation reveals equal breath sounds plus scattered wheezing over both lung fields. His abdomen is slightly distended, with nonlocalized pain on palpation, without peritoneal signs. Peristalsis sounds are minimal.

His medical history is significant for coronary artery disease, hypertension, chronic obstructive pulmonary disease (COPD), insulin-dependent diabetes type II and hyperlipidemia. About 12 months ago, he had sustained an acute inferior myocardial infarction (MI) and pulmonary edema. The right and marginal coronary arteries received stents. ECG shows atrial fibrillation (AF), frequent ventricular premature beats (VPBs), right bundle branch block (RBBB) and left ventricular (LV) hypertrophy. Echocardiographic examination reveals akinesia of the LV inferior wall, LV hypertrophy, left atrial (LA) dilation, mild-to-moderate mitral regurgitation (MR), and an ejection fraction (EF) of 40%.

The tentative diagnosis of acute mesenteric ischemia (AMI) is confirmed by abdominal contrast-enhanced CT with mesenteric angiography, which reveals occlusion of the superior mesenteric artery (SMA) and the left colic artery (LCA). Thrombectomy of the SMA and LCA is performed, and papaverine intra-arterial infusion begun. Six hours thereafter, the patient's condition worsens with his abdomen now diffusely

Department of Anesthesiology and Pain Medicine, University of Washington, 1959 NE Pacific Street, Seattle, WA 98195-6540, USA
* Corresponding author.
*E-mail address:* vitin@u.washington.edu (A. A. Vitin).

Anesthesiology Clin 27 (2009) 551–567
doi:10.1016/j.anclin.2009.07.017
1932-2275/09/$ – see front matter. Published by Elsevier Inc.

tender and rigid, with an absence of bowel sounds. His vitals are now: BP 90/45 mm Hg, HR 122, AF, RR 22, $Sa_{O_2}$ with oxygen mask is 93%. He is scheduled for an emergent exploratory laparotomy, with SMA and LCA exploration/thrombectomy and possible bowel resection.

AMI is caused by a critical reduction in intestinal blood flow that is of sufficient magnitude to compromise metabolic requirements. The result is cellular anoxia that may lead to intestinal necrosis.[1] Mortality rates of AMI range between 60% and 100%,[2,3] and the survival rate has not improved in recent decades. AMI accounts for approximately 0.1% of admissions for abdominal pain. The elderly are the most prone, with patients 80 years or older accounting for 67% of the events.[2,3] With the current trend of greater life expectancy, one can anticipate an increasing population of elderly patients with advanced cardiovascular disease leading to an increased incidence of AMI. AMI can be subcategorized (**Fig. 1**).

## PATHOPHYSIOLOGY

The splanchnic circulation receives approximately 25% of the resting cardiac output. Multiple extrinsic and intrinsic mechanisms help regulate splanchnic blood flow.[2,4] Pressure-flow autoregulation, hypoxic vasodilatation, and reactive hyperemia are components of that regulation, and oxygen delivery, rather than blood flow, is the more important stimulus for adaptive changes in the mesenteric circulation. Splanchnic vascular resistance is believed to be regulated by arteriolar wall tension receptors, whose degree of activation is directly proportional to the transmural pressure.[2]

Mesenteric blood flow is highly responsive to the adrenergic limb of the autonomic nervous system (**Fig. 2**). Catecholamines, specifically norepinephrine and high levels of epinephrine, produce vasoconstriction through $\alpha$-adrenergic receptor stimulation and decrease mesenteric blood flow.[2,5–7] Some nonadrenergic substances are also able to produce potent vasoconstriction. Cysteinyl leukotrienes, and C4 in particular, cause vasoconstriction of the liver and splanchnic vascular beds by exaggerating the response to angiotensin-II.[8,9] Thromboxane A2 and TxA2 analogues are also potent vasoconstrictors.[10–12]

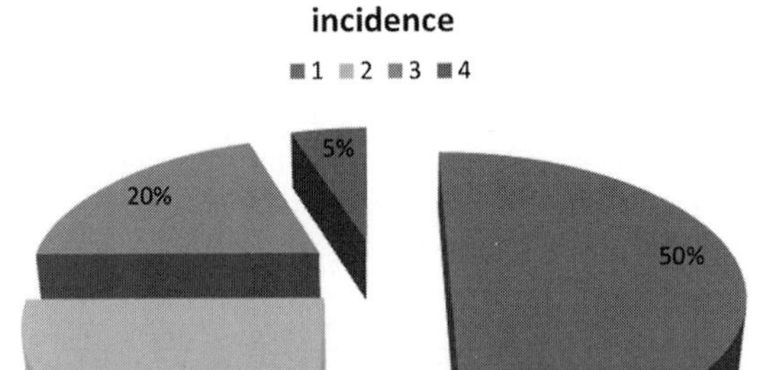


**Fig. 1.** AMI classification and incidence:[2–5] (1) SMA embolism; (2) SMA thrombosis; (3) nonocclusive; (4) MVT.

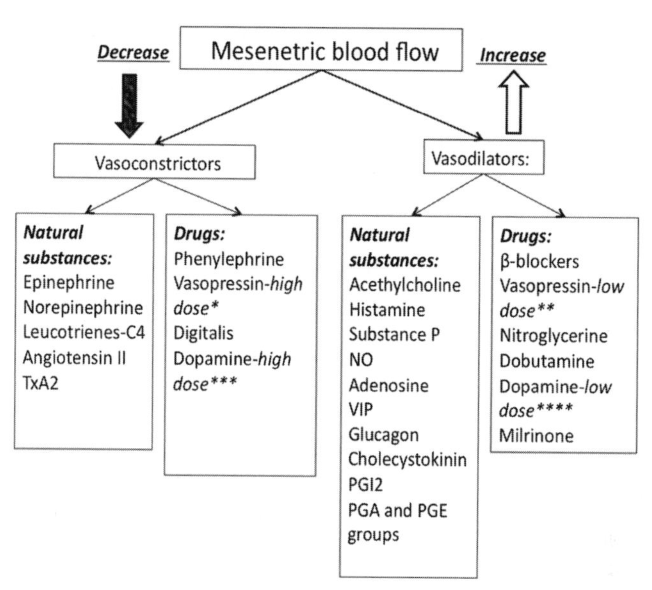


**Fig. 2.** Mesenteric blood flow regulation: role of natural components and drugs. Vasopressin, (*) >3 U/h; (**) 0.04 U/min to 2.4 U/h; dopamine, (***) 10 μg/kg/min;(****) 3 μg/kg/min.

In contrast to α-adrenergic vasoconstriction, β-adrenergic receptor stimulation causes vasodilatation with consequent increase in splanchnic blood flow (see **Fig. 2**). A variety of other substances can also produce vasodilatation.[2] Acetylcholine induces a hyperemic response in that mesenteric blood flow increases in the absence of any increase in intestinal oxygen consumption.[13] Histamine $H^3$ receptor stimulation markedly increases mesenteric and mucosal intestinal blood flow, but, in addition, increases mesenteric oxygen uptake, despite a decrease in mean BP.[14] Histamine and substance P also produce relaxation of isolated segments of small mesenteric arteries.[15] Overproduction of nitric oxide (NO) is an important factor that mediates the excessive arterial vasodilatation observed in portal hypertension.[16] Adenosine also dilates mesenteric resistance vessels.[17] Vasoactive intestinal peptide (VIP) is also a systemic and splanchnic vasodilator and 50 to 100 times more potent than acetylcholine.[18] The vasodilatory effect of VIP is believed to be attributed to the intracellular activation of adenylyl cyclase, increased NO production, increased guanosine monophosphate (GMP) and other signaling agents.[19] Glucagon increases cardiac output, mainly by increasing portal and mesenteric artery blood flow, despite minimal changes in systemic vascular resistance. However, the overall increase in mesenteric blood flow is not correlated with an increase in intestinal oxygen uptake.[20,21] Cholecystokinin (CCK) peptides have been shown to cause vasodilatation in central and mesenteric vessels. Such an effect is believed to be mediated by NO and seems to be presynaptic.[22] Prostaglandins are known to cause a potent vasodilatation action on coronary, pulmonary, and splanchnic vascular structures. Prostacyclin (PGI2) causes a profound reduction of systemic vascular resistance that decreases mean BP despite an increase in cardiac output.[23] Prostaglandins A- and E-subgroups reduce vascular responsiveness to a variety of vasoconstrictors, thus producing vasodilatation.[24]

Critical reduction of mesenteric blood flow occurs as a result of either vessel occlusion by thrombus or embolus, or a decrease in splanchnic blood flow caused by general hemodynamic instability or pharmacologically compromised mesenteric vascular tone.[1–3] Extensive collateralization between splanchnic vascular structures and a network of intramural submucosal vessels helps preserve some blood supply even if extramural arterial inflow is severely affected.[25] It has been shown that the bowels can endure up to a 75% decrease in blood flow for up to 12 hours without significant injury.[26] That may be possible because normally only about 20% of the mesenteric capillaries are functioning, and occlusion of the major mesenteric artery and subsequent distal arterial pressure reduction triggers the opening of collaterals and an adaptive increase in oxygen extraction by intestinal cells.[5,25] After several hours, however, vasoconstriction of these distal arterial vessels begins, with subsequent blood flow reduction, and may lead to cell death if blood flow cannot be reestablished.[4,5]

Embolic occlusion of the SMA is responsible for approximately 50%[2,3,5,6] of all cases of intestinal ischemia. Typically, emboli originate from an akinetic or aneurysmal portion of the left ventricle after MI or from the left atrium in patients with chronic AF.[6] Congestive heart failure, aortic aneurysm and dissection, bacterial endocarditis, rheumatic valve disease, cardiomyopathies, and intracardiac right-to-left shunt with paradoxic embolization are less frequent causes of SMA embolism. Catheter angiography or any other intra-arterial manipulation may also serve as precipitating factors.[2,5,6] The abrupt character of vessel occlusion does not usually allow any time for collateral circulation development.

Mesenteric artery thrombosis occurs most commonly in the setting of severe atherosclerosis. Slowly progressing arterial stenosis with significantly reduced flow and periods of arterial hypotension can create the conditions for thrombus formation at the SMA origin.[2,6] Other predisposing factors are hypovolemia/dehydration with diminished and tardy mesenteric blood flow and hypercoagulability. Rupture of an atherosclerotic plaque, commonly located at or near the vessel bifurcation, likely precedes the thrombus formation. In most cases, chronic mesenteric ischemia (abdominal angina) is present. In the event a stenosis forms slowly, extensive collateral circulation will develop and make it possible to tolerate even major artery occlusion for a considerable time. However, in the face of acute proximal mesenteric arterial thrombosis, even a well-developed collateral network may prove insufficient and result in bowel infarction.[2,5]

Nonocclusive mesenteric ischemia (NOMI) makes up to 20% of overall incidence, with a mortality rate of about 50%.[27] The major predisposing factors are: low cardiac output status, hypovolemia, hypotension, CHF, aortic valve insufficiency/regurgitation,[2] acute aortic dissection,[28] major abdominal and cardiovascular surgery, and cardiopulmonary bypass.[29,30] Some vasoactive agents, specifically norepinephrine and epinephrine, seem to divert blood flow away from mesenteric circulation (mesenteric steal syndrome).[31] High-dose vasopressin infusion decreases mesenteric blood flow with concomitant reduction of intestinal and liver $Po_2$ to a hypoxic level.[32] It also reduces collateral flow.[33] However, recent studies demonstrated no detrimental effect of low-dose infusions of vasopressin and terlipressin on mesenteric blood flow in endotoxemia and septic shock models.[34,35] Digitalis produces mesenteric vasoconstriction in the presence of proximal SMA stenosis[36] and exerts deleterious effects on vascular resistance and oxygen uptake as a result of a heightened myogenic response to acute venous hypertension.[37] Nonselective β-blockers (propranolol and, to some extent, carvedilol), and selective β-blockers (methoprolol, esmolol), may cause a decline in splanchnic blood flow and portal pressure by decreasing cardiac output,[38–43] and by selective inhibition of vasodilatory receptors in the splanchnic circulation.[2,44] However, β-blockers and angiotensin-converting enzyme (ACE) inhibitors stabilize the myogenic tone of splanchnic vessels and, in so doing, demonstrate a protective influence on gut microcirculation.[45]

Mesenteric venous thrombosis (MVT) is an uncommon cause of mesenteric ischemia, representing 5% to 15% of all cases.[6,46] Predisposing factors include abdominal malignancy (liver and pancreas), liver cirrhosis with portal hypertension, abdominal trauma and surgery, morbid obesity, various hypercoagulable states (thrombophilia, protein C and S deficiency, lupus, prothrombin mutations), coronary artery disease, history of coronary artery bypass graft (CABG),[47,48] genetic causes (hyperhomocysteinemia), and advanced age.[49] Increased D-dimer plasma levels seem to be the most consistent finding with MVT,[47,50] with other laboratory tests demonstrating insufficient specificity and sensitivity.[47]

AMI creates significant deleterious systemic effects (**Fig. 3**). SMA occlusion leads to a reduction of cardiac index (CI), along with increases in the arterial-portal vein lactate gradient and splanchnic oxygen extraction.[51] Moreover, critical splanchnic arterial hypoperfusion can provoke systemic shock through enkephalin-induced hyperactivation of δ-opioid receptors, which leads to increased plasma levels of NO,[52] systemic hyperlactatemia, and a severe anion gap acidosis.[53] It has been hypothesized that production of tumor necrosis factor-α (TNF-α) and other mediators triggers a systemic inflammatory response that ultimately leads to multiorgan failure.[54]

Intestinal ischemia-reperfusion injury may cause catastrophic systemic reactions. Oxygen free radicals, produced during ischemia and reperfusion, contribute to lipid peroxidation of cell membranes and increase the intestinal mucosal permeability with severe damage to, or complete loss of, barrier function. These changes potentiate bacterial translocation and promote a septic state.[55–57] Increased lung vascular permeability, elicited by gut ischemia-reperfusion, leads to interstitial fluid accumulation, further aggravating lung tissue hypoperfusion and hypoxia and leading to severe

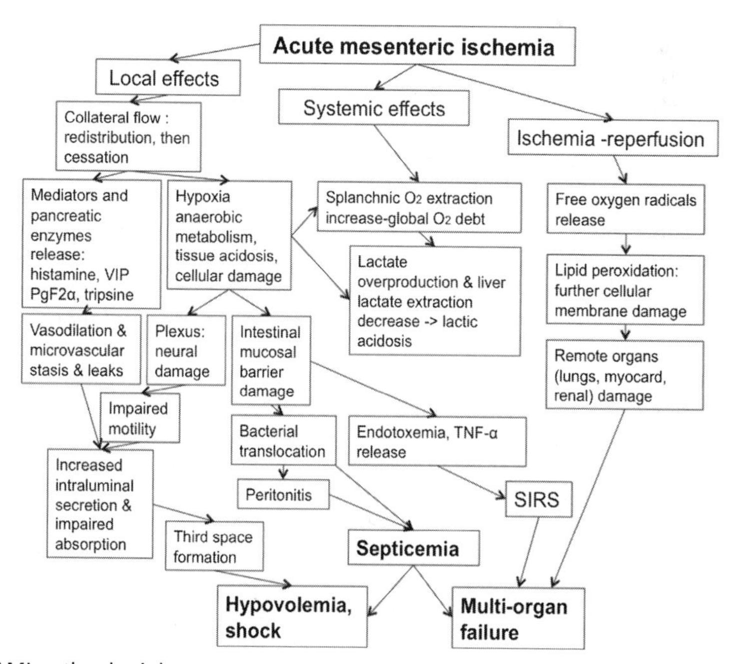


**Fig. 3.** AMI pathophysiology.

lung injury.[55,58] Significant impairment of renal function occurs as a result of severe intestinal ischemia-reperfusion. This deterioration in renal function is most likely caused by toxic metabolite free oxygen radicals, which occur in the milieu of an altered prostaglandins/thromboxane A2 ratio, such that eicosanoids with vasoconstrictor effects prevail.[59,60] In short, the pathogenesis of AMI is complex, and there is still a great deal that is poorly understood and under debate.

## DISCUSSION

Mesenteric ischemia is a well-recognized clinical entity of the elderly. Average age seems to be approximately 70 years, with a range of 57 to 96 years.[61–63] Predisposing factors include advanced arteriosclerosis, arterial hypertension, coronary artery disease and acute MI, congestive heart failure, arrhythmias (especially chronic AF), diabetes, and morbid obesity. Early diagnosis is critically important for successful preservation of bowel viability, reduction of the effect of ischemic injury, and eventually reduction in mortality among AMI patients. However, some elderly patients might have clinically atypical late presentation, or may be confused and, therefore, unable to articulate their complaints, which apparently may preclude early diagnosis. Moreover, some patients may seek medical attention for other problems, and abdominal pain may not be interpreted as a symptom suggestive for AMI. Clinical presentation can be characterized by an initial discrepancy between severe abdominal pain and apparent paucity of clinical findings.[2,6] When symptoms suggestive of abdominal catastrophe are present, bowel infarction has, most likely, already occurred, which dramatically reduces chances of survival.[6] However, apparent hemodynamic stability in vaguely symptomatic patients may obscure the true gravity of the situation. Soon after uneventful anesthesia, in the middle of the laparotomy, these patients show rapid deterioration, becoming profoundly hypotensive and acidotic, developing a full-blown septic state, which leads to early multiorgan failure with eventual unfavorable outcome.

The earlier case presentation combines AMI with a catastrophic abdominal emergency, and results in peritonitis, sepsis, and hemodynamic instability in an elderly patient with significant cardiac comorbidity.

## TREATMENT OPTIONS

Treatment options depend on the cause of the ischemia, ischemia time, presence of peritoneal signs, sepsis, overall hemodynamic stability, and severity of comorbid medical conditions. The presence of peritoneal signs is an indication for exploratory laparotomy. In cases in which no such symptoms are present, nonsurgical treatment options may be considered. These include thrombolytic therapy and various additional pharmacologic interventions.

Thrombolytic therapy includes streptokinase, urokinase, or recombinant plasminogen activator via intra-arterial infusion.[5,30,60,64] Thrombolysis seems to be most effective when started within 12 hours of the onset of abdominal symptoms, and is successful mainly for distal clots. Thrombolysis using percutaneous trans-hepatic catheter-directed infusion of urokinase[65] or operatively placed catheter for recombinant tissue plasminogen activator (rt-PA) infusion [66] has been reported to be highly effective for acute superior MVT,[67,68] and systemic anticoagulation is, for now, considered the best option for this condition.[60,69]

Vasodilator therapy for acute intestinal ischemia seems beneficial in clinical and experimental studies. Vasoconstriction not only contributes to the ischemia, but may persist even after the initial cause of the occlusion (thrombus or emboli) has been eliminated. Vasodilatation, such as provided by papaverine, reverses this vasoconstriction.[3,6,70] Not all experimental ischemia models support the positive effects of papaverine, however. In one rat study, papaverine not only failed to improve bowel viability but also redirected blood flow away from ischemic tissue, creating a steal effect.[71] Nevertheless, vasodilator therapy is still recommended to reduce splanchnic vasoconstriction after revascularization or for NOMI.[6]

If the diagnosis of acute intestinal ischemia is made on angiography, intra-arterial infusion of papaverine at a dose of 30 to 60 mg/kg into the SMA may be attempted. This intervention is feasible only if no peritoneal signs are present and the patient remains hemodynamically stable.[2,3,5,70] In rats, glucagon improves ileal mucosal viability if given early during reperfusion after segmental ischemia.[5,72] The authors could not find any studies involving human subjects.

Surgical treatment remains the mainstay of management of most case of acute intestinal ischemia.[6] The goals of surgical intervention are to first confirm the diagnosis of intestinal ischemia, then assess the viability of affected bowel, and finally to perform revascularization, if feasible. This part may involve thromboembolectomy, mesenteric bypass grafting, patch angioplasty, reimplantation, or endarterectomy.[63] Resection of infarcted bowel or abdominal washout in cases of advanced peritonitis may also be required.[6,73]

Laparoscopy as a diagnostic procedure or as a second-look technique[74,75] has its advantages as a shorter, much less invasive procedure, and may obviate the conventional open second-look laparotomy. However, laparoscopic assessment of bowel viability is limited to the serosal surface of the intestine, and does not guarantee the avoidance of laparotomy.[70]

## PREOPERATIVE CONSIDERATIONS

Regardless of the pathogenesis of intestinal ischemia, when the patient presents with acute peritoneal signs, which are a late but strong indicator of bowel infarction, emergent surgical intervention is warranted. It is well recognized that emergency abdominal surgery significantly increases morbidity and mortality rates in the elderly.[76] Comorbid diseases, particularly those affecting the cardiovascular, endocrine, renal, and pulmonary systems, are often present, further exacerbating the risk of surgery.[77] Although a thorough preoperative preparation combined with optimization of pre-existent diseases has been shown to decrease poor outcome in the aged,[78] the time constraints imposed by the emergency nature of the surgery makes this approach difficult if not impossible. Nevertheless, it is imperative to control life-threatening conditions, such as unstable arrhythmias, congestive heart failure, and severe electrolyte/metabolic disorders before proceeding to the operating room. Ideally, resuscitative efforts should be started as soon as the diagnosis is suspected, in the emergency room or intensive care unit, and continued in the operating room. The major goal is to optimize oxygen delivery and preserve intestinal blood flow primarily by treating hypovolemia, hypotension, and low cardiac output. Management steps to follow are given in **Table 1**.

## FLUID RESUSCITATION

Early manifestations of intestinal ischemia include sequestration of a large amount of extracellular fluid within the bowel wall, effectively creating circulatory hypovolemia. If uncorrected, circulatory failure and shock will ensue. Because there is no way to measure the volume of fluid retained by the ischemic bowel, estimation of actual fluid deficit and the adequacy of replacement can prove extremely difficult, demanding

**Table 1**
**Management steps**

| Optimization of $O_2$ Delivery | Preservation of Intestinal Blood Flow | Initiate Prophylaxis or Treatment of Sepsis, Multiorgan Failure, and Reperfusion Injury |
|---|---|---|
| Administer supplemental oxygen | Dynamic goal-directed fluid resuscitation | Administer broad-spectrum antibiotics to avoid bacterial translocation |
| Intubate and mechanically ventilate the patient who is obtunded or shows symptoms of respiratory distress or shock | Selective use of vasoactive/inotropic agents, primarily to improve cardiac output | Avoid vasopressors/use vasodilators if possible |
| Transfuse blood to achieve hematocrit of 30% | | Consider free oxygen scavengers |

rigorous monitoring. A variety of options for monitoring volume status in the elderly during major abdominal surgery are available.

## TRADITIONAL AND STATIC VARIABLES

Traditional clinical signs and hemodynamic variables, such as HR, positive tilt test, BP, or central venous pressure (CVP) and pulmonary capillary wedge pressure (PCWP), although important and still used in daily practice, are not always reliable monitors of volume status or tissue perfusion.[79,80] Moreover, in the elderly, baroreceptor-mediated HR control and β-receptor responsiveness to adrenergic stimulation are diminished, thereby limiting the ability of the patient to increase cardiac output by increasing HR and contractility. These changes leave the older patient more dependent on an adequate preload, making the restoration of an adequate blood volume especially important in the elderly.[81] Also, a "normal" BP may represent covert hypovolemia in an elderly patient who is chronically hypertensive. Multiple studies have shown that measurements of filling pressures (CVP, PCWP) are poor predictors of fluid status, particularly in the elderly, who often have diastolic dysfunction and a stiff ventricle.[81,82] These measures are invasive, and do not seem to improve outcome.[83,84] For instance, Sandham's multicenter[85] trial showed that in old and high-risk patients randomized to management with pulmonary-artery catheter (PAC) and an optimization filling pressure/oxygen delivery regimen versus standard care, there was no difference in overall outcome. However, the PAC group experienced a small but statistically significant increased total complication rate related to PAC insertion.

## DYNAMIC GOAL-DIRECTED FLUID RESUSCITATION

Based on the recent literature, accurate replacement of fluid deficits may be achieved using a targeted approach in which hemodynamic and clinical end points are well defined.[82] Growing evidence shows that dynamic goal-directed fluid therapy (GDFT) by means of esophageal Doppler derived parameters (cardiac output, stroke volume [SV], flow velocity, and so forth) may be superior to the previously described static variables at appreciating fluid responsiveness. Abbas and Hill,[86] in a recent review of five studies of intraoperative fluid management in patients undergoing major abdominal surgery, compared the role of esophageal Doppler monitoring with standard practice (CVP, arterial BP, and urine output). All these studies had similar algorithms using fluid challenge with colloids to augment SV and improve oxygen delivery. A significant increase in SV after fluid challenge represents a functional definition of hypovolemia, whereas minimal improvement or, worse, a decrease in SV, means that more fluid may produce ventricular overload. The studies demonstrated shorter hospital stay, reduced use of inotropes, earlier return of bowel function, and overall lower complication rates in the Doppler group. In a study performed by Noblett and colleagues[87] on patients having colorectal surgery, the reduced morbidity and hospital stay by Doppler-based GDFT therapy was also associated with reduced interleukin-6 levels, suggesting less inflammatory response and possible better outcome with GDFT.

## DYNAMIC MEASUREMENT OF SYSTOLIC AND PULSE PRESSURE VARIATION

A simple, noninvasive technique that may be more suitable for routine clinical use in emergency settings involves the evaluation of systolic pressure variation (SPV) or pulse pressure variation (PPV) that is generated by positive pressure ventilation and measured via an arterial line or plethysmograph.[88] The physiologic explanation of SPV has been fully described elsewhere.[89,90] During the inspiratory phase of mechanical ventilation, intrathoracic pressure increases leading to a temporary increase in LV preload (by squeezing blood out of the lung), and also a decrease in venous return to the right heart. The onset of exhalation therefore creates a transient decrease in LV preload and an associated decrease in SV. The cyclical variations in SV are reflected by changes in the arterial waveform ($\Delta$ up and $\Delta$ down for systolic pressure, changes in pulse pressure) that are particularly accentuated in hypovolemic patients. Many studies have proven that PPV is more reliable than conventional filling pressures as a predictor of volume status. For example, Michard[90] showed that, in mechanically ventilated patients, a change of more than 13% in pulse pressure was a much better predictor of an increase in cardiac index of greater than 15% than the absolute value of the CVP or PCWP.

## GLOBAL MEASURES OF TISSUE PERFUSION

Recently, continuous analysis of central venous oxygen saturation ($Scvo_2$) using a fiberoptic central venous catheter has become available. Targeting an $Scvo_2$ of greater than 70% in septic patients, Rivers and colleagues[91] demonstrated improvement in mortality in the GDFT group compared with a standard protocol.

Another global measurement of tissue perfusion is lactate. A lactate level greater than 2.5 mmol/L is believed to be a marker of negative outcome in patients with sepsis and low BP. Although the sensitivity of this serum marker is high, approaching 100% when bowel infarction is present, it has a disappointing specificity, ranging from 42% to 87% in varying series.[92] The parameters mentioned earlier assess global tissue perfusion, and are consequently poor indicators of the tissue oxygen level in the splanchnic bed.

Regardless of the technique chosen, the goal should be preservation of adequate tissue oxygenation and perfusion, end points that are hard to achieve with the current methods. At present, optimization of volume status in major abdominal surgery relies on integrating multiple variables potentially including filling pressures, BP, PPV, urine output, acid-base and lactate levels. The authors' personal opinion is that keeping the mean arterial pressure reasonably close to the patient's normal pressure and performing judicious fluid challenges while monitoring SPV or PPV may be the best method to avoid hypovolemia and preserve perfusion.

Given the paucity of literature regarding the choice of fluids in the elderly with mesenteric ischemia, it is difficult to state that colloid or crystalloid is superior. However, the response to a volume challenge may be easier to assess with colloid, so perhaps colloid is a better choice when performing a fluid challenge for optimization of SV. Crystalloid could then be used for fluid maintenance and third space volume. Balanced crystalloid solutions, such as Ringer lactate or Plasma-Lyte are superior to saline 0.9%, which, in large amounts, may cause hyperchloremic metabolic acidosis. Although there are no clear guidelines regarding specific transfusion thresholds in the elderly, it seems that older patients with coexistent cardiac and respiratory diseases may tolerate anemia less well,[93] therefore it is probably appropriate to target hemoglobin to at least 8 to 10 g/dL in the elderly surgical patient.

When administering fluids to the elderly, one should be aware that hypervolemia may be just as poorly tolerated as hypovolemia. A stiff, noncompliant aged heart may demonstrate abrupt increases in end-diastolic pressure from volume challenges that could lead to frank pulmonary edema and cardiac failure.[77,81] Furthermore, overzealous hydration may exacerbate bowel edema, decrease splanchnic blood flow, and lead to postoperative abdominal compartment syndrome, which in turn may promote multiple organ failure and sepsis.[93,94]

## CONTROL OF BLOOD PRESSURE

Some patients with bowel ischemia may remain persistently hypotensive despite adequate fluid replacement. In this situation vasoactive agents are indicated; however, the use of vasopressors may worsen bowel ischemia and exacerbate the condition.[2,95] Epinephrine and phenylephrine may decrease splanchnic blood flow and their use should be restricted.[96,97] If hypovolemia has been corrected, norepinephrine combined with dobutamine increases gastric mucosal perfusion and oxygen delivery in elderly septic patients, and may therefore be a reasonable choice of therapy.[98,99] Dopexamine was superior to dopamine in protecting the splanchnic circulation and increasing gastric pH during sepsis in one study.[100] The use of vasopressin is controversial, because it may exert a negative effect on the hepatosplanchnic bed, so its use should be reserved for when other drug regimens fail.[93,101,102] New drugs with combined inotropic and vasodilator effects (levosimendan and olprinone) have shown promising effects on gut mucosal perfusion in animal studies.[103,104] Recently, it has been suggested that the suppression of NO activity by methylene blue administration might constitute a valuable option for the treatment of vasopressor refractory septic state.[105] Whether this treatment translates into preservation of intestinal blood flow and reduced morbidity remains to be ascertained.

## ANESTHETIC CONSIDERATIONS

As discussed earlier, bowel ischemia is a surgical emergency and there is limited time for preoperative assessment and optimization. However, a hypoperfusional state manifested by altered mental status, low BP and urine output, significant metabolic acidosis, and other symptoms, such as electrolyte and coagulation abnormalities, indicates severe illness and deserves particular attention. In this situation, the induction of anesthesia should proceed only after the patient has been stabilized. The aggressiveness of preparation and monitoring is largely dependent on the nature of the presenting symptoms and underlying medical history. Nonetheless, a large-bore intravenous access for rapid fluid infusion and an intra-arterial catheter for blood sampling, and continuous BP and SPV monitoring are the standard of care, as major fluid shifts and hemodynamic instability are common during the surgery. Central access for infusion of vasoactive drugs and invasive hemodynamic monitoring may prove beneficial and particularly indicated in patients with severe systemic disease, sepsis, and left or right heart dysfunction. Baseline data from the invasive monitors (mean aortic pressure [MAP], CVP, PCWP, SV, $Svo_2$, and so forth) should be obtained and, ideally, the impact of fluid challenge on these variables observed. Arterial and venous blood gases and lactate may be useful to estimate global tissue perfusion. Hourly urine output of greater than 0.5 mL/kg/h may suggest, but not prove, the adequacy of end-organ perfusion.

To prevent pulmonary aspiration, a rapid sequence induction (RSI) with cricoid pressure should be performed. Old age is associated with many changes in pulmonary function, and desaturation can occur quickly during RSI. Thus, thorough preoxygenation is highly recommended. To prevent acute reduction in BP, as can be seen with even low doses of propofol, consideration should be given to etomidate or even ketamine for induction. To date, no data are available to indicate which anesthetic technique to select for the maintenance of anesthesia in elderly patients with bowel ischemia. One study could not demonstrate a significant difference in the hemodynamic effects on splanchnic circulation in patients who received either sevoflurane or total intravenous anesthesia with propofol.[106] Isoflurane and desflurane are comparable in preserving tissue oxygenation during colorectal surgery.[107] At moderate doses, morphine and likely all narcotic drugs seem to have beneficial effects by improving splanchnic blood flow and decreasing intestinal oxygen demand.[108] When choosing a maintenance technique, it is important to recognize that the spectrum of drug choice might be seriously hampered by the patient's condition and tolerance. Practically speaking, this group of patients may exhibit formidable hemodynamic intolerance to the potent inhalational agents or to propofol infusion. Often, light anesthesia is deemed necessary, which would include subanesthetic doses of inhaled anesthetics, or, at worst, no more than a small dose of amnestic (midazolam or scopolamine), a muscle relaxant, opioid, or ketamine as tolerated. Awareness is likely to occur, thus the use of a cerebral function monitor is advisable. Bispectral index (BIS) monitoring is easily applicable and widely used in clinical practice. In addition, to decrease the incidence of awareness in high-risk patients,[109] BIS-guided anesthetic titration may reduce the risk of overdosing in this compromised group of patients.[110]

Thermoregulation may already be impaired in the elderly. A prolonged procedure on an open abdomen yields significant heat loss. Accurate monitoring of core temperature and perioperative aggressive rewarming are necessary to avoid hypothermia, which may worsen already existent splanchnic vasoconstriction, impair coagulation, and increase the incidence of wound infection.[111]

As a general rule, patients scheduled for a second look, those with acidosis, severe edema after fluid resuscitation, or those who are hypoxemic and unstable, should be kept intubated and ventilated and admitted to the intensive care unit (ICU) for further stabilization.

## POSTOPERATIVE COMPLICATIONS

Resuscitation of an elderly patient with bowel ischemia invariably continues in the ICU. Sepsis with multiple organ dysfunction including acute respiratory and renal failure, abdominal compartment syndrome, or recurrence of bowel ischemia may develop and lead to adverse outcomes. If reperfusion injury is suspected, ACE inhibitors, allopurinol, and other free oxygen scavengers may ameliorate this syndrome.

## SUMMARY

The management of the elderly patient with ischemic bowel is extremely challenging, requiring an aggressive multidisciplinary approach with active participation of the surgeon, radiologist, and anesthesiologist. Elderly patients with a clinical picture suggestive of this life-threatening condition require prompt diagnosis by means of angiography followed by revascularization and resection of necrotic bowel. The major role of the anesthesiologist in this setting is to coordinate the resuscitative efforts by judicious use of crystalloids, colloids, and vasoactive drugs in combination with continuous and intensive monitoring of the hemodynamic status and tissue oxygenation.

## REFERENCES

1. Berland T, Oldenburg WA. Acute mesenteric ischemia. Curr Gastroenterol Rep 2008;10(3):341–6.
2. Oldenburg WA, Lau LL, Rodenberg TJ, et al. Acute mesenteric ischemia. A clinical review. Arch Intern Med 2004;164:1054–62.
3. Lock G. Acute mesenteric ischemia: classification, evaluation and therapy. Acta Gastroenterol Belg 2002;65(4):220–5.
4. McFadden DW, Rongione AJ. Intestinal circulation and vascular disorders. In: Miller TA, editor. Modern surgical care: physiologic foundation & clinical applications. 2nd edition. St Louis (MO): Quality Medical Publishing; 1998. p. 443–63.
5. Kozuch PL, Brandt LJ. Review article: diagnosis and management of mesenteric ischemia with an emphasis on pharmacotherapy. Aliment Pharmacol Ther 2005; 21:201–15.
6. Sternbach Y, Perler BA. Acute mesenteric ischemia. In: Zuidema GD, Yeo CJ, editors. Surgery of the alimentary tract. 5th edition, Mesenteric circulation, hernia, small intestine, vol. 5. Philadelphia: WB Saunders Company; 2001. p. 17–31.
7. Takenaga M, Kawasaki H. Neuronal control of mesenteric circulation. Nippon Yakurigaku Zasshi 1999;113(4):249–59.
8. Myers SI, Hernandez R. Leukotriene C4 regulation of splanchnic blood flow during ischemia. Am J Surg 1994;167(6):566–9.
9. Shasti S, McNeill JR, Wilson TW, et al. Cysteinyl leukotrienes mediate enhanced vasoconstriction to angiotensin II but not endothelin-1 in SHR. Am J Physiol Heart Circ Physiol 2001;281(1):H342–9.
10. Ruan Z, Shibamoto T, Shimo T, et al. Effects of platelet-activating factor and thromboxane A2 on isolated perfused guinea pig liver. Prostaglandins Other Lipid Mediat 2004;73(1–2):73–85.
11. Yokoyama Y, Nimura Y, Nagino M, et al. Role of thromboxane in producing hepatic injury during hepatic stress. Arch Surg 2005;140(8):801–7.
12. Cui S, Shlamboto T, Zhao Z, et al. Effects of L-NAME on thromboxane A2-induced vasoconstriction in isolated perfused livers from rat, guinea pig and mouse. Vascul Pharmacol 2007;47(4):215–21.
13. Jacobson ED, Gallavan RH Jr, Fonadacaro JD. A model of mesenteric circulation. Am J Phys 1982;242(6):G541–6.
14. Obuchowicz R, Pawlik MW, Brzozowski E, et al. Involvement of central and peripheral histamine H(3) receptors in the control of vascular tone and oxygen

uptake in the mesenteric circulation of the rat. J Physiol Pharmacol 2004;55(1 Pt 2):255–67.
15. Tottrup A, Kraglund K. Endothelium-dependent response in small human mesenteric arteries. Physiol Res 2004;53(3):255–63.
16. Iwakiri Y. The molecules: mechanisms of arterial vasodilatation observed in the splanchnic and systemic circulation in portal hypertension. J Clin Gastroenterol 2007;41(Suppl 3):S288–94.
17. Jakobson ED, Pawlik WW. Adenosine mediation of mesenteric blood flow. J Physiol Pharmacol 1992;43(1):3–19.
18. Somien G, Fletcher DR, Shuikes A, et al. Experimental mesenteric ischaemia in sheep: gut peptide release and haemodynamic changes. J Gasroenterol Hepatol 1989;4(3):251–8.
19. Henning RJ, Sawmiller DR. Vasoactive intestinal peptide: cardiovascular effects. Cardiovasc Res 2001;49(1):27–37.
20. Benyo I, Benyo Z, Szalal G, et al. The relationship between splanchnic oxygen consumption and blood supply. Acta Physiol Hung 1991;78(3):211–9.
21. Shapiro DM, Cronenwett JL, Lindenauer SM, et al. Effects of glucagon and prostacyclin in acute occlusive and postocclusive canine mesenteric ischemia. J Surg Res 1984;36(6):535–46.
22. Ruiz-Gayo m, Gonzalez MC, Fernandes-Alfonso S. Vasodilatory effects of cholecystokinin: a new role for an old peptide? Regul Pept 2006;137(3):179–84.
23. Vanlersberghe c, Lauwers MH, Camu F. Prostaglandin synthetase inhibitor treatment and the regulatory role of prostaglandins on organ perfusion. Acta Anaesthesiol Belg 1992;43(4):211–25.
24. Messina EJ, Weiner R, Kalev G. Prostaglandins and local circulatory control. Fed Proc 1976;36(12):2367–75.
25. Patel A, Kaleva RN, Sammartano RJ. Pathophysiology of mesenteric ischemia. Surg Clin North Am 1992;72(1):31–41.
26. Boley SJ, Brandt LJ, Veith FJ. Ischemic disorders of the intestine. Curr Probl Surg 1978;15(4):1–85.
27. Trompeter M, Brazda T, Remy CT, et al. Non-occlusive mesenteric ischemia: etiology, diagnosis, and interventional therapy. Eur Radiol 2002;12(5):1179–87.
28. Neri E, Sassi C, Massetti M, et al. Nonocclusive intestinal ischemia in patients with acute aortic dissection. J Vasc Surg 2002;36(4):738–45.
29. Schütz A, Eichinger W, Breuer M, et al. Acute mesenteric ischemia after open heart surgery. Angiology 1998;49(4):267–73.
30. Abboud B, Daher R, Boujaoude J. Acute mesenteric ischemia after cardiopulmonary bypass. World J Gastroenterol 2008;14(35):5361–70.
31. Krejci V, Hiltebrand LB, Sigurdsson GH. Effects of epinephrine, norepinephrine and phenylephrine on microcirculatory blood flow in the gastrointestinal tract in sepsis. Crit Care Med 2006;34(5):1456–63.
32. Korsbäck C, Höckerstedt K. Small bowel and liver $pO_2$ during intravenous vasopressin infusion. Ann Chir Gynaecol 1982;71(2):112–6.
33. Bulkley GB, Womack WA, Downey JM, et al. Collateral blood flow in segmental intestinal ischemia: effects of vasopressive agents. Surgery 1986;100(2):157–66.
34. Kopel T, Losser MR, Faivre V, et al. Systemic and hepatosplanchnic macro- and microcirculatory dose response to arginine vasopressin in endotoxic rabbits. Intensive Care Med 2008;34(7):1313–20.
35. Asfar P, Bracht H, Radermacher P. Impact of vasopressin analogues on the gut mucosal microcirculation. Best Pract Res Clin Anaesthesiol 2008;22(2):351–8.

36. Levinsky RA, Lewis RM, Bynum TE, et al. Digoxin-induced intestinal vasoconstriction. The effects of proximal arterial stenosis and glucagon administration. Circulation 1975;52(1):130–6.
37. Kim EH, Geweretz BL. Chronic digitalis administration alters mesenteric vascular reactivity. J Vasc Surg 1987;5(2):382–9.
38. Köksal AS, Usküdar O, Köklü S, et al. Propranolol-exacerbated mesenteric ischemia in a patient with hyperthyroidism. Ann Pharmacother 2005;39(3):559–62.
39. Westaby D, Bihari DJ, Gimpson AES, et al. Selective and non-selective beta receptor blockade in the reduction of portal pressure in patients with cirrhosis and portal hypertension. Gut 1984;25(2):121–4.
40. Sekiyama T, Komeichi H, Nagano T, et al. Effects of the alpha-/beta-blocking agent carvedilol on hepatic and systemic hemodynamics in patients with cirrhosis and portal hypertension. Arzneimittelforschung 1997;47(4):353–5.
41. Bañares R, Moitinho E, Matilla A, et al. Randomized comparison of long-term carvedilol and propranolol administration in the treatment of portal hypertension in cirrhosis. Hepatology 2002;36(6):1367–73.
42. Bauer LA, Horn JR, Maxon MS, et al. Effect of metoprolol and verapamil administered separately and concurrently after single doses on liver blood flow and drug disposition. J Clin Pharmacol 2000;40(5):533–43.
43. Masuda R, Takeda S. Responses of hemodynamics and splanchnic organ blood flow to esmolol during inhalation of volatile anesthetics in dogs. Masui 2008;57(1):69–75.
44. Schwarzkopff B, Hennersdorf M. Influence of cardiac circulation and medication on the perfusion of the intestine. Zentralbl Chir 2005;130(3):218–22.
45. Ghisietta N, von Flüe M, Eichllsberger E, et al. Mesenteric venous thrombosis (MVT): a problem in diagnosis and management. Swiss Surg 1996;2(5):223–9.
46. Acosta S, Alahald A, Svensson P, et al. Epidemiology, risk and prognostic factors in mesenteric venous thrombosis. Br J Surg 2008;95:1245–51.
47. Hedayati N, Riha CM, Kougias P, et al. Prognostic factors and treatment outcome in mesenteric vein thrombosis. Vasc Endovascular Surg 2008;42(3):217–24.
48. Hotoleanu C, Andersou O, Andersou A. Mesenteric venous thrombosis: clinical and therapeutical approach. Int Angiol 2008;27(6):462–5.
49. Cong L, Yu JC, Liu CW, et al. Acute mesenteric venous thrombosis: experience of 27 cases. Zhonghua Wai Ke Za Zhi 2008;46(6):423–6.
50. Heino A, Hartikainen J, Merasto ME, et al. Systemic and regional effects of experimental gradual splanchnic ischemia. J Crit Care 1997;12(2):92–8.
51. Carmignani M, Zucchetti F, Sacco R, et al. Shock induction by arterial hypoperfusion of the gut involves synergetic interactions between the peripheral enkephalin and nitric oxide systems. Int J Immunopathol Pharmacol 2005;18(1):33–48.
52. Jacob SM, Merasto-Minkkinen M, Tenhunen JJ, et al. Prevention of systemic lactatemia during splanchnic ischemia. Shock 2000;14(2):123–7.
53. Landow L, Andersen LW. Splanchnic ischemia and its role in multiple organ failure. Acta Anaesthesiol Scand 1994;38(7):626–39.
54. Horton JW, Walker PB. Oxygen radicals, lipid peroxidation, and permeability changes after intestinal ischemia and reperfusion. J Appl Phys 1993;74(4):1515–20.
55. Nakagawa H, Tsunooka N, Yamamoto Y, et al. Intestinal ischemia/reperfusion – induced bacterial translocation and lung injury in atherosclerotic rats with hypoadiponectinemia. Surgery 2009;145(1):48–56.

56. Khanna A, Rossman JE, Fung HL, et al. Intestinal and hemodynamic impairment following mesenteric ischemia/reperfusion. J Surg Res 2001;99(1): 114–9.
57. Uchida K, Mishima S, Otha S, et al. Inhibition of inducible nitric oxide synthase ameliorates lung injury in rats after gut ischemia-reperfusion. J Trauma 2007; 63(3):603–7.
58. Heino A, Merasto ME, Koski EM, et al. Effects of fluid and dobutamine treatment on renal function during partial superior mesenteric artery occlusion and reperfusion. Scand J Urol Nephrol 2002;36(1):5–13.
59. Rothenbach P, Turnage RH, Iglesias J, et al. Downstream effects of splanchnic ischemia-reperfusion injury on renal function and eicosanoid release. J Appl Phys 1997;83(2):530–6.
60. Barakate MS, Cappe I, Curtin A, et al. Management of acute superior mesenteric artery occlusion. ANZ J Surg 2002;72(1):25–9.
61. Kougias P, Lau D, El Sayed HF, et al. Determinants of mortality and treatment outcome following surgical interventions for acute mesenteric ischemia. J Vasc Surg 2007;46(3):467–74.
62. Heidinger D, Trommer E, Weichselberger A, et al. An 82 year old patient with severe abdominal pain and air in the portal vein. Internist (Berl) 2009;50(3): 368–73.
63. Savassi-Rocha PR, Veloso LF. Treatment of superior mesenteric artery embolism with a fibrinolytic agent: case report and literature review. Hepatogastroenterology 2002;49(47):1307–10.
64. Schoots IG, Levi MM, Reekers JA, et al. Thrombolytic therapy for acute superior mesenteric artery occlusion. J Vasc Interv Radiol 2005;16(3):317–29.
65. Lee H, Kim TH, Oh HJ, et al. Portal and superior mesenteric venous thrombosis treated with urokinase infusion via superior mesenteric artery. Korean J Gastroenterol 2006;48(1):46–50.
66. Kaplan JL, Weintraub ST, Hunt JP, et al. Treatment of superior mesenteric and portal vein thrombosis with direct thrombolytic infusion via operatively placed mesenteric catheter. Am Surg 2004;70(7):600–4.
67. Kim HS, Patra A, Khan J, et al. Transhepatic catheter-directed thrombectomy and thrombolysis of acute superior mesenteric venous thrombosis. J Vasc Interv Radiol 2005;16(12):1685–91.
68. Zhou W, Choi L, Lin PH, et al. Percutaneous transhepatic thrombectomy and pharmacological thrombolysis of mesenteric venous thrombosis. Vascular 2007;15(1):41–5.
69. Kassahun WT, Schultz T, Richter O, et al. Unchanged high mortality rates from acute occlusive intestinal ischemia: six years review. Langenbecks Arch Surg 2008;393:163–71.
70. Meilahn JE, Morris JB, Ceppa EP, et al. Effect of prolonged selective intramesenteric arterial vasodilator therapy on intestinal viability after acute segmental mesenteric vascular occlusion. Ann Surg 2001;234(1):107–15.
71. Gangadharan SP, Wagner RJ, Cronenwett JL. Effect of intravenous glucagon on intestinal viability after segmental mesenteric ischemia. J Vasc Surg 1995;21(6): 900–7.
72. Park WM, Glovicski P, Cherry KJ Jr, et al. Contemporary management of acute mesenteric ischemia: factors associated with survival. J Vasc Surg 2002;35(3): 445–52.
73. Ruotolo RA, Evans SR. Mesenteric ischemia in the elderly. Clin Geriatr Med 1999;15(3):527–57.

74. Sauerland S, Agresta F, Bergamaschi R, et al. Laparoscopy for abdominal emergencies: evidence-based guidelines of the European Association for Laparoscopic Surgery. Surg Endosc 2006;20(1):14–29.
75. Anadol AZ, Ersoy E, Taneri F, et al. Laparoscopic "second-look" in the management of mesenteric ischemia. Surg Laparosc Endosc Percutan Tech 2004;14(4):191–3.
76. John AD, Sieber FE. Age associated issues: geriatrics. Anesthesiol Clin North America 2004;22(1):45–58.
77. Story DA. Postoperative complications in elderly patients and their significance for long-term prognosis. Curr Opin Anaesthesiol 2008;21(3):375–9.
78. Jin F, Chung F. Minimizing perioperative adverse events in the elderly. Br J Anaesth 2001;87(4):608–24.
79. Kumar A, Anel R, Bunnell E, et al. Pulmonary artery occlusion pressure and central venous pressure fail to predict ventricular filling volume, cardiac performance, or the response to volume infusion in normal subjects. Crit Care Med 2004;32:691–9.
80. Gelman S. Venous function and central venous pressure: a physiologic story. Anesthesiology 2008;108(4):735–48.
81. Rooke GA. Autonomic and cardiovascular function in the geriatric patient. Anesthesiol Clin North America 2000;18(1):31–46.
82. Grocott MP, Mythen MG, Gan TJ. Perioperative fluid management and clinical outcomes in adults. Anesth Analg 2005;100(4):1093–106.
83. Harvey S, Harrison DA, Singer M, et al. Assessment of the clinical effectiveness of pulmonary artery catheters in management of patients in intensive care (PAC-Man): a randomised controlled trial. Lancet 2005;366:472–7.
84. Pulmonary Artery Catheter Consensus conference: consensus statement. Crit Care Med 1997;25:910–25.
85. Sandham JD, Hull RD, Brant RF, et al. A randomized, controlled trial of the use of pulmonary-artery catheters in high-risk surgical patients. N Engl J Med 2003;348:5–14.
86. Abbas SM, Hill AG. Systematic review of the literature for the use of oesophageal Doppler monitor for fluid replacement in major abdominal surgery. Anaesthesia 2008;63(1):44–51.
87. Noblett SE, Snowden CP, Shenton BK, et al. Randomized clinical trial assessing the effect of Doppler-optimized fluid management on outcome after elective colorectal resection. Br J Surg 2006;93:1069–76.
88. Reuter DA, Felbinger TW, Kilger E, et al. Optimizing fluid therapy in mechanically ventilated patients after cardiac surgery by on-line monitoring of left ventricular stroke volume variations. Comparison with aortic systolic pressure variations. Br J Anaesth 2002;88:124–6.
89. Rooke GA, Schwid HA, Shapira Y. The effect of graded hemorrhage and intravascular volume replacement on systolic pressure variation in humans during mechanical and spontaneous ventilation. Anesth Analg 1995;80(5):925–32.
90. Michard F. Changes in arterial pressure during mechanical ventilation. Anesthesiology 2005;103:419–28.
91. Rivers E, Nguyen B, Havstad S. et al. Early Goal-Directed Therapy Collaborative Group. Early goal-directed therapy in the treatment of severe sepsis and septic shock. N Engl J Med 2001 8;345(19):1368–77.
92. Lange H, Jackel R. Usefulness of plasma lactate concentration in the diagnosis of acute abdominal disease. Eur J Surg 1994;160:381–4.
93. Brandstrup B, Tonnesen H, Beier-Holgersen R, et al. Effects of intravenous fluid restriction on postoperative complications: comparison of two perioperative fluid

regimens: a randomized assessor-blinded multicenter trial. Ann Surg 2003; 238(5):641–8.
94. Holte K, Sharrock NE, Kehlet H. Pathophysiology and clinical implications of perioperative fluid excess. Br J Anaesth 2002;89(4):622–32.
95. Woolsey CA, Coopersmith CM. Vasoactive drugs and the gut: is there anything new? Curr Opin Crit Care 2006;12(2):155–9.
96. Meier-Hellmann A, Reinhart K, Bredle DL, et al. Epinephrine impairs splanchnic perfusion in septic shock. Crit Care Med 1997;25:399–404.
97. Levy B, Bollaert PE, Charpentier C, et al. Comparison of norepinephrine and dobutamine to epinephrine for hemodynamics, lactate metabolism, and gastric tonometric variables in septic shock: a prospective, randomized study. Intensive Care Med 1997;23:282–7.
98. Duranteau J, Sitbon P, Teboul JL. Effects of epinephrine, norepinephrine, or the combination of norepinephrine and dobutamine on gastric mucosa in septic shock. Crit Care Med 1999;27(5):893–900.
99. Sun Q, Tu Z, Lobo S, et al. Optimal adrenergic support in septic shock due to peritonitis. Anesthesiology 2003;98(4):888–96.
100. Lisbon A. Dopexamine, dobutamine, and dopamine increase splanchnic blood flow: what is the evidence? Chest 2003;123(Suppl 5):460S–3S.
101. Krejci V, Hiltebrand LB, Jakob SM, et al. Vasopressin in septic shock: effects on pancreatic, renal, and hepatic blood flow. Crit Care 2007;11(6):R129.
102. Klinzing S, Simon M, Reinhart K, et al. High-dose vasopressin is not superior to norepinephrine in septic shock. Crit Care Med 2003;31(11):2646–50.
103. Schwarte LA, Picker O, Bornstein SR, et al. Levosimendan is superior to milrinone and dobutamine in selectively increasing microvascular gastric mucosal oxygenation in dogs. Crit Care Med 2005;33(1):135–42.
104. Satoh T, Morisaki H, Ai K, et al. Olprinone, a phosphodiesterase III inhibitor, reduces gut mucosal injury and portal endotoxin level during acute hypoxia in rabbits. Anesthesiology 2003;98(6):1407–14.
105. Kwok ES, Howes D. Use of methylene blue in sepsis: a systematic review. J Intensive Care Med 2006;21(6):359–63.
106. Salihoğlu Z, Demiroluk S, Görgün E, et al. Effects of sevoflurane versus TIVA on gastric intramucosal pH and hemodynamic status in colon cancer surgery. Middle East J Anesthesiol 2003;17(3):359–69.
107. Müller M, Schindler E, Roth S, Schürholz A, et al. Effects of desflurane and isoflurane on intestinal tissue oxygen pressure during colorectal surgery. Anaesthesia 2002;57(2):110–5.
108. Tverskoy M, Gelman S, Fowler KC, et al. Influence of fentanyl and morphine on intestinal circulation. Anesth Analg 1985;64(6):577–84.
109. Myles PS, Leslie K, McNeil J, et al. Bispectral index monitoring to prevent awareness during anaesthesia: the B-Aware randomised controlled trial. Lancet 2004; 363:1757–63.
110. Punjasawadwong Y, Phongchiewboon A, Bunchungmongkol N. Bispectral index for improving anaesthetic delivery and postoperative recovery. Cochrane Database Syst Rev 2007;(4):CD003843.
111. Kongsayreepong S, Chaibundit C, Chadpaibool J, et al. Predictor of core hypothermia and the surgical intensive care unit. Anesth Analg 2003;96:826–33.

# Informed Consent and the Ethical Management of the Older Patient

Yulia Ivashkov, MD[a,*], Gail A. Van Norman, MD[a,b]

**KEYWORDS**

• Informed • Consent • Older • Ethical • Elderly • Management

*A 79-year-old man presents with left femoral fracture for repair. His previous medical history is significant for hypertension, adult-onset diabetes, hyperlipidemia, cerebrovascular accident with residual right hemiplegia and hearing loss. He is oriented to place and person, yet appears somewhat confused and agitated, producing unclear mumbling, and sometimes not responding to questions. There are two consent forms on the patient's chart, one for a research protocol for an experimental hip prosthesis and the other for the surgical procedure and anesthesia. An 'X' is scribbled on the signature lines of both consent documents. The operating room nurse is processing the universal protocol and asks you if this represents adequate documentation for the surgery and spinal anesthesia.*

Elderly patients are particularly vulnerable in the informed consent process. Not only are they more likely to suffer from medical conditions that can impair cognition by virtue of age, but they may also suffer from physical disabilities (such as hearing loss) that impair communication even when cognition is intact. Coercive social factors, such as physical dependency, financial impoverishment, restricted health care resources, and family pressures, can play important roles in preventing elderly patients from formulating or expressing truly autonomous decisions with regard to their health care. The anesthesiologist must bear two important questions in mind when obtaining consent from any patient: (1) Is this patient able to give informed consent?; (2) Is there a way I can promote this patient's ability to give informed consent?

Until recently, physicians all over the world held God-like authority over patients. That authority originated during ancient times when blind faith was often the primary instrument and prayer a principle option for treatment. Disclosure of medical

[a] Department of Anesthesiology and Pain Medicine, Harborview Medical Center, University of Washington, 325 9th Avenue, Seattle, WA 98104, USA
[b] Department of Biomedical Ethics, University of Washington, 110 37th Avenue E, Seattle, WA 98112, USA
* Corresponding author.
*E-mail address:* ivashy@u.washington.edu (Y. Ivashkov).

Anesthesiology Clin 27 (2009) 569–580
doi:10.1016/j.anclin.2009.07.016 anesthesiology.theclinics.com
1932-2275/09/$ – see front matter 

information (eg, revealing a diagnosis of cancer) was considered by physicians to be excessive, unnecessary, and potentially harmful. In 1961, for example, only 12% of physicians would consider informing their oncological patients of the diagnosis.[1] By tradition, medical care was prescribed for the patient, but not really discussed with him or her.

This trust in doctors was compromised in the middle of the 20th century when Western society was shocked by information concerning human experimentation in Nazi concentration camps. Advances in medical technology were causing patients to question whether sustaining life at all costs was appropriate. As a result, primary assumptions regarding physician authority began to change. Today, when human rights are a priority in Western society, and ethical values in medicine have shifted from paternalism toward respect for patient autonomy, patients may no longer passively accept the decisions and advice of physicians, preferring to participate actively in making health care decisions. The concept of autonomy was brought to life by the ancient Greeks, who stated that people, unlike animals, are capable of ruling their own lives with responsibility and reason. Autonomy remained primarily a theoretical concept until the development of democracy as a political system, when autonomy acquired the meaning of the personal right to self-determination.

Modern Western medical ethics are based on principles of beneficence, nonmaleficence, respect for patient autonomy, and justice. Health care aims first to do good and promote well-being, and second to avoid causing harm and remove existing harm. In the framework of current medical ethics, promoting well-being is no longer necessarily measured by saving lives, but by preserving and promoting quality of life, a concept that relies on the patient's determination of what quality of life is. Thus, fulfilling the principle of beneficence also requires respecting the patient's wishes: in other words, respecting patient autonomy.

In the patient-doctor relationship, ethical principles state that a competent patient has the right to decide what should or should not be done to him or her. This principle was first firmly established as a legal right in the United States in the case of *Schloendorff v Society of New York Hospital*.[2] A woman who had agreed to undergo anesthesia for examination but had specifically refused surgery was nevertheless operated on while unconscious. She suffered a brachial plexus injury that eventually led to the amputation of fingers on one hand. She argued that she had not consented to the procedure, and that she would not have been injured if her wishes had been followed. Citing constitutional protection against noninterference and in favor of protection of privacy, the court sided with her. The decision was classically expressed by Justice Benjamin Cordozo: "Every human being of adult years and sound mind has a right to determine what shall be done with his own body; and a surgeon who performs an operation without his patient's consent commits an assault for which he is liable in damages." It is particularly relevant to the readers that that the original case regarding medical consents in the United States was related to anesthesia and surgery.

The personal values of patients may differ significantly from the medical goals of treatment. For some Jehovah's Witness patients, for example, the medical goals of transfusion may be in direct and irresolvable conflict with spiritual values. Because physicians were resistant to accepting the rights of patients to refuse blood transfusions, the courts intervened, and the law has now long recognized the rights of competent adult Jehovah's Witnesses to refuse blood.

In fact, any competent patient now has a legal right to refuse any medical intervention, for any reason, including no reason at all, even if that refusal appears to be absurd or harmful from a doctor's point of view. The law requires that medical treatment or research be preceded by the informed consent of the patient, and failure to obtain informed consent is not only illegal, but also constitutes malpractice. Courts and public opinion have also defended the interests of infirm elderly people for whom a surrogate or health care proxy is making decisions. State regulations defining legally authorized representatives differ widely, with some jurisdictions failing to provide clear guidance.

**ELEMENTS OF INFORMED CONSENT**

"Informed consent" is a legal term that implies an autonomous, informed authorization by a patient to undergo a medical procedure or treatment. The physician cannot make medical decisions for a competent patient, but is obliged to provide the patient with accurate, meaningful, and relevant information so that the patient can make informed medical choices. The ethical principle of respect for autonomy further requires that physicians do whatever is possible to promote patient autonomy. Thus, when a patient suffers from reversible conditions that impair autonomy the physician has a duty to treat those conditions, provided treatment can be accomplished in a time frame that still allows anesthesia and surgical care to be meaningful.

Informed consent includes a proper discussion between a physician and a patient, and covers all relevant aspects of a proposed treatment. This discussion is usually documented in the patient's chart, although the note or signed consent form does not substitute for the conversation between the physician and patient. The formal signed consent form in the chart is not a universal legal requirement, but the discussion is considered mandatory.

The important elements of valid informed consent are:

1. Voluntarism. The consent to medical treatment should be given exclusively by the patient's free will, without coercion or undue influences and pressures.
2. Disclosure. The presentation of relevant and accurate information, including the nature of his or her illness, the proposed treatment and its risks and benefits, and all reasonable alternatives to proposed treatment, including no treatment at all.
3. Competence (the legal term for decision-making capacity; in medical texts, "capacity" is often used). To be considered competent, a person should be capable of the following: understanding the provided information, appreciating the remote consequences of the treatment, and making and expressing a reasoned medical choice.

Every adult patient is legally assumed to be competent of making informed medical care decisions, unless there is evidence to the contrary. It is important to realize that competence for medical consent is not a global but a task-specific quality. A person may not be competent to live independently, for example, but still be competent to decide whether or not he or she wants to receive a blood transfusion.

Although the informed consent process is usually straightforward, it nevertheless can have hidden pitfalls. For example, the physician, led by his own understanding of good and reason, may persuade the patient to make a choice that does not reflect the patient's true values. The patient's consent to treatment or to research may be given not by free will, but under influence of pain or anxiety, fear of bad treatment, or loss of independence. The patient may not be fully informed of the nature of treatment and may remain unaware of risks that he or she would not otherwise be willing to undertake. All these factors may violate respect for patient autonomy, or undermine autonomy itself.

## SPECIAL PROBLEMS FACING ELDERLY PATIENTS IN THE CONSENT PROCESS

What constitutes old age is changing as patients remain healthier later in life. Elderly people of the 21st century may be healthier than ever, but they are also older than ever, and their number is growing. It is estimated that by 2030 one in five people will be older than 65 years, and that in 2050 in the United States the number of people who are 85 years and older will approximate 8.0 million.[3]

In the early 20th century an elective operation for inguinal hernia in a patient older than 50 years was frowned upon; nowadays people in their 70s may undertake cosmetic surgery, and octogenarians commonly undergo elective joint replacements and cardiac surgeries to improve their quality of life. As the population gets older, geriatric problems become common in all areas of modern medicine. Agism (discrimination or prejudice against the elderly population[4]), previously so common in society and medicine, has no place in modern health care.

Age is not a disease, and increase in biologic age per se does not indicate decreased brain function or neuronal loss. Nevertheless, aging is associated with a variety of changes. Advanced age is accompanied by increased risk of severe cognitive changes, such as those caused by Alzheimer's disease, Parkinson's disease, and organic brain damage following long-standing cardiovascular disorders. Almost 11% of those over the age of 65 years may suffer from Alzheimer's disease, and that number will continue to grow.[5]

Mental illness that affects decision-making capacity also creates significant difficulties in the process of informed consent. However, cognitive deficits and mental illness do not automatically indicate that a patient is unable to participate in his or her health care decisions. In fact, most patients with some degree of mental impairment are still capable of participating in medical decision-making and should not be treated against their will.

Many psychiatric disorders common in geriatric patients, such as depression, may affect understanding and the ability to express oneself, but studies in depressed patients reveal that decision-making capacity of these patients is usually intact, even if it appears otherwise.[6] The same is true regarding memory impairment. A patient may have difficulties recalling the details of the process of informed consent, but that does not mean that he or she did not understand the information given during consent, or that the decision was not a competent one. Studies reveal a strong desire among hospitalized aging patients to receive detailed information regarding their health care,[7] and efforts should be made to deliver that information in the most effective way.

Many elderly patients face difficult end-of-life problems and choices, such as the choice between palliative care and life-extending therapies. There may also be significant differences between their own desires and the interests of loved ones, who may suffer significant moral and financial burdens to care for the individual or who may stand to benefit emotionally or financially. The choice made by a geriatric patient might be perfectly reasoned in the settings of his or her specific personal values. However, this choice may appear unreasonable to a medical practitioner, especially if it contradicts the physician's understanding of "good," and opposes medical advice. Studies show that physicians often believe such patients to be incompetent, when that is actually not the case.[6]

Research shows that many terminally ill elderly patients prefer treatment that palliates suffering and provides comfort over life-extending therapies.[8,9] On the other hand, physicians frequently underestimate the desire of aging patients to receive life-prolonging therapies. Patients also often rate their quality of life higher than do caregivers or family members,[10] and may be interested in intensive and aggressive treatment.[11] Such therapies, if they are desired, should not be denied to the patient based on his or her advanced age, but should be considered in light of the benefits and burdens imposed by the therapy. Physicians must avoid under treatment of elderly patients, as well as unwanted over treatment.

## ASSESSING COMPETENCE OF A GERIATRIC PATIENT

Assessing competence in the geriatric patient population is complicated by many factors. Patients who are capable of making medical decisions may suffer communication difficulties because of their level of education, hearing or visual impairment, fear of the financial burdens of treatment, anxiety, or pain. While these problems also occur in younger patients, elderly patients more frequently suffer from medical comorbidities that contribute to such problems.

The unfamiliar environment of the hospital, noise and artificial lighting of the hospital wards, disturbance of routine sleeping and eating habits, and underlying disease might all contribute to significant confusion and agitation on the part of the patient. Specific problems such as expressive aphasia can cause great challenges in communication during the process of consent. When reversible problems impede the informed consent process, physicians are ethically obliged to try to reverse or mitigate these factors. Assessing understanding is also problematic. If a patient's ability to understand information is questionable, and the situation allows time for additional testing, quick cognitive assessment may be performed using simple tests such as the Mini-Mental State Examination (MMSE) or the Mini-Cog. However, even relatively low scores on these examinations do not preclude ability to undertake treatment-related decisions,[7] and psychiatric consultation and competence assessment may be necessary. Many attempts to determine capacity have rested on retrospective instruments that inquire of the patient what they have been told, and many practitioners continue to use this as the standard. Thus, if it is clear that the patient does not understand what has been explained, then the physician has to try again or make the determination that the patient is not competent.

## PROMOTING PATIENT AUTONOMY DURING THE INFORMED CONSENT PROCESS

In the informed consent process, the physician has an ethical obligation to promote autonomy and participation in medical decision-making to the degree that the patient is capable. Because different patients have different capabilities and challenges, the informed consent process requires an individualized approach, appropriate for the patient's level of education and understanding. Clearly there is no standard protocol for informed consent that will suit all.[12]

Barriers to communication, such as language differences, hearing loss, pain, anxiety, decreased mental capacity, and impaired ability to communicate should be specifically addressed, because they may mask a patient's ability to consent.[13] If the patient is not fluent in the doctor's language, a medical interpreter may be necessary, and is often preferable to relying on a family member to interpret. Family members may have language limitations of their own, may not understand medical terms, and may also have conflicts relating to family culture and lines of authority.[14] They may desire to soften important facts, and critical information may be deliberately or accidentally omitted. Furthermore, interpreting technically difficult and emotionally charged information for a sick family member imposes additional and unfair burdens upon loved ones during already difficult times. In some areas, professional translation services have become mandatory so that even bilingual staff members cannot serve as translators.

Use of clear and slow speech with pauses between key phrases, understandable language, short sentences, and simple grammar are always useful in communicating complex information. A short but comprehensive explanation has a greater chance of being understood than one that is long and overly detailed.[15] The physician should position him- or herself directly in front of the patient so that the patient can see the physician's face. Pain medications and anxiolytics should not be withheld in the setting of informed consent. Pain and anxiety can interfere with a patient's ability to process critical information. Withholding such therapies may result in a situation in which a patient who is suffering from pain appears to have been, or may actually have been, unduly influenced into consenting to obtain relieving medication.[16] A consent obtained in this way violates the ethical and legal principles of informed consent. Providing aids to vision and hearing during the consent process, by allowing the patient to better see the physician's face and hear his or her voice, may aid communication and understanding. Aphasic or demented patients may require nontraditional methods of communication; gestures, pictures, and written key words might work better than spoken words.[13,17] Involvement of family members in the discussion can be valuable; they might enhance consent quality by asking relevant questions that an aphasic patient is not able to articulate.[17] Severe aphasia may necessitate consultation with a speech and language specialist.[18] If aphasia presents a problem in the informed consent process, postponement of surgery and anesthesia may be necessary to obtain the necessary help in communication.

## MANAGING THE INCOMPETENT PATIENT

Research indicates that patients are more likely to be referred for competency evaluation if they refuse treatment, rather than for obvious signs of incompetence.[6] This tendency reflects physicians' biases rooted in the principle of beneficence and saving lives. Refusal per se should not automatically trigger a psychiatric consultation; only the lack of decision-making capacity is an indication for such referral. Agreement to treatment by an incompetent patient is equally problematic. Even if a patient consents to treatment, if decision-making capacity is in question, consideration should be given to obtaining a competency evaluation and possibly seeking an appropriate surrogate decision-maker.

If the patient is deemed incompetent and incompetence is likely to persist, the physician might have to rely on a surrogate decision-maker. Proxy consent for incapable individuals is thought to promote autonomy.[19] Some patients, incapable of deciding about medical treatment, may still retain capacity to appoint a proxy agent, and in this case their choice should be respected.[20] Mechanisms for surrogate decision-making include advance directives, legal guardians, and family members in a strict hierarchy that varies considerably from state to state. The anesthesiologist needs to be aware of state and local regulations regarding who is a legitimate surrogate for specific purposes.

If the patient is clearly incompetent (ie, unconscious or delirious) and needs emergency care, the state law may permit a life-saving treatment in the absence of consent. The care should be directed at goals that, in the opinion of the physician, are in the patient's best interest. The physician should not use this circumstance to circumvent a valid, written advance directive. This emergency exception to informed consent is based on the "reasonable man" standard, in which the law assumes that if the patient were competent, he or she would accept a life-saving treatment, because it is in his or her best interests.[21] What constitutes an emergency, however, varies in different states, and the type of documentation needed to support such a decision will probably be clearly defined in hospital policies and procedures. An "emergency" does not give a physician permission to ignore a competent patient's decisions, or, in the case of an incapacitated patient, previously expressed health care directives. An emergency exception applies only when the patient's desires are unknown and have not previously been expressed, and time will not permit the location of an appropriate surrogate decision-maker.

Legally and ethically, this emergency exception does not apply to the patient who has refused treatment when conscious and clearly competent, but has lost consciousness or the ability to communicate later. If that were true, then all physicians would have to do would be to wait for a patient to lose consciousness, and then do whatever they think is best, a course of action that completely usurps autonomy. The rights of unconscious patients to have their previously expressed choices followed have been confirmed in many court cases, including the cases of Karen Ann Quinlan,[22] Nancy Cruzan,[23] and most recently, Terri Schiavo.[24] Each of these women had become permanently unconscious and dependent on medical care consisting of mechanical ventilation (Quinlan) and artificial nutrition (Cruzan and Schiavo). Family members sued to have medical interventions stopped in accordance with each patient's previously expressed wishes. In all cases, court decisions confirmed the rights of these patients to refuse even life-saving therapy through surrogate decision-makers. In 1990, the Patient Self-Determination Act passed by the US Congress confirmed these rights and established the process of advance directives.[25] These cases also pointed to how different potentially legitimate surrogates may have very different perspectives on the patient's wishes, making it important that the anesthesiologist understands and acts in accordance with the relevant policies and procedures.

Advance directives are statements regarding future medical decision-making created by a person while still competent and may be written or oral. Two types of written advanced directives include living wills and Durable Powers of Attorney for Health Care Decisions (DPOAs). Living wills allow caregivers to understand the patient's wishes and philosophy, and address a limited number of specific decisions. However, it is impossible to foresee all future situations, and living wills may lack specific instructions for dealing with many complex situations. For that reason, a DPOA may be used. A DPOA authorizes a designated person to act as a health care proxy when the patient is not competent to decide. The circumstances under which a DPOA becomes effective may vary in different states.

In cases in which a patient has never been competent or has become incompetent without providing advance care directives, state law may designate a hierarchy of persons to make medical decisions for the patient. A common hierarchy is the patient's spouse or domestic partner, followed by the patient's children over 18 years old if all are in agreement, followed by the patient's parents if both are in agreement, followed by the patient's siblings if all are in agreement. A legal guardian may be appointed by court as a surrogate decision-maker when appropriate surrogates are not available, or if surrogates cannot agree. The law assumes that surrogate decision-makers will make medical decisions on behalf of the patient by the principle of substituted judgment. Substituted judgment means that the proxy presumably is familiar with the patient's values and desires, has had discussions about possible future illness, knows what the patient would like, and will make the same decisions regarding health care that the patient would make for him- or herself.[26] The weakness of this approach is that in reality many family members do not discuss illness-related and end-of-life issues, and do not know what the patient would really want. Even worse, some proxies may give consent even if they believe that the cognitively impaired patent would not do so if he or she were capable.[27] If the patient's desires are not known, and there is no proxy decision-maker available, then care should be instituted in the patient's best interests, based on what a "reasonable person" would decide.

Anesthesiologists should be aware that in some cases state law prevents anyone but a court from consenting for specific procedures. In the state of New York, for example, electroconvulsive therapy cannot be consented to by a surrogate decision-maker such as a spouse or parent, even if one is available. Such treatment requires a court order.[28] Laws vary from state to state.

### *Surrogate Consent for Research*

Regulations regarding the protection of human research subjects are found primarily in federal regulations and guidelines (45 Code of Federal Regulations [CFR] 46, 21 CFR 50). These regulations specifically refer to a "legally authorized representative" but leave to state law how that is defined. The Secretary's Advisory Committee on Human Research Protections (an advisory body to the Secretary of Health and Human Services) has recently recommended that federal regulation address these definitions (http://www.hhs.gov/ohrp/sachrp/mtgings/mtg03-09/mtg03-09.html).

## INFORMED REFUSAL AND DO NOT RESUSCITATE ORDERS

The principle of respect for patient autonomy is rendered nonsensical if informed patients are not allowed to refuse therapy, because this invalidates the essential voluntary aspect of consent. Decisions to forego or terminate life-saving therapy such as mechanical ventilation in the intensive care unit (ICU) have become commonplace. But what about refusals of life-saving therapy in the operating room? Geriatric patients facing critical procedures near the end of life may have important wishes regarding their medical care during anesthesia and surgery. They do not a priori surrender their rights at the operating room doors to have such decisions guide their care while under anesthesia.

Do not resuscitate (DNR) orders can present substantial difficulty to operating room personnel, who may feel that principles of nonmaleficence and beneficence are compromised if a cardiac arrest during surgery cannot be treated.[29–31] Surgical stress and bleeding, purposeful pharmacological respiratory depression, extensive use of fluids and vasoactive drugs all contribute to the perception of surgery with anesthesia as a process of ongoing resuscitation. Many argue that acute events that happen during surgery are often reversible, carry favorable prognosis, and should always be treated. Consequently, perioperative care providers are inclined to initiate resuscitation promptly and to do everything that is possible to save a patient's life. As many as 50% of anesthesiologists assume that DNR orders are automatically suspended during surgery.[29]

The argument that anesthesia and surgery are a process of ongoing resuscitation is specious, because cardiopulmonary resuscitation (CPR) is something that anesthesiologists try to avoid in the operating room, rather than being a part of routine anesthesia care. Simply because some of the aspects of routine anesthesia care, such as mechanical ventilation, resemble some aspects of CPR does not make them the same, any more than one would describe a patient being ventilated in the ICU as undergoing ongoing resuscitation.

However, many of the concerns of operating room health care workers are justified. CPR does carry a somewhat more favorable prognosis in the operating room than in other hospital locations.[32] This is likely because cardiac arrest in the operating room is witnessed and due to specific and generally reversible causes, and treatment is therefore directed to a specific cause and initiated earlier in the arrest. But while these facts change the prognosis of the treatment, and are important to present to patients who have DNR orders, they do not alter the obligation of physicians to obtain consent from the patient to suspend a DNR order, or to respect the DNR order if the patient does not wish to suspend it for surgery.

CPR may prolong life, but for terminally ill elderly patients it may not necessarily represent "doing good" and can cause significant harm. Resuscitation may bring about prolongation of dying and suffering instead, such as prolonged stay in the ICU, long-term mechanical ventilation, tube feedings, multiple intravenous lines, and loss of control over end-of-life issues. Up to 44% of all survivors of in-hospital CPR have significant residual functional impairment,[33] and few patients fully recover to the previous state of health. The prognosis is even worse for older patients. While survival after CPR in the operating room is better than that in other hospital settings, significant numbers of patients will still suffer painful injuries, residual disabilities, and death.[34–36]

Surgical patients have the right, based on law, to refuse any medical treatment, including life-sustaining treatment.[37] Surveys indicate that patients who are older and functionally impaired are more likely to decline CPR.[38] Many terminally ill elderly patients seek surgical palliation of their conditions. Requiring them to suspend their DNR orders and potentially undergo CPR to obtain the desired palliation is inhumane, and does not appropriately recognize their right to make health care decisions.

Many institutions have policies by which DNR orders are automatically, presumably temporarily, suspended when a patient enters the operating room. Most medical ethicists and medical professional organizations associated with surgical care of patients now agree that automatic suspension of DNR orders in the setting of anesthesia and surgery does not appropriately recognize the ethical principle of respecting patient autonomy. However, continuing DNR orders in the operating room without discussing the risks and benefits does not address patient rights to make informed decisions. Professional guidelines of the American Society of Anesthesiologists,[39] American College of Surgeons,[40] Association of Operating Room Nurses,[41] and Joint Commission on Accreditation of Healthcare Organizations (JCAHO)[42] all state that "Rediscussion of DNR orders and consent/refusal should be documented before the patient enters the operating room."

Because the reasons for, and prognosis of, CPR in the operating room are different from those of other hospital locations, the anesthesiologist has an ethical obligation to provide patients and their surrogate decision-makers with DNR orders with the relevant information, and determine what their wishes would be under these altered circumstances. This discussion should include determining the patient's goals for therapy, and which aspects of resuscitation from cardiac arrest would be acceptable. Therapies common to resuscitation that cannot be avoided because of the nature of the surgery should be carefully explained. It may be impossible, for example, to undertake thoracotomy if the patient utterly refuses intubation. Discussion of specific therapies is often necessary, but the goal of such discussions is to establish the patient's general goals with regard to resuscitation, rather than providing an exhaustive "checklist" of therapies to the patient for approval or disapproval.

Now let us go back to the case described at the beginning of this article.

Do the consent forms attached to the chart of that patient represent valid consent to surgery and anesthesia?

The best way to verify the validity of the consent is to talk to the patient. Although he appears to be confused, his appearance may be the result of discomfort, pain, anxiety, or hearing impairment, and not true confusion. After the anesthesiologist ensures that the patient is positioned in the bed comfortably with his hearing aids in, and has provided treatment for pain or anxiety if necessary, he or she should ask the patient in a clear voice, using simple vocabulary, whether he understands what is happening. The conversation may then help to reassure the health care team that the patient understands his current situation, and that he has indeed provided a valid consent for surgical procedure.

Even if, after these measures, the patient still appears confused, it does not necessarily mean that he was not competent when the consent was given. Witnesses to the signing of the patient's "X" may be able to state whether the patient understood what he was signing. If the signature on the consent form was not witnessed, then the consent might not be valid. If the surgery is not emergent, options include delaying surgery for a competency evaluation or until an appropriate surrogate decision-maker can be found. If the surgery is emergent, then the physicians should proceed with their best understanding of the patient's best interests, and the likely decisions a reasonable patient would make.

If the patient is deemed not competent to have consented for surgery, then he was also not competent to consent for a clinical research study. Depending on the research protocol and Institutional Review Board (IRB) approval, a surrogate decision-maker may be able to consent for the patient to be included in the study, but this should be verified and not assumed. In such cases, if a surrogate decision-maker cannot be found, the patient should not receive an experimental implant and should be removed from the study protocol.

## SUMMARY

Informed consent in elderly patients presents many ethical and legal challenges. However, aging should not be viewed as a disease, and physicians should avoid biases with regard to aging patients and their wishes. The purpose of informed consent is to promote autonomy, to protect a patient from undesired treatment, and to help the patient to make appropriate medical care decisions that correlate with his or her personal values. Informed consent is a process of shared decision-making, not merely an act of obtaining a signature on a consent form. Most aging patients are competent to provide consent for medical care. Physicians should facilitate the consent process by clear communication and by relieving obstacles such as pain, undue anxiety, and language barriers. A surrogate decision-maker should be sought for an incompetent patient. If the care is emergent and no surrogate decision-maker is available, regulation may permit the physician to undertake treatment with appropriate documentation. Advance directives are legally and ethically binding tools by which patients can express their decisions regarding medical care before they lose capacity to do so. DNR orders should not be automatically suspended for anesthesia and surgery. Discussion of these orders is part of informed consent, and the patient's wishes regarding resuscitation in the operating room should be respected. Surrogate consent for participation in research is not necessarily allowed by IRB approval and research protocols. The acceptability of enrolling an incompetent patient in a research protocol via surrogate consent should be verified before doing so.

## REFERENCES

1. Oken D. What to tell cancer patients. A study of medical attitudes. JAMA 1961;175:120–8.

2. Schloendorff V. Society of New York hospital, in 211 N.Y. 125, 105 N.E. 92 1914. Court of appeals of New York.
3. U.S. Census Bureau, 2000. Available at: http://www.census.gov/.
4. American Psychological Association (APA). Resolution on ageism, 2002. Available at: http://www.apa.org/pi/aging/ageism.html.
5. Evans DA. Estimated prevalence of Alzheimer's disease in the United States. Milbank Q 1990;68(2):267–89.
6. Weinstock R, Copelan R. Competence to give informed consent for medical procedures. Bull Am Acad Psychiatry Law 1984;12(2):117–25.
7. Paillaud E, Ferrand E. Medical information and surrogate designation: results of a prospective study in elderly hospitalised patients. Age Ageing 2007;36(3):274–9.
8. Somogyi-Zalud E, Zhong Z. The use of life-sustaining treatments in hospitalized persons aged 80 and older. J Am Geriatr Soc 2002;50(5):930–4.
9. Yellen S, Cella D. Age and clinical decision making in oncology patients. J Natl Cancer Inst 1994;86(23):1766–70.
10. Epstein AM, Hall JA, Tognetti J, et al. Using proxies to evaluate quality of life. Can they provide valid information about patients' health status and satisfaction with medical care? Med Care 1989;27(3 Suppl):S91–8.
11. Penson RT, Daniels KJ, Lynch TJ Jr. Too old to care? Oncologist 2004;9(3): 343–52.
12. Appelbaum PS, Grisso T. Assessing patients' capacities to consent to treatment. N Engl J Med 1988;319(25):1635–8.
13. Kagan A. Revealing the competence of aphasic adults through conversation: a challenge to health professionals. Top Stroke Rehabil 1995;2(1):15–28.
14. Bezuidenhout L, Borry P. Examining the role of informal interpretation in medical interviews. J Med Ethics 2009;35:159–62.
15. Epstein L. Obtaining informed consent. Form or substance. Arch Intern Med 1969;123(6):682–8.
16. Van Norman GA, Palmer SK. The ethical boundaries of persuasion: coercion and restraint of patients in clinical anesthesia practice. Int Anesthesiol Clin 2001; 39(3):131–43.
17. Stein J, Brady Wagner LC. Is informed consent a "yes or no" response? Enhancing the shared decision-making process for persons with aphasia. Top Stroke Rehabil 2006;13(4):42–6.
18. Penn C, Frankel T. Informed consent and aphasia: evidence of pitfalls in the process. Aphasiology 2009;23(1):3–32.
19. Eyler L, Jeste D. Enhancing the informed consent process: a conceptual overview. Behav Sci Law 2006;24(4):553–68.
20. Kim SY, Appelbaum PS. The capacity to appoint a proxy and the possibility of concurrent proxy directives. Behav Sci Law 2006;24(4):469–78.
21. Richards EP, Rathbun KC. Medical risk management: preventive legal strategies for health care providers. The medical and public health law site; 1982.
22. In the Matter of Karen Quinlan. 70 NJ 10, in 355 A 2d 647 (1976, supreme court of New Jersey).
23. Cruzan v. Director. Missouri Dept. of Health, in 497 U.S. 261 (1990, Supreme Court of the United States).
24. Jeb Bush v. Michael Schiavo (2004, Florida Supreme Court).
25. Patient Self-Determination Act, in 42, C.o.t. United States of America, Editor. 1990. p. 101–508.
26. Emanuel EJ, Emanuel LL. Proxy decision making for incompetent patients. An ethical and empirical analysis. JAMA 1992;267(15):2067–71.

27. Warren JW, et al. Informed consent by proxy. An issue in research with elderly patients. N Engl J Med 1986;315(18):1124–8.
28. Sundrum SJ, Stavis PF. Obtaining informed consent for treatment of mentally incompetent patients. A decade under New York's innovative approach. Int J Law Psychiatry 1999;22(2):107–23.
29. Ewanchuk M, Brindley PG. Perioperative do-not-resuscitate orders – doing 'nothing' when 'something' can be done. Crit Care 2006;10(4):219.
30. Margolis JO, et al. Do not resuscitate (DNR) orders during surgery: ethical foundations for institutional policies in the United States. Anesth Analg 1995;80(4): 806–9.
31. VanNorman GA. Who speaks for the patient? Ethical principles in assessing patient competence and appropriate use of proxy decision-makers in the practice of anesthesiology. In: Waisel D, Van Norman G, editors. ASA syllabus on ethics: informed consent. Park Ridge (IL): ASA publications; 1998.
32. Brindley PG, et al. Predictors of survival following in-hospital adult cardiopulmonary resuscitation. CMAJ 2002;167(4):343–8.
33. Zoch TW, et al. Short- and long-term survival after cardiopulmonary resuscitation. Arch Intern Med 2000;160(13):1969–73.
34. Elshove-Bolk J, Guttormsen AB, Austlid I. In-hospital resuscitation of the elderly: characteristics and outcome. Resuscitation 2007;74(2):372–6.
35. Newland MC, et al. Anesthetic-related cardiac arrest and its mortality: a report covering 72,959 anesthetics over 10 years from a US teaching hospital. Anesthesiology 2002;97(1):108–15.
36. Sprung J, et al. Predictors of survival following cardiac arrest in patients undergoing noncardiac surgery: a study of 518,294 patients at a tertiary referral center. Anesthesiology 2003;99(2):259–69.
37. Burns JP, et al. Do-not-resuscitate order after 25 years. Crit Care Med 2003;31(5): 1543–50.
38. Phillips R, Wenger N. Choices of seriously ill patients about cardiopulmonary resuscitation: correlates and outcomes. Am J Med 1996;100:128–37.
39. Ethical guidelines for the anesthesia care of patients with do-not-resuscitate orders or other directives that limit treatment. Park Ridge (IL): American Society of Anesthesiologists; 2008.
40. American College of Surgeons. Statement on advance directives by patients: "do not resuscitate" in the operating room. Bull Am Coll Surg 1994;79(9):29.
41. American Society of Perianesthesia Nurses. A position statement on the perianesthesia patient with a do-not-resuscitate advance directive. Denver (CO): AORN; 1996.
42. Joint Commission on Accreditation of Health Care Organizations. Manual of the joint commission on accreditation of health care organizations. Chicago (IL): Patient Rights Chapter; 1994.

# Perioperative Use of β-Blockers in the Elderly Patient

Stefan A. Lombaard, MBChB, FANZCA*, Reinette Robbertze, MBChB, FANZCA

**KEYWORDS**

• Perioperative • β-Blockers • Elderly
• Comorbidities • Drug interactions

An 85-year-old man presented for a nephrectomy for renal cell carcinoma. His medical history included smoking (150 pack years), significant obstructive pulmonary disease requiring $O_2$ at 2 L/min at night, stable infrarenal abdominal aortic aneurysm involving both common iliac arteries, a history of supraventricular tachycardia, and type 2 diabetes that was well controlled on glyburide. The patient was seen by the medical consult service and thought to be in optimal condition for surgery. However, he was not on regular β-blocker therapy at the time he was seen in the clinic. Slow-release metoprolol 25 mg PO daily was prescribed, which the patient started taking 3 days before surgery. The plan was to continue with 2.5 mg intravenously every 4 hours postoperatively. Multiple premature ventricular complexes (PVCs) were noted on his electrocardiograph (ECG) in the preoperative holding area. Anesthesia was induced with fentanyl 90 μg, etomidate 10 mg, and rocuronium 30 mg. The patient underwent endotracheal intubation. Phenylephrine was used in 50-μg increments to maintain an acceptable blood pressure. The surgeon completed a cystoscopy and during repositioning for the nephrectomy, the patient became bradycardic with a rate down to 30 beats per minute, and hypotensive with a systolic blood pressure of 50 mm Hg. The ECG showed a new first-degree heart block with slight ST segment changes and multifocal PVCs. He responded to intravenous glycopyrrolate 0.5 mg. After discussion with the surgeon, it was decided not to proceed with surgery. The anesthetic was discontinued and the patient was extubated. He was then transferred to the postanesthesia care unit without further incident. The patient was referred for further cardiac evaluation to assess the first-degree heart block. Serial ECGs did not indicate signs of ischemia and he did not have raised troponin levels. The β-blocker was thought to have been contributory to his first-degree block and bradycardia. The brief period of profound hypotension did not result in any neurologic or other sequelae.

Department of Anesthesiology and Pain Medicine, Box 356540, University of Washington Medical Center, 1959 NE Pacific Street, Seattle, WA 98195-6540, USA
* Corresponding author.
*E-mail address:* lombaard@u.washington.edu (S.A. Lombaard).

Anesthesiology Clin 27 (2009) 581–597
doi:10.1016/j.anclin.2009.07.015 **anesthesiology.theclinics.com**
1932-2275/09/$ – see front matter 

Elderly patients are increasingly referred for complex surgery. Elderly patients are, however, at particular risk for coronary artery disease. The incidence doubles in men aged 65 to 94 compared with ages 35 to 64 years, whereas it triples in women.[1] Rankin and colleagues[2] found advanced age to be only second to emergency surgery as a variable that independently influenced operative mortality. This finding can to a significant extent be attributed to cardiovascular disease. Therefore, the elderly stand to benefit the most from strategies to prevent perioperative cardiac events. One strategy is to employ perioperative β-blockade, but doing so has the potential to increase the incidence of congestive heart failure (CHF),[3] perioperative hypotension, bradycardia, and stroke.[4,5]

Prescription of β-blockers is complicated by the fact that the most widely quoted β-blocker trials showed different outcomes.[5–7] A recent meta-analysis found that the trials promoting the beneficial effects had a high risk of bias.[4] The optimal timing of initiation of perioperative β-blockade, and dosage and duration of β-blockade remains to be elucidated. In addition, even the choice of β-blocker agent may make a difference, with some randomized controlled trials showing no beneficial effect with metoprolol.[8–10] The significance of this finding is difficult to determine in light of there being a large heterogeneity in the heart rate response to β-blockade, specifically with metoprolol.[3]

The American College of Cardiology (ACC) and the American Heart Association (AHA) have identified subgroups in which there is level I and IIa evidence that perioperative β-blockade is beneficial[11] (**Table 1**). Physicians may withhold therapy in elderly patients who meet these criteria because of safety concerns arising from comorbidity, tolerability,[12] potential drug contraindications with age, alterations in drug clearance, and the lack of follow-up after initiating perioperative medication.[13,14]

Trials in which the heart rate was controlled the most (maximal heart rate less than 100 beats per minute) were associated with a reduced incidence of postoperative myocardial infarction. It has been suggested that in the elderly the optimal dose should be the highest dose that the patient can tolerate without adverse symptoms.[15]

## COMMON COMORBIDITIES IN THE ELDERLY THAT MAY BENEFIT FROM THE CHRONIC USE OF β-BLOCKERS

β-Blockers play a role in the therapy for a variety of chronic medical conditions that are common in the elderly. β-Blockers are indicated for the prevention of myocardial infarction, ventricular and atrial arrhythmias, migraine, essential tremor, and symptomatic treatment of hypertrophic obstructive cardiomyopathy. These patients, as with

**Table 1**
**Patients to whom β-blockers should be administered perioperatively**

| | |
|---|---|
| Class I | Currently on β-blocker therapy to treat angina, symptomatic arrhythmias, hypertension, or other AHA/ACC Class I guideline indications |
| Class I | Patients undergoing vascular surgery with ischemia on preoperative testing |
| Class IIa | Patients undergoing vascular surgery in whom preoperative assessment identifies coronary heart disease but without documented ischemic changes on testing |
| Class IIa | Patients undergoing vascular surgery in whom preoperative assessment identifies multiple clinical risk factors |
| Class IIa | Patients with known coronary heart disease or at high cardiac risk as defined by the presence of multiple clinical risk factors, undergoing intermediate- or high-risk procedures |

*Data from* Ref.[11]

any patient on chronic β-blocker therapy, should have their therapy continued in the perioperative period. In addition, if patients with these conditions are found not to be on chronic β-blocker therapy, consideration should be given to starting such therapy.

The AHA/ACC guidelines for secondary prevention of myocardial infarction and death recommend β-blockers for all postmyocardial infarction patients, to be continued indefinitely.[16] Patients in whom preoperative testing indicates the presence of coronary artery disease or patients with multiple clinical risk factors for coronary artery disease may benefit from remaining on β-blocker therapy indefinitely.[17]

### *Atrial Fibrillation in Cardiac Surgery*

The prevalence of atrial fibrillation dramatically increases with age.[18] It is estimated that atrial fibrillation occurs in approximately 30% of patients following cardiothoracic surgery.[19] Various studies have reported that postoperative atrial fibrillation is associated with increased early and late mortality after cardiac surgery, increased incidence of stroke, and prolonged hospital length of stay.[20,21] Overall, the risk for death is increased by 9.7% (range 3%–33.3%) in patients who develop postoperative atrial fibrillation.[22]

Risk factors identified with postoperative atrial fibrillation include advanced age, valvular heart surgery, chronic obstructive pulmonary disease (COPD), stenosis of the right coronary artery, reduced left ventricular ejection fraction, left atrial enlargement, autonomic dysfunction (with a higher incidence in diabetic patients), and perioperative withdrawal of chronic β-blocker therapy.[23,24] Obesity in older patients (older than 50 years) was also a risk factor.[23] β-Blockers are considered by a 2004 Cochrane database review to be the best class of drug at preventing postoperative atrial fibrillation in patients undergoing cardiac surgery.[25] β-Blockers significantly reduced the incidence and seemed to prevent occurrence of atrial fibrillation in patients with systolic heart failure.[26–28] The results of the Atrial Fibrillation and Congestive Heart Failure trial indicate that a routine strategy of rhythm control does not reduce rate of death, and suggest that rate control should be considered a primary approach for patients with atrial fibrillation and heart failure.[27]

### *Congestive Heart Failure*

The incidence of CHF increases threefold between the ages of 65 and 85 years.[29] In 1999 the CIBIS II (Cardiac Insufficiency Bisoprolol Study II),[28] MERIT-HF (Metoprolol CR/XL Randomised Intervention Trial in Congestive Heart Failure),[30] and SENIORS[31] studies found that β-blocker use demonstrated a significant reduction in morbidity and mortality in patients with mild to moderate, stable heart failure. The mechanisms of these benefits are still disputed but may involve prevention of atrial fibrillation.[28,30] In 2001 Packer and colleagues[32] also proved a benefit from β-blockers in patients with stable severe chronic heart failure. All of the major randomized trials involving the use of β-blockers for heart failure included many elderly patients who appeared to derive similar benefit to younger patients.[30]

### *Hypertension*

Hypertension is the most common cardiovascular disease of the elderly, with an incidence that increases with age, and reaches 6.2% in men and 8.6% in women aged 70 to 79 years. Hypertension is the leading cause for congestive heart failure, accounting for 39% of heart failure events in men and 59% in women.[33] A 2007 Cochrane Database review,[12] a meta-analysis published in 2006,[34] and a large meta-analysis published in 2005[35] concluded that the available evidence does not support the use of β-blockers as first-line drugs in the treatment of hypertension.

When compared with calcium channel-blockers and rennin-angiotensin system (RAS) inhibitors, β-blockers had a 16% higher relative risk for stroke. The relative risk for stroke with β-blockers was only lower when compared with no treatment or placebo. The greatest increase in stroke was seen in the trials involving atenolol (26%) and the trials that studied combined use of diuretics and β-blockers. β-Blockers demonstrated an increase in all-cause mortality (3%) compared with other drugs, but there was no difference for myocardial infarction. Patients on β-blockers were more likely to discontinue treatment than those on diuretics or RAS inhibitors.[34]

Current European hypertension guidelines and United States national hypertension guidelines regard β-blockers as the first choice antihypertensive agent in patients postmyocardial infarction, at high risk for coronary disease, or with heart failure.[36,37]

### *Coronary Artery Disease*

Approximately 65% of myocardial infarctions occur in patients older than 65 years of age and 33% occur in patients older than 75 years.[38] Up to 80% of all deaths related to myocardial infarction occur in persons 65 years or older.[39] Elderly patients are much less likely to present with classic chest pain, and diagnosis may be delayed until cardiac markers are elevated. In the absence of a complaint of chest pain, the initial focus of care often centers on the patient's comorbidities.[40]

β-Blocker therapy constitutes first-line treatment for chronic effort-induced angina by improving the balance of myocardial oxygen supply and demand. The optimal dose should result in a resting heart rate of 55 to 60 beats per minute, with a reduction in the peak heart rate and blood pressure during exercise. This dose should not have significant side effects.[41] Atrial and ventricular arrhythmias are common after acute myocardial infarction, and are associated with a poor prognosis. The CAPRICORN trial indicated that an early treatment with carvedilol reduced the incidence of atrial arrhythmias following myocardial infarction in patients with left ventricular systolic dysfunction.[42] β-Blockers are also used in the management of acute myocardial infarction. The COMMIT/CCS2 trial (N = 45,852) showed a reduced mortality in patients who were hemodynamically stable. In contrast, there was an increased mortality in patients who presented with hemodynamic instability.[43]

## PROPHYLACTIC PERIOPERATIVE USE OF β-BLOCKERS

β-Blockers are thought to be effective in reducing perioperative cardiac events by decreasing sympathetic tone and improving the myocardial $O_2$ supply/demand balance, and preventing ventricular arrhythmias. β-Blockers are also considered important in limiting the shear stress across vulnerable atherosclerotic plaques. Atherosclerotic plaque rupture may be implicated in almost 50% of all perioperative myocardial infarctions.[17]

### *Overview of Influential Studies on Perioperative β-Blockade*

The study by Mangano and colleagues[6] was not the first to show benefit in using β-blockers. However, it was arguably one of the most influential early studies to suggest that cardiac morbidity can be reduced even up to 2 years after surgery (**Table 2**). Further support came from the study by Poldermans and colleagues,[44] published in 1999. Unfortunately, these studies had some significant limitations. In the

Mangano study, only postoperative adverse cardiac events were included in the long-term results.[45,46] If in-hospital events were included, the difference in deaths between the groups would have lost statistical significance. The number of patients was small: the overall difference in cardiac events between the placebo and treatment groups was only 16 patients. The randomization was criticized in an editorial that accompanied the original Mangano article. There was a trend toward a more severe cardiac history in the placebo group.[47] β-Blocker treatment was acutely stopped in 8 patients on chronic β-blocker therapy when they were randomized to the control group.[46] This stop may have contributed to a worse outcome in the control group. The Poldermans study was terminated early and the sample size was small. The study population was high-risk patients who underwent high-risk surgery, which may not extrapolate to a lower-risk group. Patients with severe coronary artery disease were excluded. Treatment was not blinded, and may have led to more careful treatment and monitoring postoperatively.

The DIPOM (Diabetic Postoperative Mortality and Morbidity) trial[9] evaluated β-blockade in diabetic patients, whereas the MaVS (Metoprolol after Vascular Surgery) study[10] focused on patients presenting for vascular surgery. Both of these studies did not show benefit from β-blockade. The DIPOM trial included a large percentage of low-risk procedures and the patients had few risk factors other than diabetes. The β-blocker dose was low and was not titrated to a target heart rate. The POBBLE (Perioperative Beta-Blockade)[8] trial also failed to show significant benefit. Although the study was a double-blind study, the anesthesiologists managing the cases were unblinded. The number of study subjects was relatively small. A retrospective case control study by Lindenauer and colleagues[7] in fact showed that whereas there was a benefit in higher-risk patients, β-blockade may in fact be detrimental in lower-risk groups.

The POISE (PeriOperative ISchemic Evaluation) trial[5] is the largest prospective, randomized trial to date. This trial proved that perioperative β-blockade reduced the rate of perioperative myocardial infarction; however, mortality was significantly increased in the metoprolol group due to stroke. More than 75% of the strokes were ischemic and were possibly due to the high incidence of hypotension. This study has been criticized because the starting dose was fixed and relatively large. The dose was only reduced after patients became bradycardic or developed a low blood pressure.

### *Target Population for Perioperative Prophylactic Use*

The ideal target population remains to be defined.[11] Lindenauer and colleagues[7] found that patients with a revised cardiac risk index of ≥3 (**Box 1**) benefit from β-blocker therapy and should receive a β-blocker, if not already on one. Some investigators believe that patients with even just one or two cardiac risk factors (**Box 1**) should be considered for β-blockade.[17,46]

In 2005 Lindenauer and colleagues[7] observed that low-risk patients prescribed β-blockers may be put at increased risk for complications associated with β-blocker therapy. In an article published in 2008, Kaafarani and colleagues[48] came to a similar conclusion. The Lindenauer observation has been questioned, because the β-blockers may have been prescribed in response to cardiac complications rather than as prophylaxis for cardiac complications.[49] Further randomized controlled trials are needed to explore this issue.

Black patients are known to respond less well to β-blockers when prescribed for treatment of CHF or hypertension, due to genetic polymorphism of receptors or enzyme systems. However, they do benefit from β-blockers prescribed for coronary artery disease and should receive β-blockers in this situation.[50]

**Table 2**
**Summary of influential studies**

| | Mangano et al[6] | Poldermans et al[44] | DIPOM[9] | POBBLE[8] | MaVS[10] | Lindenauer et al[7] | POISE[5] |
|---|---|---|---|---|---|---|---|
| Year | 1996 | 1999 | 2004 | 2005 | 2006 | 2005 | 2008 |
| Number of subjects | 200 | 101 | 921 | 103 | 497 | 119,632 + 216,290 controls | 8351 |
| AHA risk | Intermediate to high | High | Intermediate to high | High | High | All | Intermediate to high |
| Type of study | Prospective Randomized double-blind placebo-controlled | Prospective Randomized unblinded Multicenter | Prospective Randomized double-blind placebo-controlled Multicenter | Prospective Randomized double-blind placebo-controlled | Prospective Double-blind placebo-controlled Multicenter | Retrospective, Case-control | Prospective Randomized double-blind placebo-controlled Multicenter |
| Age range (mean) | 44–89 (68) | 61–75 (68) | 54–75.8 (64.8) | 61–79 (73.5) | 55.9–75.9 (66.1) | 47–74 (62) | (69) |
| Surgery | Mainly vascular & intra-abdominal | Major vascular surgery. | Noncardiac surgery >1 h | Infrarenal vascular surgery | Abdominal aortic surgery infrainguinal or axillofemoral revascularization | Major noncardiac surgery (length of stay >2 d) Mainly abdominal & orthopedic | Noncardiac surgery with length of stay of >24 h |
| Inclusion criteria | Two or more risk factors for CAD (patients on BB not excluded) | Positive results on dobutamine echocardiography | Diabetics Age ≥40 y | – | ASA III or less | Age >18 y RCRI ≥1 | >45 years, history of CAD, PVD, stroke, CHF, major vascular surgery, or ≥3 of 7 high-risk criteria |

| Exclusion | None listed | Extensive wall-motion abnormalities, asthma<br>Left main or severe 3-vessel CAD<br>Current BB Rx | CHF class 4, pregnancy/ breast feeding<br>Current BB Rx | Asthma<br>Aortic stenosis<br>Bradycardia<br>Hypotension<br>Documented MI<br>Unstable angina or + dobutamine stress test<br>Current BB Rx | Amiodarone<br>Asthma<br>CHF<br>Heart block<br>Current BB Rx | Bradycardia<br>Heart block<br>CHF<br>Hypotension<br>Asthma/COPD | Bradycardia<br>Heart block<br>Asthma<br>Coronary artery bypass graft surgery<br>Low-risk surgery<br>Verapamil<br>Current BB Rx |
|---|---|---|---|---|---|---|---|
| Beta-blocker | Atenolol | Bisoprolol | Metoprolol (CR) | Metoprolol | Metoprolol | Any | Metoprolol (ER) |
| Preoperative protocol | First dose 30 min before surgery 5 mg + 5 mg IV after 10 min | First dose 1 week before surgery 5 mg PO and increased to 10mg if HR > 60/min | First dose evening before surgery 50 mg PO<br>Second dose 1–2 h before surgery: Metoprolol 100 mg PO | First dose started 24 h before surgery 50 mg PO or 25 mg PO (depends on weight)<br>Second dose before intubation: 2–4 mg IV | First dose started 2 h before surgery 100 mg PO (>75 kg), 50mg PO (40–75 kg), or 25 PO mg (<40 kg) | Any | First dose 2–4 h before surgery 100 mg PO |
| Dose adjustment | Withheld if HR <55/ min; 50 mg PO/5 mg IV if HR >55 & <65; 100 mg PO/ 10 mg if HR >65 | – | Withheld if HR <55/min or SBP <100 mm Hg<br>Reduced to 50 mg PO if HR was 55–65/min and the SBP ≥100 mm Hg | No further drug given to patients who did not tolerate the test dose | (Drug withheld if HR <50/min while awake and <45/min while asleep or if SBP <100 mm Hg) | – | Withheld if HR <50/min or SBP <100 mm Hg |

(*continued on next page*)

**Table 2 (*continued*)**

| | Mangano et al[6] | Poldermans et al[44] | DIPOM[9] | POBBLE[8] | MaVS[10] | Lindenauer et al[7] | POISE[5] |
|---|---|---|---|---|---|---|---|
| Postoperative protocol | Immediately postop<br>Every 12 h thereafter starting first morning (either IV or PO) | Daily 5 mg Bisoprolol PO<br>IV metoprolol to keep HR <80 until oral bisoprolol could be started | Metoprolol 100 mg PO once daily or Metoprolol 5mg IV every 6 hours | Twice daily | Within 2 h after surgery (oral or IV), then IV every 6 h or PO twice daily | – | Within 6 hours after surgery 100 mg PO, then 200 mg PO 12 h after first postoperative dose<br>Daily 200 mg PO<br>If patient not able to take PO 15 mg IV over 60 min |
| Duration of treatment | Discharge or maximum of 7 d | 30 d postoperatively | Discharge or maximum of 7 d | 7 d postoperatively | Discharge or maximum of 5 d | – | 30 d postoperatively |
| Results | Signifi cant reduction in all-cause death, cardiac death, cardiac events | Decreased incidence of cardiac death or myocardial infarction during follow-up | No difference in all-cause mortality, cardiac events between metoprolol and control group | No difference in cardiac events in low-risk patients<br>Duration of hospitalization shorter in the metoprolol group | No difference in cardiac events at 30 days and 6 months<br>Intraoperative complications were higher with metoprolol group | Reduction in the risk of death in patients with a RCRI of $\geq 2$<br>Low-risk patients: 43% increase in risk of death | Decreased incidence of MI<br>Increased overall mortality second stroke |
| Adverse event from β-blocker therapy | None | – | None | Metoprolol group required more inotropic support | Intraoperative hypotension and bradycardia requiring treatment | – | – |

ACC, American College of Cardiology; AHA, American Heart Association; BB, β-blocker; CAD, coronary artery disease; CHF, congestive heart failure; COPD, chronic obstructive pulmonary disease; CV, cardiovascular; DM, diabetes mellitus; HR, heart rate; IV, intravenous; MI, myocardial infarction; PO, orally; PVD, peripheral vascular disease; RCRI, Revised Cardiac Risk Index; SBP, systolic blood pressure; TIA, transient ischemic attack.

**Box 1**
**Revised cardiac risk index**

- High-risk surgery
- Ischemic heart disease
- History of congestive heart failure
- History of cerebrovascular disease
- Insulin therapy for diabetes
- Preoperative serum creatinine of >2 mg/dL

*Data from* Ref.[84]

### *Treatment Effect*

Currently there is no consensus on the hemodynamic target for perioperative β-blockade. However, it is commonly believed that the target effect should be a resting heart rate of less than 60 beats per minute. One editorial felt that titrating to a resting heart rate may not be an adequate measure of β-blockade, and that β-blockade could be most accurately assessed by a response to exercise or an adrenergic challenge.[17] A recent prospective study[51] concluded that tight heart rate control in the low- to intermediate-risk patient may not be necessary. Their median heart rate was 66 beats per minute. On the other hand, a retrospective study published in 2008 found tight heart rate control essential to decrease perioperative cardiac risk.[48]

### *Timing, Dosage, and Choice of β-Blocker*

The optimal timing and protocol for instituting β-blocker therapy remains to be defined. Patients should be screened for the need of β-blocker therapy well in advance of surgery, to ensure adequate time to titrate β-blocker therapy to a target effect and to address adverse reactions to β-blockers before the day of surgery. Studies that compare β-blockers are lacking, and it is unknown which is the better β-blocker to use perioperatively. It seems that longer-acting agents are superior to the shorter-acting agents.[11] This difference may be due to a withdrawal effect that occurs with missed doses of the shorter-acting β-blockers.

Also of note is that all the studies that reported a cardiovascular benefit have used agents that are either moderately (atenolol, metoprolol) or highly (bisoprolol) β1 selective.[52] It should be kept in mind that with increasing dosage, receptor selectivity is lost.[50]

Although overall β-blockers are well tolerated in the elderly, only approximately 50% of the target dose recommended in randomized controlled trials is achieved in the elderly with congestive heart failure. This low dose may be effective in an elderly population with heart failure, but prescription of at least a medium dose (> or =50% target dose) may achieve a higher benefit. Elderly patients may not tolerate the higher doses well.[53]

Although not proven yet, there may be an adverse association with β-blockers with intrinsic sympathomimetic activity (eg, pindolol, acebutolol, oxprenolol, and penbutolol) when used in the perioperative prophylaxis of coronary events. β-Blockers with intrinsic sympathomimetic activity are not used postmyocardial infarction as they have not been demonstrated to be beneficial and are less effective than other β-blockers in the management of angina and tachyarrhythmias. The choice of β-blockers should therefore be limited to those that have been demonstrated to be more effective (eg, atenolol, bisoprolol, or metoprolol).[50]

### *Duration of Perioperative Treatment*

The optimal duration of perioperative β-blockade is still unclear. Most of the studies that showed no difference in cardiovascular events continued β-blockers for only 5 to 8 days postoperatively.[8–10] Most of the studies that showed a difference in cardiovascular events continued β-blockers for at least 30 days postoperatively.[5,44]

### *Contraindications to the Use of β-Blockers*

The absolute contraindications to the use of β-blockers are listed in **Box 2**. There are several relative contraindications that must be kept in mind by the anesthesiologists evaluating an elderly surgical patient. Care should be taken in instituting β-blocker therapy in patients with a history of cerebrovascular events and transient ischemic attacks.[5] The POISE study confirmed the reduced incidence of clinically significant atrial fibrillation and cardiac complications, but at the cost of a significantly increased risk of stroke rate, clinically significant hypotension and bradycardia, and an increase in overall mortality.[54] It should be noted that more than 75% of the strokes observed in the POISE trial were ischemic, possibly being due to the high incidence of hypotension.[54]

Sepsis is another condition for which β-blocker treatment should be undertaken with care. The POISE trial found that the only reported cause of death for which there was a significant difference between the groups was sepsis in the metoprolol group compared with the placebo group.[5,11]

Selective β-blockers can be carefully instituted in patients with some of the known relative contraindications, for example, stable CHF, COPD, and asthma. The presence of COPD has been shown to affect the treatment of CHF, as COPD is still viewed as a contraindication to β-blockers.[55] Impaired lung function seems to be an independent risk factor for arrhythmias, coronary events, and all-cause mortality, and a specific predictor of mortality resulting from cardiac causes.[56] The cumulative evidence from trials and meta-analyses indicates that cardioselective β1-blockers (exemplified by metoprolol and atenolol) should not be routinely withheld from patients with COPD because the benefits (of selective β1-blockers in patients with COPD who also have cardiac disease) far outweigh the risks.[57,58] A recent study examined 1205 patients with COPD undergoing major vascular surgery. Of these patients, 37% received cardioselective β-blockers at a dose greater than 25% of the maximum recommended therapeutic dose. This group experienced a lower 30-day and long-term mortality.[59]

**Box 2**
**Absolute contraindications for β-blocker prescription**

- Symptomatic bradycardia
- Second- or third-degree atrioventricular block (in the absence of a pacemaker)
- Severe heart failure requiring intravenous diuretics or inotropes (Class IV or ejection fraction <30%)
- Symptomatic hypotension
- Cardiogenic shock
- COPD with a strong reactive component or severe asthma requiring steroids
- Known intolerance to β-blockers
- Aortic valve stenosis

Due to limited long-term data on the safety of β-blockers in COPD, it seems prudent to use cardioselective agents and to start at a low dose and titrate up slowly, paying attention to lung function and symptoms.[60]

### *Perioperative Considerations*

β-Blockade suppresses the normal cardiac responses. This suppression may be beneficial in the context of laryngoscopy; however, it may be deleterious in situations in which tachycardia is a necessary homeostatic response, such as with isovolumic hemodilution.[61] β-Blockade may also mask the signs of light anesthesia that may increase the risk of awareness in fully paralyzed patients. β-Blockers may also enhance the risk for bradycardia and hypotension in association with vasovagal episodes, other anesthetic drugs, or techniques such as thoracic epidurals.[62,63] Another rare, but important interaction is that in the event of anaphylaxis, a β-blocked patient may be refractory to treatment.[64] β-Blocked patients may respond with vasoconstriction and bradycardia to epinephrine due to antagonism of β-mediated vasodilation. In diabetic patients, selective β-blockers are preferable due to the risk of hypoglycemia. Also, the warning signs of hypoglycemia (tachycardia and tremor) may not occur.

There is a large heterogeneity in the heart rate response to β-blockade, specifically metoprolol.[3] Polymorphisms of the gene encoding β1 receptors have been described; in one group there was a three-fold greater reduction in blood pressure in response to metoprolol.[65]

## PHARMACOLOGIC EFFECTS OF AGING

There are a variety of physiologic changes that happen with increasing age, such as changes in body composition and changes in the elimination of drugs. Pathologic factors such as heart failure of renal failure may also play a role in altering the response to a particular drug.

Most cardiovascular drugs are absorbed passively, and age-related changes such as decreased gastric emptying, reduced acid secretion, and reduced splanchnic flow does not affect oral agents in a clinically significant way.[66] Elderly patients have reduced first-pass metabolism, which can increase the bioavailability of drugs such as propranolol and labetalol.[67] Lean body mass[68] and total body water[69] deceases with age, resulting in a decrease in volume of distribution and a higher plasma concentration of the more water-soluble drugs such as digoxin.[70] Hepatic blood flow and hepatic size decreases with age, resulting in reduced phase I reactions, which can lead to increased bioavailability and increased plasma levels. Phase II reactions do not seem to be affected by age.[71]

Water-soluble β-adrenergic blockers such as sotalol, nadolol, and atenolol are not significantly metabolized in the liver. These drugs are less prone to metabolic drug interactions. The cytochrome P450 (CYP-450) system converts hydrophobic drugs to a hydrophilic form that can be eliminated by kidneys. Many of the lipophilic β-adrenergic blocking agents are metabolized by CYP2D6. Examples include bisoprolol, metoprolol, propranolol, timolol. The CYP2D6 isoenzyme is inhibited by drugs such as amiodarone, cimetidine, clomipramine, fluoxetine, haloperidol, paroxetine,[72] quinidine, ritonavir, sertraline, and thioridazine. This inhibition results in increased plasma levels. In contrast, drugs such as carbamazepine, phenobarbitol, phenytoin, rifampin, and ritonavir induce the enzyme system and may lower plasma levels.[73]

Alterations in liver blood flow may occur when calcium channel blockers and β-adrenergic blocking agents are combined. Metoprolol reduces the clearance of verapamil and conversely, verapamil increases the bioavailability of metoprolol, requiring a reduced dose of metoprolol.[74]

On average, renal function decreases from 20 years of age and is only 50% of normal function at 75 years. However, individual variation is wide, and some elderly patients have normal renal function, resulting in decreased clearance of drugs such as atenolol.[75]

Baroreceptor reflexes are diminished with age, and postural hypotension may be more frequent in elderly patients on antihypertensive therapy. There is an age-related increase in catecholamines, with a reduced responsiveness to sympathetic stimulation. Older patients have a decreased responsiveness to β-blockers.[71]

Elderly patients are more likely to be taking multiple drugs, resulting in the potential for drug interactions.[75,76] (see article elsewhere in this issue). For example, calcium antagonists (such as verapamil and amiodarone) can cause bradycardia or heart block when combined with β-blockers.[73] Bradycardia has occurred in patients undergoing dipyridamole stress testing, probably because of additive negative chronotropic effects.[77] β-Blockers prevent compensatory tachycardia due to vasodilatory drugs, and can cause syncope when given concurrently with α-antagonists.[78]

## RECOMMENDATIONS AND SUMMARY

When instituting perioperative β-blockade, a practice guideline or protocol and a multidisciplinary approach may be most effective.[79] The multidisciplinary team can ensure maintenance and adequate follow-up of perioperative β-blocker therapy.[14,80] In view of the findings of the POISE trial,[5] it can be argued that perioperative β-blocker use should be limited to patients for whom there is a Class I or IIa recommendation as defined by the ACC and AHA (see **Table 1**).[11]

Patients on β-blockers should continue with β-blockers throughout the perioperative period. The mortality rate was high among patients prescribed β-blockers and discontinuing treatment without titration. There is also an increased mortality rate among patients who should be on β-blockers chronically, but are not.[81]

In the more recent literature, many investigators have expressed the opinion that β-blockers were underprescribed in the perioperative period, especially in the elderly population.[13,14,17,82,83] However, these opinions were based on earlier guidelines for β-blocker use and were expressed despite the lack of evidence of efficacy for all patient populations. The New AHA/ACC guidelines on the perioperative use of β-blockade and findings of trials such as the POISE trial may soften this stance.[11]

Further adequately powered, randomized trials are needed to define the most effective yet safe method of perioperative β-blockade in patients who will be started on such therapy before surgery. The issues include choice of drug, the best end point for dosage, and how much time will be needed to determine a given patient's optimal dose.

## REFERENCES

1. Lerner DJ, Kannel WB. Patterns of coronary heart disease morbidity and mortality in the sexes: a 26-year follow-up of the Framingham population. Am Heart J 1986; 111(2):383–90.
2. Rankin JS, Hammill BG, Ferguson TB Jr, et al. Determinants of operative mortality in valvular heart surgery. J Thorac Cardiovasc Surg 2006;131:547–57.
3. Beattie WS, Wijeysundera DN, Karkouti K, et al. Does tight heart rate control improve beta-blocker efficacy? An updated analysis of the noncardiac surgical randomized trials. Anesth Analg 2008;106(4):1039–48.

4. Bangalore S, Wetterslev J, Pranesh S, et al. Perioperative beta blockers in patients having non-cardiac surgery: a meta-analysis. Lancet 2008;372(9654): 1962–76.
5. Devereaux PJ, Yang H, Yusuf S, et al. Effects of extended-release metoprolol succinate in patients undergoing non-cardiac surgery (POISE trial): a randomised controlled trial. Lancet 2008;371(9627):1839–47.
6. Mangano DT, Layug EL, Wallace A, et al. Effect of atenolol on mortality and cardiovascular morbidity after noncardiac surgery. Multicenter Study of Perioperative Ischemia Research Group. N Engl J Med 1996;335(23):1713–20.
7. Lindenauer PK, Pekow P, Wang K, et al. Perioperative beta-blocker therapy and mortality after major noncardiac surgery. N Engl J Med 2005;353:349–61.
8. Brady AR, Gibbs JS, Greenhalgh RM, et al. Perioperative beta-blockade (POBBLE) for patients undergoing infrarenal vascular surgery: results of a randomized double-blind controlled trial. J Vasc Surg 2005;41(4):602–9.
9. Juul AB, Wetterslev J, Kofoed-Enevoldsen A, et al. Diabetic Postoperative Mortality and Morbidity group. The Diabetic Postoperative Mortality and Morbidity (DIPOM) trial: rationale and design of a multicenter, randomized, placebo-controlled, clinical trial of metoprolol for patients with diabetes mellitus who are undergoing major noncardiac surgery. Am Heart J 2004;147:677–83.
10. Yang H, Raymer K, Butler R, et al. The effects of perioperative beta-blockade: results of the Metoprolol after Vascular Surgery (MaVS) study, a randomized controlled trial. Am Heart J 2006;152:983–90.
11. Fleisher LA, Beckman JA, Brown KA, et al. ACC/AHA 2007 guidelines on perioperative cardiovascular evaluation and care for noncardiac surgery: a report of the American College of Cardiology/American Heart Association Task Force on Practice Guidelines (Writing Committee to Revise the 2002 Guidelines on Perioperative Cardiovascular Evaluation for Noncardiac Surgery): developed in collaboration with the American Society of Echocardiography, American Society of Nuclear Cardiology, Heart Rhythm Society, Society of Cardiovascular Anesthesiologists, Society for Cardiovascular Angiography and Interventions, Society for Vascular Medicine and Biology, and Society for Vascular Surgery. Circulation 2007;116(17):e418–99.
12. Wiysonge CS, Bradley H, Mayosi BM, et al. Beta-blockers for hypertension. Cochrane Database Syst Rev 2007;(1):CD002003.
13. VanDenKerkhof EG, Milne B, Parlow JL. Knowledge and practice regarding prophylactic perioperative beta blockade in patients undergoing noncardiac surgery: a survey of Canadian anesthesiologists. Anesth Analg 2003;96(6): 1558–65.
14. Rapchuk I, Rabuka S, Tonelli M. Perioperative use of beta-blockers remains low: experience of a single Canadian tertiary institution. Can J Anaesth 2004;51(8): 761–7.
15. Fu M. Beta-blocker therapy in heart failure in the elderly. Int J Cardiol 2008; 125(2):149–53.
16. Smith SC Jr, Blair SN, Bonow RO, et al. AHA/ACC Scientific Statement: AHA/ACC guidelines for preventing heart attack and death in patients with atherosclerotic cardiovascular disease: 2001 update. A statement for healthcare professionals from the American Heart Association and the American College of Cardiology. Circulation 2001;104:1577–9.
17. Kertai MD, Bax JJ, Klein J, et al. Is there any reason to withhold beta blockers from high-risk patients with coronary artery disease during surgery? Anesthesiology 2004;100(1):4–7.

18. Abi Nasr I, Mansencal N, Dubourg O. Management of atrial fibrillation in heart failure in the elderly. Int J Cardiol 2008;125(2):178–82.
19. Taylor AD, Groen JG, Thorn SL, et al. New insights into onset mechanisms of atrial fibrillation and flutter after coronary artery bypass graft surgery. Heart 2002;88(5): 499–504.
20. Mathew JP, Fontes ML, Tudor IC, et al. A multicenter risk index for atrial fibrillation after cardiac surgery. JAMA 2004;291:1720–9.
21. Villareal RP, Hariharan R, Liu BC, et al. Postoperative atrial fibrillation and mortality after coronary artery bypass surgery. J Am Coll Cardiol 2004;43: 742–8.
22. Kaireviciute D, Aidietis A, Lip GY. Atrial fibrillation following cardiac surgery: clinical features and preventative strategies. Eur Heart J 2009;30(4):410–25.
23. Echahidi N, Pibarot P, O'Hara G, et al. Mechanisms, prevention, and treatment of atrial fibrillation after cardiac surgery. J Am Coll Cardiol 2008;51(8):793–801.
24. Burgess DC, Kilborn MJ, Keech AC. Interventions for prevention of post-operative atrial fibrillation and its complications after cardiac surgery: a meta-analysis. Eur Heart J 2006;27:2846–57.
25. Crystal E, Garfinkle MS, Connolly SS, et al. Interventions for preventing post-operative atrial fibrillation in patients undergoing heart surgery. Cochrane Database Syst Rev 2004;(4):CD003611.
26. Abi Nasr I, Bouzamondo A, Hulot JS, et al. Prevention of atrial fibrillation onset by beta-blocker treatment in heart failure: a meta-analysis. Eur Heart J 2007;28(4): 457–62.
27. Roy D, Talajic M, Dubuc M, et al. Atrial fibrillation and congestive heart failure. Curr Opin Cardiol 2009;24(1):29–34.
28. CIBIS-II Investigators and Committees. The Cardiac Insufficiency Bisoprolol Study II (CIBIS-II): a randomised trial. Lancet 1999;353(9146):9–13.
29. Alexander KP, Roe MT, Chen AY, et al. Evolution in cardiovascular care for elderly patients with non-ST-segment elevation acute coronary syndromes: results from the CRUSADE National Quality Improvement Initiative. J Am Coll Cardiol 2005; 46(8):1479–87.
30. MERIT-HF Study Group. Effect of metoprolol CR/XL in chronic heart failure: Metoprolol CR/XL Randomised Intervention Trial in Congestive Heart Failure (MERIT-HF). Lancet 1999;353:2001–7.
31. Flather MD, Shibata MC, Coats AJS, et al. Randomized trial to determine the effect of nebivolol on mortality and cardiovascular hospital admission in elderly patients with heart failure (SENIORS). Eur Heart J 2005;26(3):215–25.
32. Packer M, Coats AJ, Fowler MB, et al. Effect of carvedilol on survival in severe chronic heart failure. N Engl J Med 2001;344(22):1651–8.
33. Kannel WB. Incidence and epidemiology of heart failure. Heart Fail Rev 2000; 5(2):167–73.
34. Bradley HA, Wiysonge CS, Volmink JA, et al. How strong is the evidence for use of beta-blockers as first-line therapy for hypertension? Systematic review and meta-analysis. J Hypertens 2006;24(11):2131–41.
35. Lindholm LH, Carlberg B, Samuelsson O. Should beta blockers remain first choice in the treatment of primary hypertension? A meta-analysis. Lancet 2005; 366:1545–53.
36. European Society of Hypertension/European Society of Cardiology Guidelines Committee. 2003 European Society of Hypertension/European Society of Cardiology guidelines for the management of arterial hypertension. J Hypertens 2003;21:1011–53.

37. Chobanian AV, Bakris GL, Black HR, et al. Joint National Committee on Prevention, Detection, Evaluation, and Treatment of High Blood Pressure. Seventh Report of the Joint National Committee on prevention, detection, evaluation, and treatment of high blood pressure. Hypertension 2003;42:1206–52.
38. Roger VL, Jacobsen SJ, Weston SA, et al. Trends in the incidence and survival of patients with hospitalized myocardial infarction, Olmsted County, Minnesota, 1979 to 1994. Ann Intern Med 2002;136(5):341–8.
39. Mehta RH, Rathore SS, Radford MJ, et al. Acute myocardial infarction in the elderly: differences by age. J Am Coll Cardiol 2001;38:736–41.
40. Milner KA, Vaccarino V, Arnold AL, et al. Gender and age differences in chief complaints of acute myocardial infarction (Worcester Heart Attack Study). Am J Cardiol 2004;93:606–8.
41. Gibbons RJ, Abrams J, Chatterjee K, et al. ACC/AHA 2002 guideline update for the management of patients with chronic stable angina—summary article: a report of the American College of Cardiology/American Heart Association Task Force on Practice Guidelines (Committee on the Management of Patients With Chronic Stable Angina). Circulation 2003;107(1):149–58.
42. McMurray J, Køber L, Robertson M, et al. Antiarrhythmic effect of carvedilol after acute myocardial infarction: results of the Carvedilol Post-Infarct Survival Control in Left Ventricular Dysfunction (CAPRICORN) trial. J Am Coll Cardiol 2005;45(4): 525–30.
43. Chen ZM, Pan HC, Chen YP, et al. Early intravenous then oral metoprolol in 45,852 patients with acute myocardial infarction: randomised placebo-controlled trial. Lancet 2005;366(9497):1622–32.
44. Poldermans D, Boersma E, Bax JJ, et al. The effect of bisoprolol on perioperative mortality and myocardial infarction in high risk patients undergoing vascular surgery: Dutch Echocardiography Cardiac Risk Evaluation Applying Stress Echocardiography Study Group. N Engl J Med 1999;341(24): 1789–94.
45. Beattie WS. Evidence-based perioperative risk reduction. Can J Anaesth 2005; 52(Suppl 1):R17–27.
46. Priebe HJ. Perioperative myocardial infarction—aetiology and prevention. Br J Anaesth 2005;95(1):3–19.
47. Eagle KA, Froehlic JB. Reducing cardiovascular risk in patients undergoing noncardiac surgery. N Engl J Med 1996;335(23):1761–3.
48. Kaafarani HMA, Atluri PV, Thornby J, et al. Beta-blockade in noncardiac surgery: outcome at all levels of cardiac risk. Arch Surg 2008;143(10): 940–4.
49. Poldermans D, Boersma E. Beta-blocker therapy in noncardiac surgery. N Engl J Med 2005;353:412–4.
50. London MJ, Zaugg M, Schaub MC, et al. Perioperative beta-adrenergic receptor blockade: physiologic foundations and clinical controversies. Anesthesiology 2004;100:170–5.
51. De Virgilio C, Yaghoubian A, Nguyen A, et al. Peripheral vascular surgery using targeted beta blockade reduces perioperative cardiac event rate. J Am Coll Surg 2009;208(1):14–20.
52. Auerbach AD, Goldman L. Beta-blockers and reduction of cardiac events in noncardiac surgery: scientific review. JAMA 2002;287(11):1435–44.
53. Dobre D, Haaijer-Ruskamp FM, Voors AA, et al. Beta-adrenoceptor antagonists in elderly patients with heart failure: a critical review of their efficacy and tolerability. Drugs Aging 2007;24(12):1031–44.

54. Sear JW, Giles JW, Howard-Alpe G, et al. Perioperative beta-blockade, 2008: what does POISE tell us, and was our earlier caution justified? Br J Anaesth 2008;101(2):135–8.
55. Le Jemtel TH, Padeletti M, Jelic S. Diagnostic and therapeutic challenges in patients with coexistent chronic obstructive pulmonary disease and chronic heart failure. J Am Coll Cardiol 2007;49(2):171–80.
56. Sin DD, Man SF. Chronic obstructive pulmonary disease: a novel risk factor for cardiovascular disease. Can J Physiol Pharmacol 2005;83:8–13.
57. Huiart L, Erns P, Suissa S. Cardiovascular morbidity and mortality in COPD. Chest 2005;128:2640–6.
58. Albouaini K, Andron M, Alahmar A, et al. Beta-blockers use in patients with chronic obstructive pulmonary disease and concomitant cardiovascular conditions. Int J Chron Obstruct Pulmon Dis 2007;2:535–40.
59. Van Gestel YR, Hoeks SE, Sin DD, et al. Impact of cardioselective beta-blockers on mortality in patients with chronic obstructive pulmonary disease and atherosclerosis. Am J Respir Crit Care Med 2008;178:695–700.
60. Cazzola M, Noschese P, D'Amato G, et al. The pharmacologic treatment of uncomplicated arterial hypertension in patients with airway dysfunction. Chest 2002;121:230–41.
61. Beattie S, Karkouti K, Mitsakakis N, et al. Beta blockers increase perioperative risk in acute anemia surgery. Can J Anaesth 2008;55(Suppl 1):4745621–2.
62. Tripathi M, Singh PK. Complete heart block after epidural anaesthesia in a patient on beta-blocker. J Indian Med Assoc 1994;92(2):53–4.
63. Fikkers BG, Damen J, Scheffer GJ, et al. Thoracic epidural analgesia and antihypertensive therapy: a matter of timing? Eur J Anaesthesiol 2006;23(10): 893–5.
64. Mueller UR. Cardiovascular disease and anaphylaxis. Curr Opin Allergy Clin Immunol 2007;7(4):337–41.
65. Johnson JA, Zineh I, Puckett BJ, et al. Beta 1-adrenergic receptor polymorphisms and antihypertensive response to metoprolol. Clin Pharmacol Ther 2003;74: 44–52.
66. Cusack BJ, Vestal RE. Clinical pharmacology: special considerations in the elderly. In: Calkins E, Davis PJ, Ford AB, editors. Practice of geriatric medicine. Philadelphia: WB Saunders; 1986. p. 115–34.
67. Castleden CM, George CF. The effect of aging on the hepatic clearance of propranolol. Br J Clin Pharmacol 1979;7:49–54.
68. Novak LP. Aging, total body potassium, fat-free mass and cell mass in males and females between the ages of 18 and 85 years. J Gerontol 1972;27: 438–43.
69. Vestal RE, Norris AH, Tobin JD, et al. Antipyrine metabolism in man: influence of age, alcohol, caffeine and smoking. Clin Pharmacol Ther 1975;18:425–32.
70. Cusack B, Kelly J, O'Malley K, et al. Digoxin in the elderly: pharmacokinetic consequences of old age. ClinPharmacol Ther 1979;25(6):722–6.
71. Williams BR, Kim J. Cardiovascular drug therapy in the elderly: theoretical and practical considerations. Drugs Aging 2003;20(6):445–63.
72. Goryachkina K, Burbello A, Boldueva S, et al. Inhibition of metoprolol metabolism and potentiation of its effects by paroxetine in routinely treated patients with acute myocardial infarction (AMI). Eur J Clin Pharmacol 2008;64(3):275–82.
73. Anderson JR, Nawarskas JJ. Cardiovascular drug-drug interactions. Cardiol Clin 2001;19(2):215–34.

74. Flockhart DA, Tanus-Santos JE. Implications of cytochrome P450 interactions when prescribing medication for hypertension. Arch Intern Med 2002;162: 405–12.
75. Rang HP, Dale MM, Ritter JM, et al. In: Hunter L, editor. Pharmacology. 5th edition. Churchill Livingstone; 2003. p. 713–4.
76. Johnson JF. Considerations in prescribing for the older patient. Scottsdale (AZ): PCS Health Systems; 1998. 1/98.
77. Roach PJ, Magee MA, Freedman SB. Asystole and bradycardia during dipyridamole stress testing in patients receiving beta-blockers. Int J Cardiol 1993;42: 92–4.
78. Elliott HL, McLean K, Sumner DJ, et al. Immediate cardiovascular responses to oral prazosin: effects of concurrent beta-blockers. Clin Pharmacol Ther 1981; 29:303–9.
79. Weller J, Karim Z. Perioperative beta-blockade: guidelines and practice in New Zealand. Anaesth Intensive Care 2005;33(5):645–50.
80. Hepner DL, Correll DJ, Beckman JA, et al. Needs analysis for the development of a preoperative clinic protocol for perioperative beta-blocker therapy. J Clin Anesth 2008;20(8):580–8.
81. Hoeks SE, Scholte Op Reimer WJ, van Urk H, et al. Increase of 1-year mortality after perioperative beta-blocker withdrawal in endovascular and vascular surgery patients. Eur J Vasc Endovasc Surg 2007;33(1):13–9.
82. Schmidt M, Lindenauer PK, Fitzgerald JL, et al. Forecasting the impact of a clinical practice guideline for perioperative beta-blockers to reduce cardiovascular morbidity and mortality. Arch Intern Med 2002;162(1):63–9. This group also suggested practice guidelines to institute perioperative beta blockade.
83. Siddiqui AK, Ahmed S, Delbeau H, et al. Lack of physician concordance with guidelines on the perioperative use of beta-blockers. Arch Intern Med 2004; 164(6):664–7.
84. Lee TH, Marcantonio ER, Mangione CM, et al. Derivation and prospective validation of a simple index for prediction of cardiac risk of major noncardiac surgery. Circulation 1999;100:1043–9.

# Anesthetic Care for Patients with Skin Breakdown

Daniel K. O'Neill, MD[a,*], Jason Maggi, MD[b]

**KEYWORDS**

- Pressure ulcer • Regional • General • Local • Sedation
- Diabetes • Skin

S.C. was an 84-year-old man with a history or noninsulin-dependent diabetes mellitus well controlled on oral therapy, who was admitted with acute cholecystitis for antibiotics therapy and eventual surgery. Before this illness, S.C. was active, living with his spouse, traveling frequently, and playing tennis 2 to 3 times per week. He had undergone a right hip replacement 8 years earlier. On his third hospital day he underwent a laparoscopic cholecystectomy and endoscopic ductal exploration for stones. The patient was placed in a supine position with the legs split. Due to difficulty removing a distal stone, the operation required 5.5 hours.

Postoperatively the patient complained bitterly about pain in his right hip, and did not get out of bed. On the second postoperative day, he was noted to have Stage II breakdown of the skin over both of his ischial tuberosities. He was transferred to an air mattress and the areas were dressed, but the skin became necrotic after another 2 days. The patient was scheduled for wound debridement in the operating room. He was extremely concerned about waking up with pain in his hip again. His wife claimed the wounds were the fault of the first anesthesiologist and wanted details concerning the anesthetic approach to her husband for this procedure.

## ANATOMY OF DECUBITUS ULCERS

Despite advances in awareness and caring for pressure ulcers, they continue to be prevalent in epidemic proportions. It is estimated that prevalence of pressure ulcers in acute care settings is approximately 15%, in long-term care settings from 2.3% to 28%, and in home care from 0% to 29%.[1–3] No single cause can be attributed to the development of pressure ulcers, but contributing factors include pressure per unit area, friction, shearing stress, and moisture. In addition, associated factors, such as nutrition, physiologic status, body mass index (BMI; calculated as the weight

[a] Department of Anesthesiology, New York University School of Medicine, New York, NY, USA
[b] Division of Wound Healing and Regenerative Medicine, Department of Surgery, NYU Langone Medical Center, 550 First Avenue, IRM 605, New York, NY 10016, USA
* Corresponding author.
*E-mail address:* Daniel.ONeill@nyumc.org (D.K. O'Neill).

Anesthesiology Clin 27 (2009) 599–603
doi:10.1016/j.anclin.2009.07.014 anesthesiology.theclinics.com

in kilograms divided by height in meters squared), and other medical conditions all play a part in the development of skin breakdown. Of these factors the most important is pressure, which is of utmost concern in the operative setting. Frequent turning and pressure reduction techniques have been repeatedly proven to be beneficial in reducing incidence of pressure ulcer development.[4] Increased tissue pressure, above the normal pressures of 12 to 32 mm Hg, can impede circulation and oxygenation in the local tissue. Pressures as high as 150 mm Hg can be generated over bony prominences while the patient is positioned on an operating table.[5] These bony prominences are the primary sites of pressure ulcer development, the majority of which are found in the pelvic area and below. Primary sites include the ischium, the sacral promontory, the gluteal area, and the heel.

As pressure is a primary cause for the development of skin breakdown, it follows that the operating room is an ideal location for the development of an ulcer. Incidence of pressure ulcers in surgical patients is often difficult to define, as few studies have addressed this specific group. Indeed, it is difficult to assess the exact incidence of purely operating room acquired pressure ulcers, due to the temporally associated nature. In addition, the use of grading scales, most notably the Braden Scale, is of little use intraoperatively, as all patients would be identified as at risk.[6] These scales are useful in identifying patients at risk, for whom additional preventative measures need to be taken. Furthermore, Scott and colleagues[7] found that the American Society of Anesthesiologists classification can be a possible preoperative predictor of pressure ulcer development.

Pressure ulcers are classified according to stages, from I to IV. In addition, the National Pressure Ulcer Advisory Panel has recognized deep tissue injury as a contributing factor in the development of pressure ulcers.[8–12] Deep tissue injury is a term denoting local tissue injury, and denotes an area at risk for development of a pressure ulcer. This injury may be represented as an area of erythema, pain, and rapid evolution to a pressure ulcer. Pressure ulcers that develop intraoperatively are primarily stage I to II. Stage I ulcers are an area of nonblanching erythema, primarily over a bony prominence. The tissue, even at this early stage, may be painful and different in texture from surrounding tissue. Stage II ulcers represent a partial thickness loss of the dermis, with visual evidence of skin breakdown. This stage may manifest as an open ulcer, or as a blister overlying the tissue breakdown. For ulcers recognized early in the postoperative period, these ulcers will often show a base of granulation tissue, with necrosis and frank purulence reserved for those of longer duration. Stage III ulcers denote full-thickness tissue loss, to the level of the subcutaneous fat. Depth of ulcer varies according to anatomic location. Stage IV pressure ulcers represent wounds that extend to muscle, tendon, or bone. Stage III and IV ulcers are often much more complex, with variable amounts of undermining, and pockets of fibrinous and purulent material. In the authors' experience, it is rare to develop intraoperatively acquired stage III to IV pressure ulcers without prior tissue injury at the site.

What, then, are the identifiable factors associated with intraoperative acquired pressure ulcers? In a prospective follow-up study of 208 patients, including operative times of 4 hours or greater, Schoonhoven and colleagues[13] found length of surgery as the only reliable predictor of development of a pressure ulcer. Rates of pressure ulcers acquired in the operating room vary widely, ranging from 4.7%[14] to 45%.[15] Part of this increased incidence has been attributed to the inability of patients to feel pain caused by prolonged pressure, thus not allowing them to change position when not under general anesthesia.[16] This problem, in addition to the stress of the operative procedure itself, would lead one to believe that surgery could be an independent risk factor.

The depth of a pressure ulcer is hard to determine from the external appearance. In planning for these cases, the operating room team should be aware that a small skin lesion may overlie extensive necrotic tissue that will require debridement down to, and sometimes including, bone.

## ANESTHETIC CARE OF THE PATIENT WITH A CHRONIC WOUND

### *Transfers and Positioning*

Some patients with chronic wounds are on specialized beds, some of which are extremely heavy. These beds can be brought to the operating room if it would be too difficult for the patient to be placed on a stretcher. Chronic wound patients can be fragile and debilitated. More than normal, this shifts the responsibility for a safe transfer to the bed onto the operating room staff. If contact precautions are required, appropriate barrier protection should be worn by all staff members. The number of staff members doing the transfer should be sufficient to divide the workload to a safe biomechanical load to prevent occupational associated musculoskeletal injury to the workers and providers. Vigilance needs to be maintained to prevent unintentional patient injury or line removal.

The operating position should be known before performing blocks or surgery. For example, surgery on sacral wounds can be done in either the lateral or prone positions. Each has its issues with airway management, ventilation, and pressure point protection. The supine and lithotomy positions are commonly used for foot, heel, and leg wounds, including those which are circumferential. Airway management is easier in these positions for the provider. The entire body should always be checked for risks of undesirable pressure injury, especially eyes, ears, elbows, and knees.

Patients with severe arthritis or prosthetic joints may have a limited range of motion in one or more areas. These cases are best managed, when possible, by determining a comfortable position for the patient, including placement in stirrups, before the induction of anesthesia.

### *Neuropathy*

The nervous system can have impaired axonal conduction secondary to degenerative disease, trauma, or neurotoxins. For example, spinal cord injury can cause complete or incomplete paraplegia or quadriplegia. Stroke can cause hemiplegia. Diabetes that is associated with microangiopathy can lead to peripheral neuropathies in a stocking-glove pattern. The degree of neuropathy varies from patient to patient.

When planning an anesthetic using local anesthetics for subcutaneous injection or regional block, insensate regions may require less need for sodium channel blockade. The diagnosis of diabetes, for example, does not guarantee that a neuropathy is present or extensive enough to preclude the need for anesthesia. Spinal cord injury similarly may be incomplete and associated with chronic pain syndromes. A spinal anesthetic may be indicated to cover breakthrough pain from surgical stimulation and to minimize the risk of autonomic hyperreflexia associated with spinal cord neuropathy. Therefore, a good history and physical examination would be needed to formulate an appropriate anesthetic plan.

### *Limits of Local Anesthetics*

The sodium channel blockade of local anesthetics is dependent on the neuroanatomy in the region of distribution subcutaneously, regionally, or centrally (spinal or epidural). The dermatosomal distribution of the drug effect would determine the antinociceptive efficacy during the surgical stimulus. The physical characteristics of the local anesthetics (pKa, molecular weight, lipid solubility, protein binding, tissue pH) and the histology of the nerves determine pharmacologic effects: lidocaine (pKa = 7.9, protein binding = 64%), mepivacaine (pKa = 7.7, protein binding = 77%), bupivacaine (pKa = 8.2, protein binding = 96%). The onset, duration of action, and toxicity depend on site of injection and the associated rate of absorption into the bloodstream. Potency of local anesthetics increases with increasing molecular weight and increasing lipid solubility.

Abscesses that are usually caused by coagulase-positive *Staphylococcus aureus* have classically been resistant to the antinociceptive prosperities of local anesthetics. Although the acidic tissue pH may be a factor, cellular mediators and macromolecular debris may physically bind the weakly basic local anesthetic and effectively inactivate it.

## SELECTING AN ANESTHETIC REGIMEN

### *Local with Sedation*

Patients presenting for decubitus ulcer debridement frequently suffer from multiple comorbid conditions and are frequently depressed. Failure to mobilize increases the risk of pneumonia as well. Finally, these wounds are both visually and olfactorily challenging. These issues have frequently been raised as an argument for use of the least anesthesia possible, local without any sedation, or with minimal sedation. This choice may be appropriate; however, the limitation of local anesthetic agents in the vicinity of devitalized tissue along with the difficulty in determining the depth to which the debridement will be performed make local anesthetic with sedation a potentially inadequate approach to preventing pain and maintaining stable vital signs. The choice of sedative medications should be guided to the extent appropriate by the physical condition and age of the patient. For elderly patients, who comprise many of those with chronic wounds, meperidine should be avoided. Short-acting benzodiazepines can be used with caution, with the understanding that some patients may develop paradoxic agitation. Analgesic medication is of paramount importance.

### *Spinal*

For wounds within the anatomic scope of spinal anesthesia, this technique can be very effective. Both spinal and general provide the depth of analgesia necessary to conduct deep and wide debridement, if needed. Spinal anesthesia must be accomplished by placing the needle through normal, noninflamed tissue, so if the area of inflammation extends up the back, this technique is probably complicated. However, the mere presence of a decubitus ulcer is not a contraindication to spinal anesthesia.

### *General*

Operating time for wound debridement cases is usually short. The better the operating conditions for the surgeon, the faster and more complete the procedure will be. It is worth emphasizing that the anesthesia team can greatly facilitate an adequate debridement by providing optimal operating conditions. Airway management for such cases can be simple, using a well-fit mask or laryngeal mask airway. Many, if not most of these patients are elderly. Ketamine, in combination with a short-acting benzodiazepine, is a formulation that can be used successfully in this situation.

## SUMMARY

Wound patients commonly have multiple comorbidities, which should be optimized before anesthesia. These factors contribute not only to skin breakdown but also to other causes of mortality and morbidity. Skin becomes more vulnerable to damage from pressure, friction, shear, and moisture when the skin is dry, less elastic, and less perfused. Careful assessment and implementation of an anesthetic plan using regional or general techniques can improve outcomes. Deeper wounds are more likely to be associated with osteomyelitis. Bone resection, which has anesthetic implications, may be required to control the infection. Sharp debridement in the operating room with anesthesia, an aseptic technique, illumination, and instrumentation allows the removal of necrotic and infected tissue, sampling for microbiology and pathology, and advanced wound care strategies to optimize the likelihood of wound healing. The anesthesiologist plays a vital role in maintaining homeostasis during the surgically stressful perioperative period of the wound patient.

Globally speaking, aggressive wound management in the early stages is likely to prevent wound progression to deeper levels. Nationally, policies are being implemented to decrease the risk of pressure ulcers through prevention. The operating room anesthesiologist certainly is expected to prevent skin breakdown during anesthesia time.

## REFERENCES

1. Wolff K, Goldsmith LA, Katz SI, et al. Skin changes due to mechanical and physical factors: decubitus (pressure) ulcers and venous ulcers. In: Freedberg IM, editor. Fitzpatrick's dermatology in general medicine. New York: McGraw-Hill Professional; 2003. p. 1256.
2. Kanj LF, Wilking SVB, Phillips TJ, et al. Pressure ulcers. J Am Acad Dermatol 1998;38:517–83.
3. Grey JE, Enoch S, Harding KG. Pressure ulcers. BMJ 2006;332:472–5.
4. Krapfl L, Gray M. Does regular repositioning prevent pressure ulcers. J Wound Ostomy Continence Nurs 2008;35(6):571–7.
5. Phillips Tania J, Odo Lilian M, Chapter 99. Decubitus (Pressure) Ulcers. (chapter) Wolff K, Goldsmith LA, Katz SI, et-al, Fitzpatrick's dermatology in general medicine, 7th edition: Available at: http://www.accessmedicine.com/content.aspx?aID=2980481.
6. Byers P, Carta S, Mayrovitz H. Pressure ulcer research issues in surgical patients. Adv Skin Wound Care 2000;13(3):115–21.
7. Scott EM, Leaper DJ, Clark M, et al. Effect of warming therapy on pressure ulcers—a randomised trial. AORN J 2001;73:921–38.
8. National Pressure Ulcer Advisory Panel's Updated Pressure Ulcer Staging System. The National Pressure Ulcer Advisory Panel (NPUAP). Available at: http://www.npuap.org.
9. Butterworth JF IV, Strichartz GR. Molecular mechanisms of local anesthesia: a review. Anesthesiology 1990;72:711–34.
10. Hadzic, Admir. Textbook of regional anesthesia and acute pain management. McGraw-Hill Company; 2007.
11. Sanchez V, Arthur GR, Strichartz GR, et al. Fundamental properties of local anesthetics I. The dependence of lidocaine's ionization and octanol:buffer partitioning on solvent and temperature. Anesth Analg 1987;66:159–65.
12. Strichartz GR, Sanchez V, Arthur GR, et al. Fundamental properties of local anesthetics II. Measured octanol:buffer partition coefficients and pKa values of clinicallly used drugs. Anesth Analg 1990;71:158–70.
13. Schoonhoven L, Defloor T, Van der Tweel I, et al. Risk indicators for pressure ulcers during surgery. Appl Nurs Res 2002;15(3):163–73.
14. Lewicki L, Mion L, Splane K, et al. Patient risk factors for pressure ulcers during cardiac surgery. AORN J 1997;65(5):933–42.
15. Grous CA, Reilly NJ, Gift AG. Skin integrity in patients undergoing prolonged operations. J Wound Ostomy Continence Nurs 1997;24(2):86–91.
16. Vermillion C. Operating room acquired pressure ulcers. Decubitus 1990;3(1):26–30.

# Index

*Note:* Page numbers of article titles are in **boldface** type.




Anesthesiology Clin 27 (2009) 605–615
doi:10.1016/S1932-2275(09)00086-X
**anesthesiology.theclinics.com**

## D

# Moving?

## *Make sure your subscription moves with you!*

To notify us of your new address, find your **Clinics Account Number** (located on your mailing label above your name), and contact customer service at:

**Email: journalscustomerservice-usa@elsevier.com**

**800-654-2452** (subscribers in the U.S. & Canada)
**314-447-8871** (subscribers outside of the U.S. & Canada)

**Fax number: 314-447-8029**

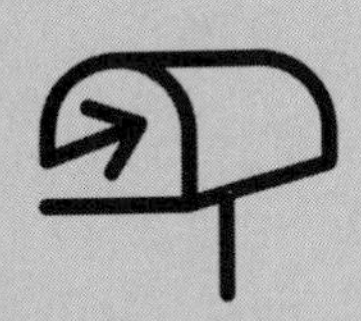

**Elsevier Health Sciences Division**
**Subscription Customer Service**
**3251 Riverport Lane**
**Maryland Heights, MO 63043**

*To ensure uninterrupted delivery of your subscription, please notify us at least 4 weeks in advance of move.

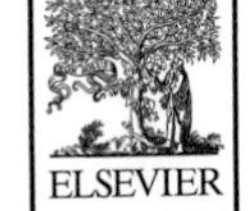